Practical
Microbiology

Second Edition

Practical
Microbiology

Bharti Arora MD

Professor & Head, Department of Microbiology,
Maharaj Agrasen Medical College,
Agroha, Hisar, Haryana (India)

DR Arora MD PhD MNAMS

Ex-Professor & Head, Department of Microbiology,
Postgraduate Institute of Medical Sciences, Rohtak, Haryana (India), and
Maharaja Agarsen Medical College, Agroha, Hisar, Haryana (India)

Ex-Professor & Head, Department of Microbiology,
Medical Superintendent, and Dean Faculty of Allied Health Sciences,
SGT University, Gurugram, Haryana (India)

Ex-WHO Fellow; and Visiting Professor, University of Mauritius

Lead Assessor and Member, Accreditation Committee,
National Accreditation Board for Testing and Calibration Laboratories (NABL),
Gurugram, Haryana (India)

Principal Assessor, National Accreditation Board for Hospitals &
Healthcare Providers (NABH), New Delhi (India)

Assessor, National Accreditation Board for
Education and Training (NABET), New Delhi (India)

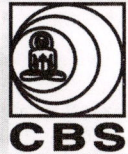

CBS

CBS Publishers & Distributors Pvt Ltd

New Delhi • Bengaluru • Chennai • Kochi • Kolkata • Mumbai
Bhopal • Bhubaneswar • Hyderabad • Jharkhand • Nagpur • Patna • Pune
• Uttarakhand • Dhaka (Bangladesh) • Kathmandu (Nepal)

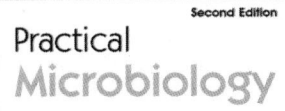

ISBN: 978-93-89396-60-7

Copyright © Authors

Second Edition: 2020
First Edition: 2007
Reprint: 2007, 2009, 2012, 2013, 2014, 2015, 2017, 2018

Published by Satish Kumar Jain and produced by Varun Jain for

CBS Publishers & Distributors Pvt Ltd

4819/XI Prahlad Street, 24 Ansari Road, Daryaganj, New Delhi 110 002, India
Ph: 011-23289259, 23266861, 23266867   Website: www.cbspd.com
Fax: 011-23243014   e-mail: delhi@cbspd.com; cbspubs@airtelmail.in

Corporate Office: 204 FIE, Industrial Area, Patparganj, Delhi 110 092
Ph: 011-49344934   Fax: 011-49344935   e-mail: publishing@cbspd.com; publicity@cbspd.com

Branches

- **Bengaluru:** Seema House 2975, 17th Cross, K.R. Road,
  Banasankari 2nd Stage, Bengaluru 560 070, Karnataka
  Ph: +91-80-26771678/79   Fax: +91-80-26771680   e-mail: bangalore@cbspd.com
- **Chennai:** 7, Subbaraya Street, Shenoy Nagar, Chennai 600 030, Tamil Nadu
  Ph: +91-44-26680620, 26681266   Fax: +91-44-42032115   e-mail: chennai@cbspd.com
- **Kochi:** 42/1325, 1326, Power House Road, Opposite KSEB Power House,
  Ernakulam 682 018, Kochi, Kerala
  Ph: +91-484-4059061-65   Fax: +91-484-4059065   e-mail: kochi@cbspd.com
- **Kolkata:** 6/B, Ground Floor, Rameswar Shaw Road, Kolkata-700 014, West Bengal
  Ph: +91-33-22891126, 22891127, 22891128   e-mail: kolkata@cbspd.com
- **Mumbai:** 83-C, Dr E Moses Road, Worli, Mumbai-400018, Maharashtra
  Ph: +91-22-24902340/41   Fax: +91-22-24902342   e-mail: mumbai@cbspd.com

Representatives

• Bhopal	0-8319310552	• Bhubaneswar	0-9911037372	• Hyderabad	0-9885175004	• Jharkhand	0-9811541605
• Nagpur	0-9421945513	• Patna	0-9334159340	• Pune	0-9623451994	• Uttarakhand	0-9716462459
• Dhaka (Bangladesh)	01912-003485	• Kathmandu (Nepal)	977-9818742655				

Printed at:

City Printer, Delhi (India)

to

Maharaja Agrasen

Preface to the Second Edition

For qualifying an examination, a microbiology student has to get through in theory and practical separately. Though a large number of theory books in microbiology are available, no good book covering practical aspects is available. Keeping in view the above, a simple and comprehensive book on practical aspects of all sections of microbiology has been devised. Rapidly increasing information in medical science requires that textbooks be revised and updated to keep pace. Earlier edition of the *Practical Microbiology* has received an overwhelming response from undergraduate and postgraduate students, and the teachers. This has played a vital role in bringing out the second edition of the book. Each chapter has been carefully updated and expanded. The text is presented in a simple and lucid manner. It is illustrated with eight colour plates containing 52 figures, computer-drawn figures and photomicrographs. These make the book colourful and the readers can have a better understanding. This book has been divided into nine sections that include General Bacteriology, Serology/Immunology, Parasitology, Systemic Bacteriology, Mycology, Virology, Recent Advances, Spots and Appendices. Each practical exercise ends with important questions and their answers which help the student to prepare for theory, practical and viva voce examination.

We express our sincere thanks to Dr. Amit Arora for proofreading, invaluable suggestions and continuous encouragement. We are grateful for valuable professional help and support provided by Mr YN Arjuna (Senior Vice President—Publishing, Editorial and Publicity), Mr BM Singh and other staff at CBS Publishers & Distributers. We honestly acknowledge the most sincere and dedicated support and advice of Mr Dharmvir. This book will be highly useful to MBBS, BDS, BSc MLT, MSc MLT, MSc and MD microbiology students, and technical staff of (clinical) laboratories. It is also hoped that it will serve as a useful resource for teachers of microbiology. The readers are requested to send suggestions for improvement of the book which will be incorporated in the next edition. Shortcomings, if any, may please be communicated at *draroradr@rediffmail.com*.

Bharti Arora
DR Arora

Preface to the First Edition

For qualifying an examination, a microbiology student has to get through in theory and practical separately. Though a large number of theory books in microbiology are available, no good book covering practical aspects is available. Keeping in view the above, a simple and comprehensive book on practical aspects of all sections of microbiology has been devised. This book has been divided into nine parts that include General Bacteriology, Serology/Immunology, Parasitology, Systemic Bacteriology, Mycology, Virology, Recent Advances, Spots and Appendices. Each practical exercise ends with important questions and their answers which help the student to prepare for theory, practical and viva voce examination.

This book is meant for BDS, BSc MLT, MSc, MSC MLT students and technical staff of medical (clinical) laboratories. It is a 'bench book' containing well-tried methods. This will also help the students preparing for postgraduate entrance examination.

We express our sincere thanks to Dr. Amit Arora for proofreading, invaluable suggestions and continuous encouragement. We are deeply indebted to Dr. (Mrs.) B. Arora, Professor and Head, Department of Pathology, Postgraduate Institute of Medical Sciences, Rohtak, for contributing photomicrographs and valuable suggestions. We owe our debt of gratitude to Dr. Harender and Mr. Prabhat Ranjan for proofreading and for meticulously drawing all the figures. Thanks are also due to Mr. Dharamvir, Mr. Kuldeep and Mr. Parveen Sharma for composing this book, Mr. B.R. Sharma for encouragement and M/s CBS Publishers & Distributors for their cooperation and keen interest in the publication of this book.

Bharti Arora
DR Arora

General Instructions to the Students for Safety

- Protect your clothings in the laboratory by wearing an overall. This should not be worn outside the department.
- All microorganisms should be regarded as capable of causing disease.
- Long hair should be tied back to avoid risks from fire and accidental contamination.
- Mouth pipetting should not be done.
- Always flame the bacteriological loop before and after use.
- Do not try to smell any bacterial culture.
- Do not expose microbiological cultures longer than necessary.
- Do not shake liquid cultures.
- Do not place cotton wool plugs or other stoppers on the bench.
- Do not place contaminated pipettes on the bench top.
- Do not sit on bench top.
- Do not lick labels with tongue.
- Do not put pencils, fingers and other objects in your mouth.
- Do not eat or drink in the laboratory.
- Discard the used and contaminated slides and other material in disinfectant jar.
- Do not wander about the laboratory.
- Do not forcibly expel material from a pipette.
- Always wash your hands thoroughly at the end of your work.
- Bench tops should be disinfected immediately after experiment is over.
- All accidents like cuts and burns in the laboratory should be reported to your teacher.
- Accidental spillage of bacterial growth or other contaminated material should be reported to your teacher or laboratory technician.

Discussion

1. **Enumerate conditions which lead to accidental ingestion of microorganisms.**
   - Mouth-pipetting of specimens or liquid cultures.
   - No proper hand washing after handling cultures.
   - Eating or drinking in the laboratory.

2. **Enumerate organisms which can penetrate the normal, healthy skin.**
   - *Treponema* spp.
   - *Leptospira* spp.

3. **How aersols are formed in the laboratory?**
   - Heating a contaminated wire loop in an open Bunsen burner flame.
   - Vigorous shaking of liquid cultures.
   - Forcibly expelling an infected fluid from Pasteur pipette.
   - Dropping or spilling a culture or specimen.
   - Opening a centrifuge immediately following the breakage of a tube of infected fluid.

4. **How do you deal with spilled blood or potentially infected material on the floor?**
   It should be covered with a cloth/blotting paper soaked in 10% sodium hypochlorite solution. After 30 minutes, cloth is removed with gloved hands and discarded in infectious waste, which is incinerated.

5. **Which disinfectants are highly active against viruses?**

Chlorine-releasing disinfectants.

6. **Which disinfectants are effective against mycobacteria?**

Phenols.

7. **What should be the concentration of sodium hypochlorite for discard jars and routine surface disinfection?**

For discard jars and surface disinfection, sodium hypochlorite 2.5% and 1% should be used, respectively.

8. **Why alcohols are used at a concentration of 60 to 70% in water?**

Because water is essential for their antimicrobial action.

9. **How do you classify infective microorganisms?**

Group 1: Unlikely to cause human disease.

Group 2: May cause human disease, unlikely to spread in community and effective prophylaxis and treatment is available.

Group 3: Cause severe human disease and may pose a high risk of spread in the community, but effective prophylaxis and treatment is available.

Group 4: Same as Group 3, but there is no effective prophylaxis or treatment.

10. **Enumerate group 4 organisms.**

- Crimean/Congo haemorrhagic fever virus
- Ebola
- Marburg
- Variola
- Junin
- Machupo
- Lassa fever virus

11. **How many levels of laboratory containment are known to you?**

The levels of laboratory containment are numbered according to the category of hazard which an organism presents.

Containment level 1: Hazard group 1

Containment level 2: Group 2

Containment level 3: Group 3

Containment level 4: Group 4

12. **How do you classify safety cabinets?**

Class 1: Open fronted, deals with cultures of infective organisms.

Class 2: Open fronted, usually preferred for keeping uninoculated cell culture.

Class 3: Tightly closed, deals with group 4 organisms.

13. **What is the alternative of mouth pipetting?**

Use a rubber treat or automatic suction device.

Contents

Preface to the second edition .... *vii*
Preface to the first edition .... *ix*
General instructions to the students for safety .... *xi*

Section 1
GENERAL BACTERIOLOGY

1. The compound microscope 3
2. Gram staining 6
3. Ziehl-Neelsen staining 9
4. Albert's staining 12
5. Spore staining 14
6. Capsule staining 16
7. Motility of bacteria 18
8. Sterilization 20
9. Liquid culture media 24
10. Solid culture media 27
11. Collection and transportation of specimen 30
12. Cultivation of bacteria 34
13. Identification of bacteria (biochemical reactions) 38
14. Antimicrobial susceptibility testing 42

Section 2
SEROLOGY/IMMUNOLOGY

15. Venereal disease research laboratory (VDRL) test 49
16. Widal test 53
17. C-reactive protein (CRP) test 56
18. Rheumatoid factor (RF) test 58
19. Antistreptolysin O (ASO) test 60
20. Complement fixation test 62
21. Weil-Felix test 64
22. Paul-Bunnell test 66
23. Cold agglutination test 68
24. Brucella agglutination test 70
25. Enzyme immunoassay (EIA) 72

Section 3
PARASITOLOGY

26. Collection and preservation of stool specimen 77
27. Examination of stool 80
28. Identification of faecal eggs 87
29. Identification of faecal trophozoites, cysts and oocysts 90
30. Culture techniques 95
31. Examination of blood 100

Section 4
SYSTEMIC BACTERIOLOGY

32. *Staphylococcus* 111
33. *Streptococcus pyogenes, S. agalactiae* and enterococci 115
34. *Streptococcus pneumoniae* (Pneumococcus) 119
35. *Neisseria* 121
36. *Corynebacterium* 124
37. *Mycobacterium tuberculosis* 128
38. Diagnostic approach to anaerobes 132
39. *Clostridium* 136
40. *Escherichia coli* 140
41. *Klebsiella* 142
42. *Proteus* 144
43. *Shigella* 146
44. *Salmonella* 148
45. *Pseudomonas* 151
46. *Vibrio* 154
47. Spirochaetes 158
48. Bacteriological examination of water 160

Section 5
MYCOLOGY

49. Laboratory diagnosis of mycoses 165
50. *Candida albicans* 168
51. *Cryptococcus neoformans* 170
52. *Aspergillus* 172
53. Mucoraceae 174
54. Dermatophytes 176

Section 6
VIROLOGY

55. Diagnostic approach to viral infections 181

Section 7
RECENT ADVANCES

56. Molecular biology 191

Section 8
SPOTS

57. Spots 197

APPENDICES

Appendix I: pH indicators 207
Appendix II: Greek alphabets 207
Appendix III: International System of Units (SI)—SI prefixes 207
Appendix IV: Notifiable infectious diseases 208
               Old nomenclature of a few organisms 208
Appendix V: Characterstic colonial appearance 209
               Characteristic appearance of bacteria in stained smear 209
Appendix VI: Differentiation of bacteria of Enterobacteriaceae by biochemical tests 210
Appendix VII: Overview of microbiology, mycology and parasitology 211

PLATE I

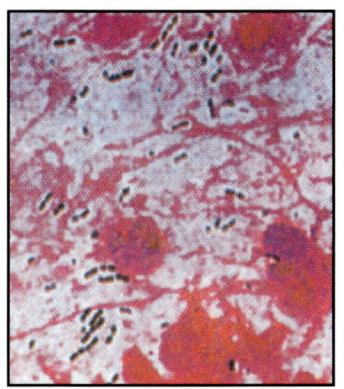

Fig. 1. Gram-stained sputum smear showing Gram-positive, encapsulated, extracellular diplococci from a patient of *pneumococcal pneumonia* (×1000).

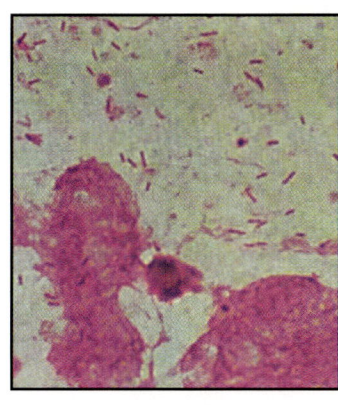

Fig. 2. Gram-stained smear showing Gram-negative bacilli (×1000).

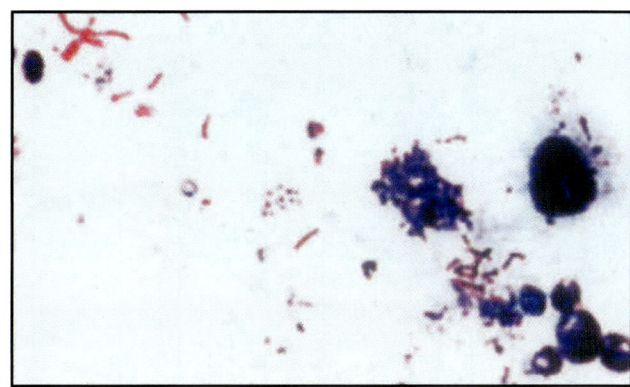

Fig. 3. Sputum smear showing acid-fast bacilli (×1000).

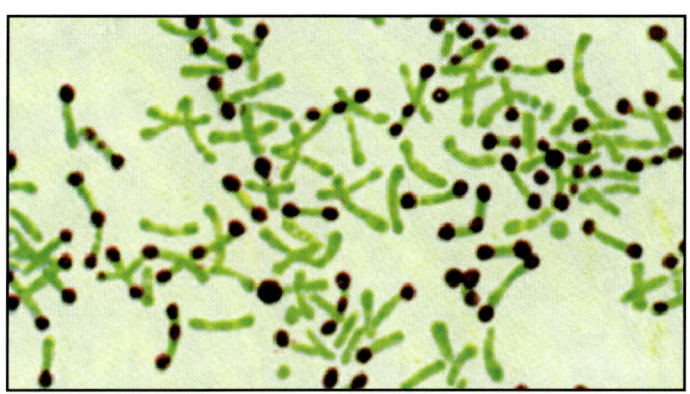

Fig. 4. *Corynebacterium diphtheriae* showing metachromatic granules (Albert's stain, ×1000).

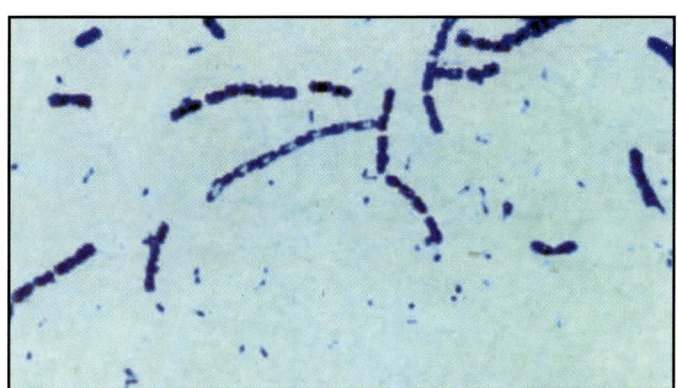

Fig. 5. Gram-stained smear of *Bacillus subtilis* showing Gram-positive bacilli in chains with spores which appear as unstained areas within the bacilli (×1000).

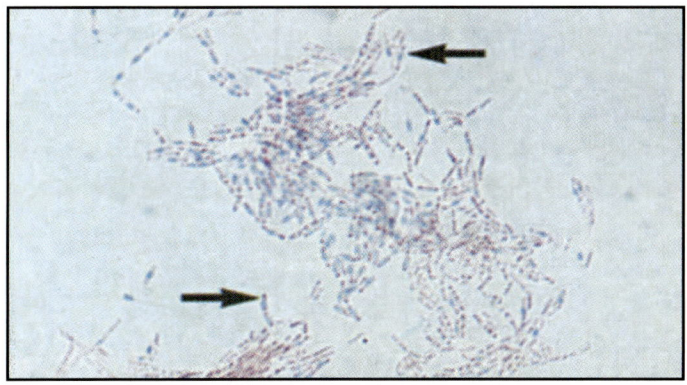

Fig. 6. Malachite green stained smear of *Bacillus cereus* showing red bacilli with green spores (×1000).

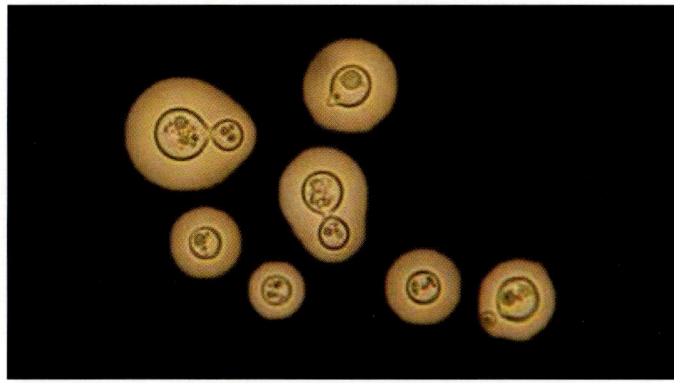

Fig. 7. An India ink wet mount of *Cryptococcus neoformans* showing encapsulated budding yeast cells (×400).

PLATE II

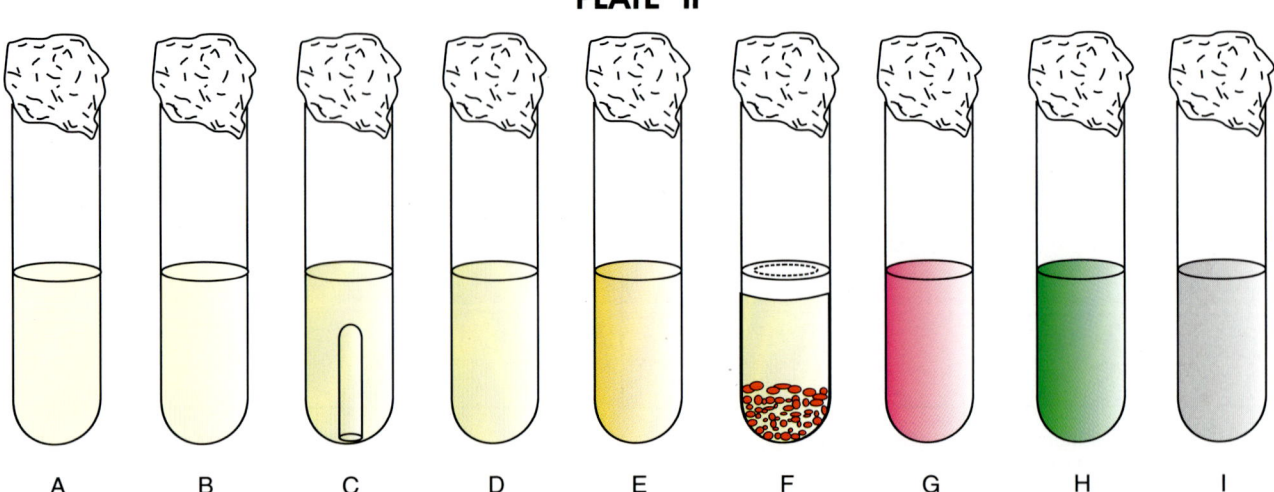

Fig. 8. **(A)** Peptone water, **(B)** Nutrient broth, **(C)** Sugar medium, **(D)** Glucose broth, **(E)** Bile broth, **(F)** Cooked meat broth, **(G)** Buffered glycerol saline, **(H)** Brilliant green tetrathionate broth, and **(I)** Selenite-F broth

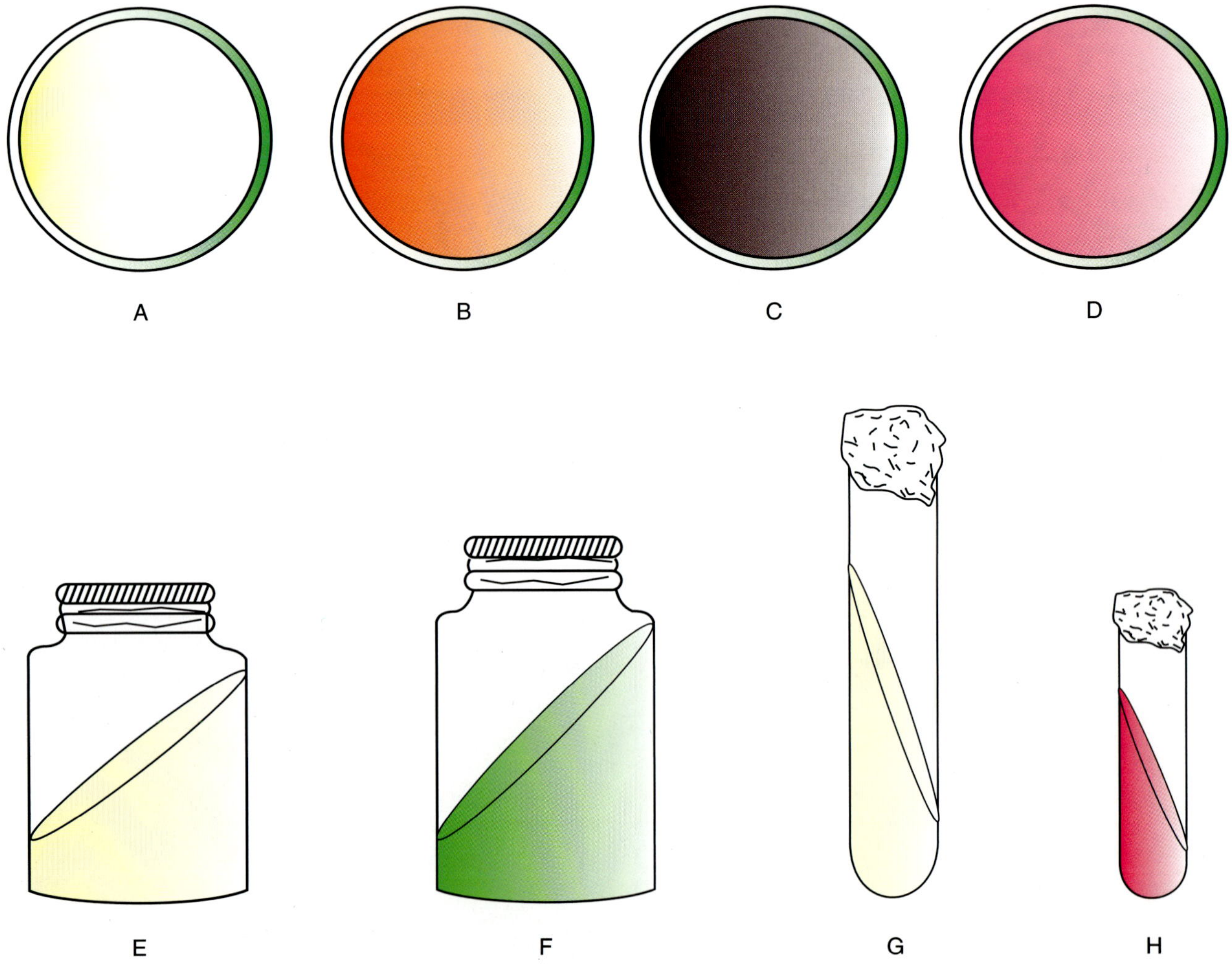

Fig. 9. **(A)** Nutrient agar, **(B)** Blood agar, **(C)** Chocolate agar, **(D)** MacConkey agar, **(E)** Loeffler's serum slope, **(F)** Lowenstein-Jensen medium, **(G)** Sabouraud's dextrose agar, and **(H)** Triple sugar iron agar.

PLATE III

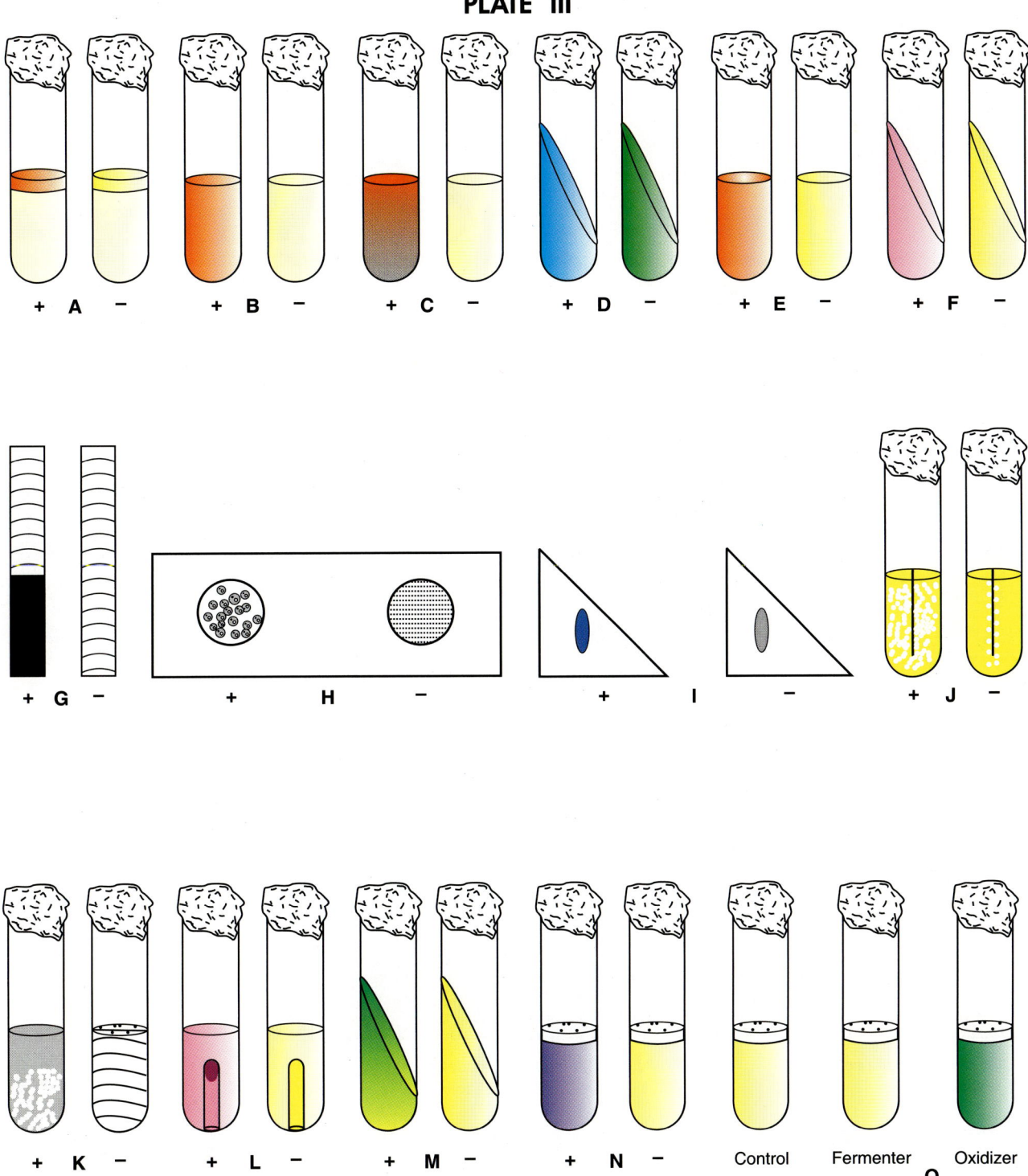

Fig. 10. **(A)** Indole test, **(B)** MR test, **(C)** VP test, **(D)** Citrate utilization test, **(E)** Nitrate reduction test, **(F)** Urease test, **(G)** H$_2$S test, **(H)** Catalase test, **(I)** Oxidase test, **(J)** Motility test, **(K)** Potassium cyanide test, **(L)** Sugar fermentation test, **(M)** PPA test, **(N)** Decarboxylase test, and **(O)** OF test.

PLATE IV

Eggs, Trophozoites, Cysts and Oocysts in the Stool of Man

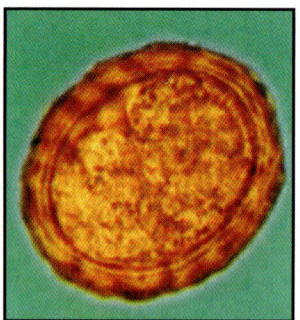

Fig. 11. Fertilized egg of *Ascaris lumbricoides* (saline wet mount, ×400).

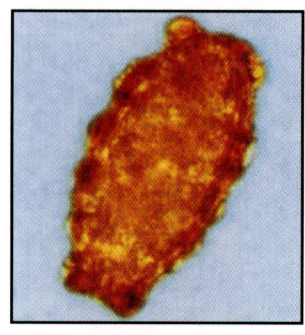

Fig. 12. Unfertilized egg of *Ascaris lumbricoides* (saline wet mount, ×400).

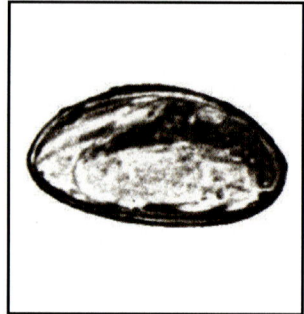

Fig. 13. Egg of *Enterobius vermicularis* (saline wet mount, ×400).

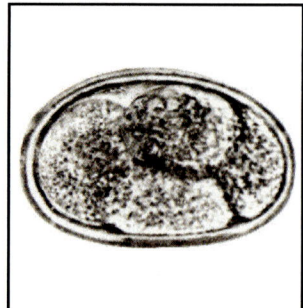

Fig. 14. Egg of *Ancylostoma duodenale* (saline wet mount, ×400).

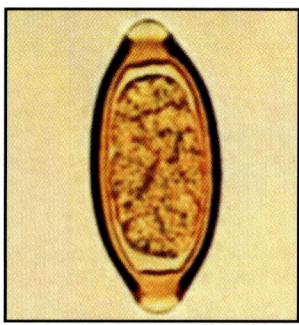

Fig. 15. Egg of *Trichuris trichiura* (saline wet mount, ×400).

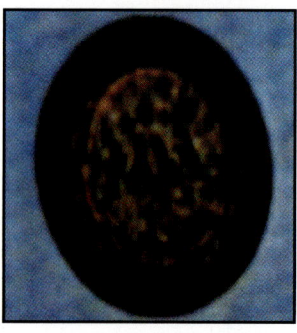

Fig. 16. Egg of *Taenia* (saline wet mount, ×400).

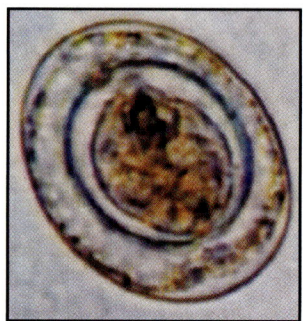

Fig. 17. Egg of *Hymenolepis nana* (saline wet mount, ×400).

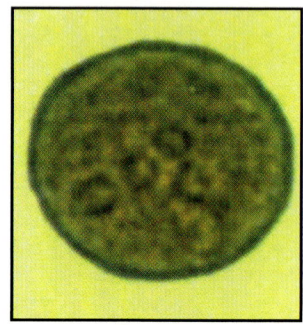

Fig. 18. Cyst of *Entamoeba histolytica* in stool (iodine wet mount, ×400).

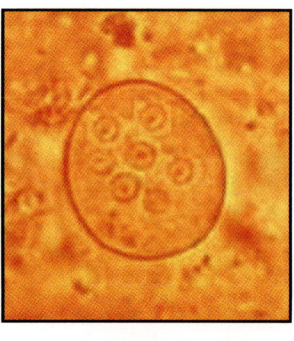

Fig. 19. Cyst of *Entamoeba coli* in stool (iodine wet mount, ×400).

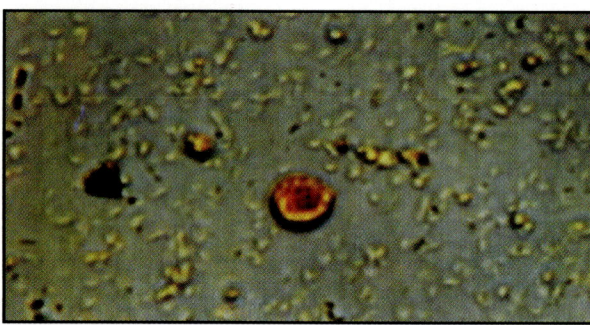

Fig. 20. Cyst of *Iodamoeba buetschlii* in stool (iodine wet mount, ×400).

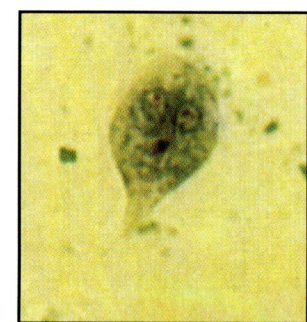

Fig. 21. Trophozoite of *Giardia lamblia* in stool (iron haematoxylin stain, ×400).

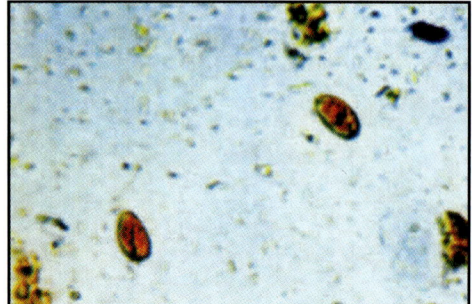

Fig. 22. Cysts of *Giardia lamblia* in stool (iodine wet mount, ×400).

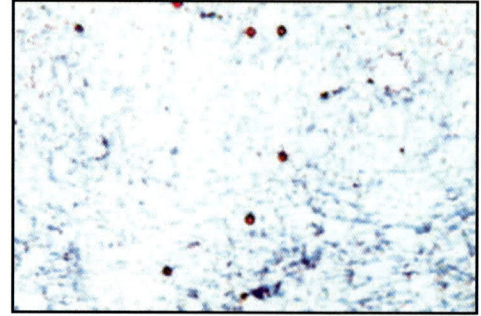

Fig. 23. Oocysts of *Cryptosporidium parvum* in faecal smear stained with modified acid-fast stain (×400).

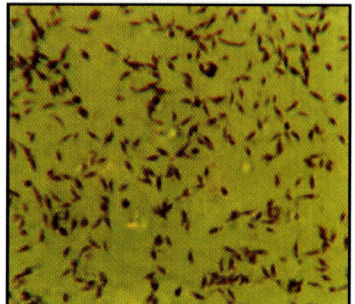

Fig. 24. Promastigote forms of *Leishmania donovani* in culture (Giemsa stain, ×400).

PLATE V

Plasmodium vivax	*Plasmodium falciparum*	*Plasmodium malariae*	*Plasmodium ovale*
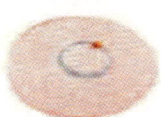 Early trophozoite (Ring stage)	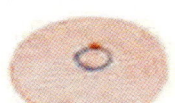 Early trophozoite (Ring stage)	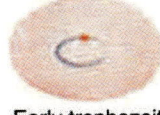 Early trophozoite (Ring stage)	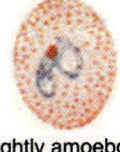 Early trophozoite (Ring stage) with Schüffner's dots
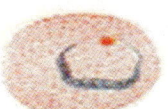 Late trophozoite with Schüffner's dots	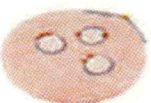 Multiple infections with accolé form	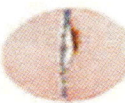 Band form	Early trophozoite (enlarged RBC)
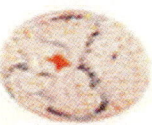 Amoeboid form with Schüffner's dots	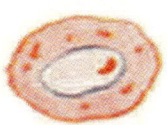 Ring with Maurer's dots	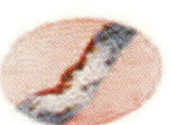 Band form	Slightly amoeboid
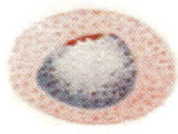 Early schizont	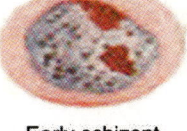 Early schizont	Early schizont	Early schizont
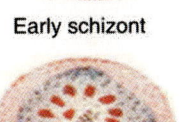 Maturing schizont	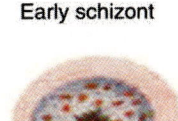 Maturing schizont	Maturing schizont	Maturing schizont
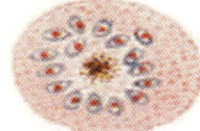 Mature schizont	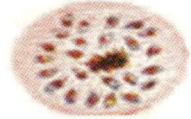 Mature schizont	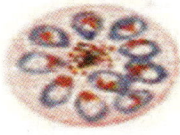 Mature schizont	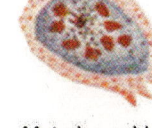 Mature schizont
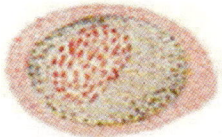 Male gametocyte	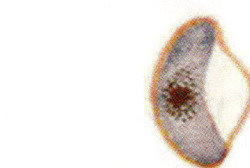 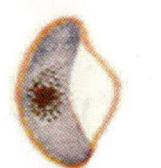 Male gametocyte	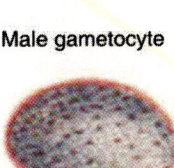 Male gametocyte	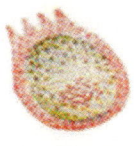 Male gametocyte
Female gametocyte	Female gametocyte	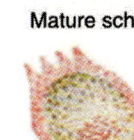 Female gametocyte	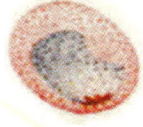 Female gametocyte

Fig. 25. Morphological forms of malaria parasites.

PLATE VI

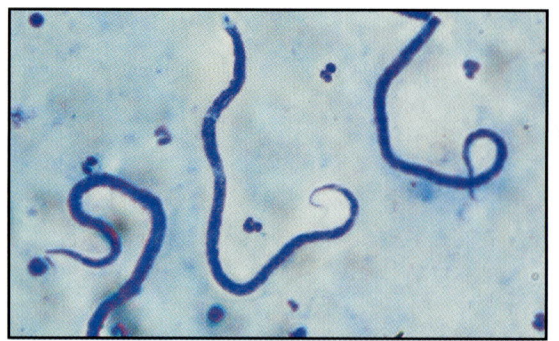

Fig. 26. *Microfilaria bancrofti* in peripheral blood (Giemsa stain, ×400).

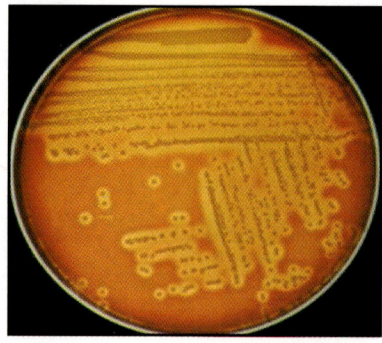

Fig. 27. Growth of *Staphylococcus aureus* on blood agar showing β-haemolysis.

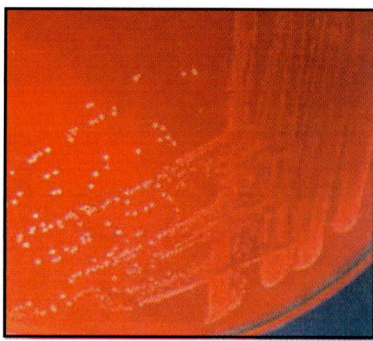

Fig. 28. Coagulase-negative staphylococci growing on blood agar.

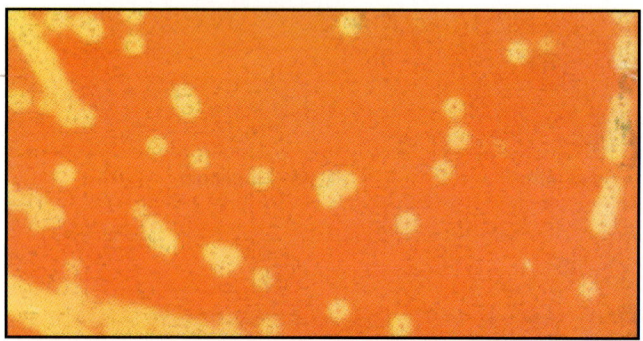

Fig. 29. *Streptococcus pyogenes* on blood agar showing β-haemolysis.

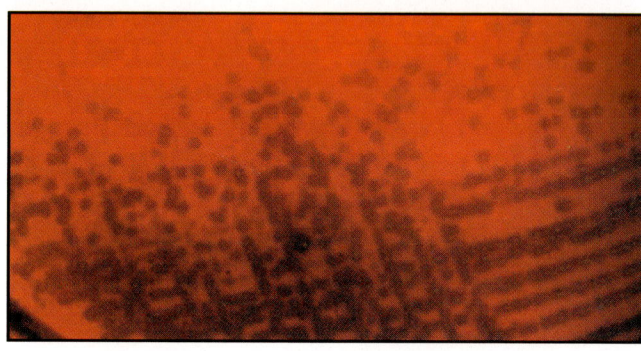

Fig. 30. *Streptococcus pneumoniae* on blood agar showing α-haemolysis.

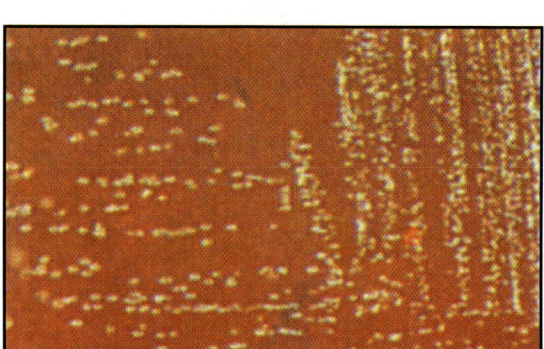

Fig. 31. *Neisseria gonorrhoeae* growing on Thayer-Martin medium.

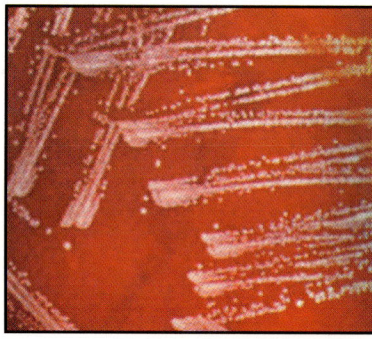

Fig. 32. *Corynebacterium diphtheriae* growing on blood agar.

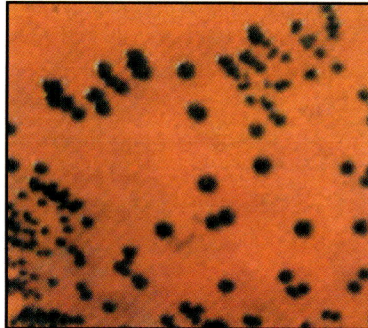

Fig. 33. *C. diphtheriae* showing black colonies on blood tellurite agar

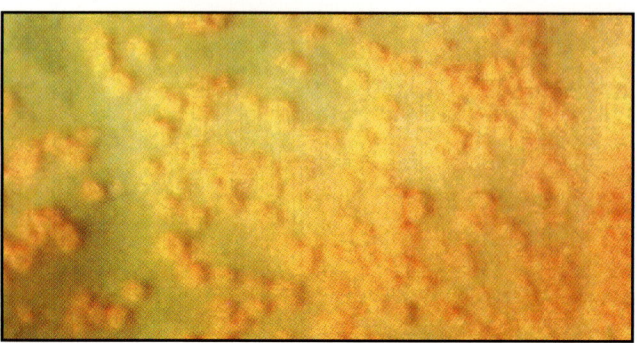

Fig. 34. Growth of *Mycobacterium tuberculosis* on Lowenstein-Jensen medium.

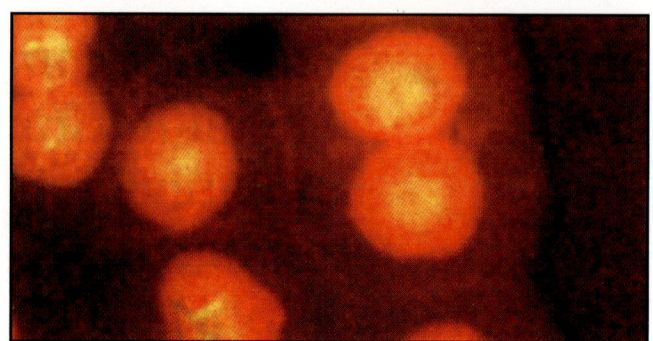

Fig. 35. *Clostridium perfringens* showing double zone haemolysis on blood agar.

PLATE VII

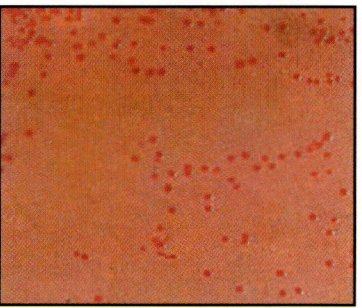

Fig. 36. *Escherichia coli* showing lactose fermenting colonies on MacConkey agar.

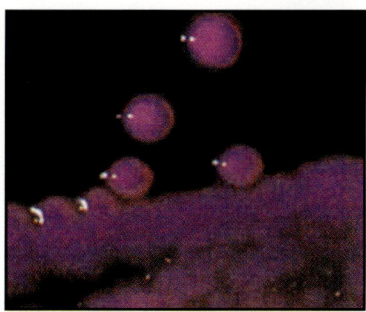

Fig. 37. *Klebsiella* spp. showing mucoid lactose fermenting colonies on MacConkey agar.

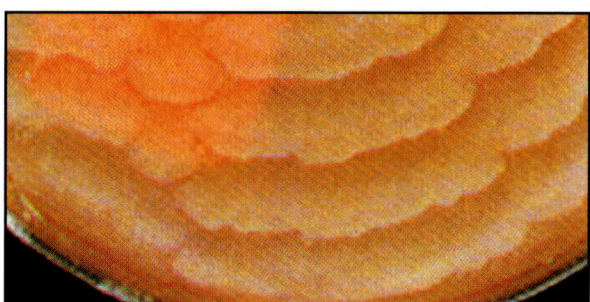

Fig. 38. *Proteus mirabilis* showing swarming on blood agar.

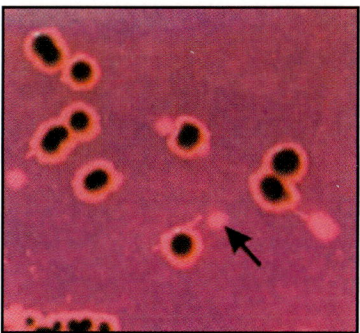

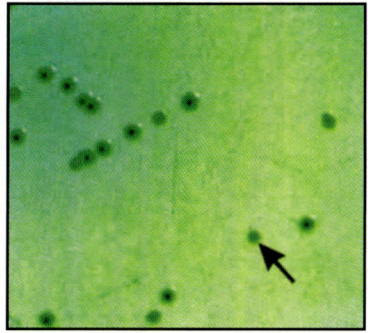

Fig. 39. *Shigella* spp. showing red colonies on xylose lysine deoxycholate agar (left), and green colonies on Hektoen enteric agar (right).

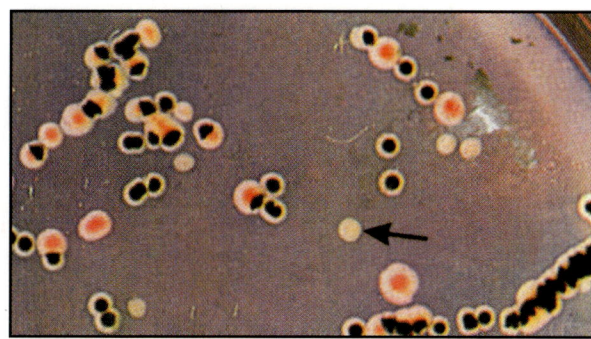

Fig. 40. *Shigella* spp. showing colourless colonies on *Salmonella-Shigella* agar.

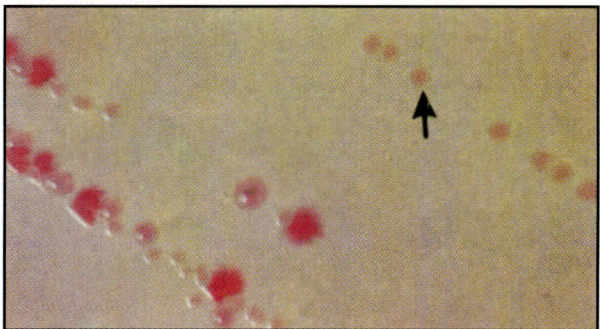

Fig. 41. *Salmonella* serotype Typhi showing colourless colonies on MacConkey agar.

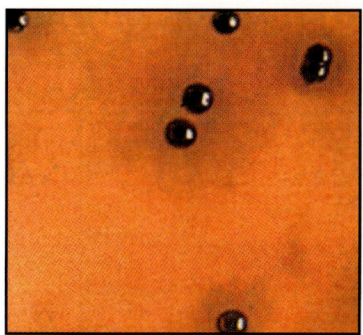

Fig. 42. *Salmonella* serotype Typhi showing black colonies on Wilson and Blair's medium (left), and red colonies with black centres on XLD agar (right).

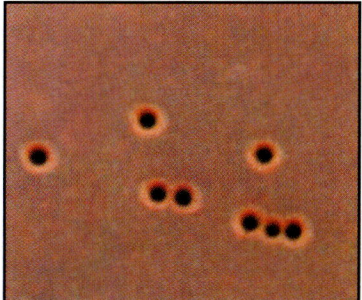

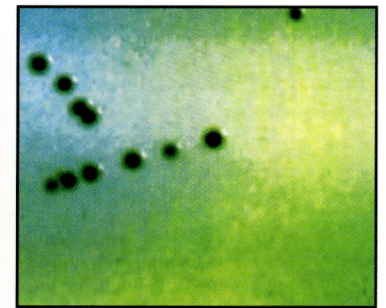

Fig. 43. *Salmonella* spp. showing colourless colonies with black centres on *Salmonella-Shigella* agar (left), and green colonies with black centres on Hektoen enteric agar (right)

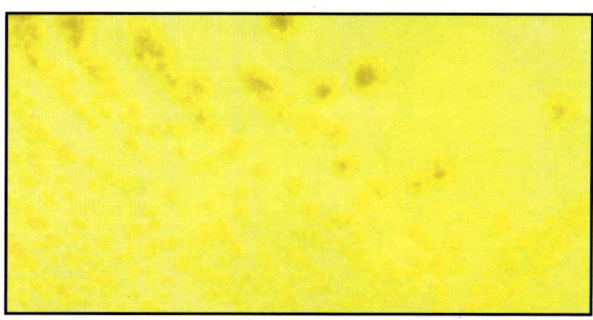

Fig. 44. *Pseudomonas aeruginosa* growing on nutrient agar.

PLATE VIII

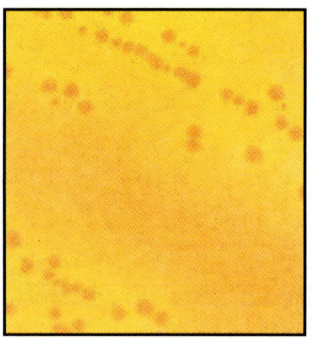 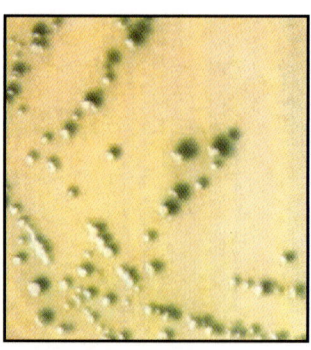

Fig. 45. *Vibrio cholerae* showing yellow colonies (left), and *V. parahaemolyticus* showing green ones (right) on TCBS agar

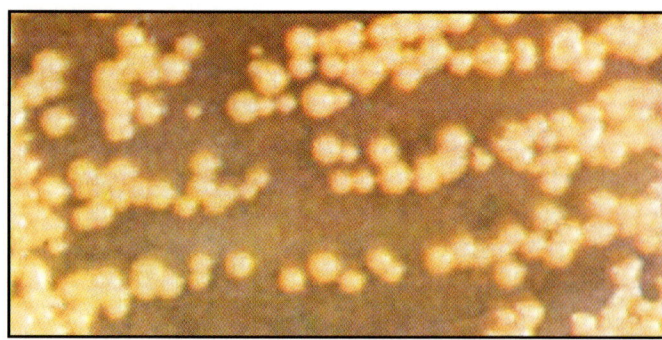

Fig. 46. *Candida albicans* showing colonies on Sabouraud's dextrose agar.

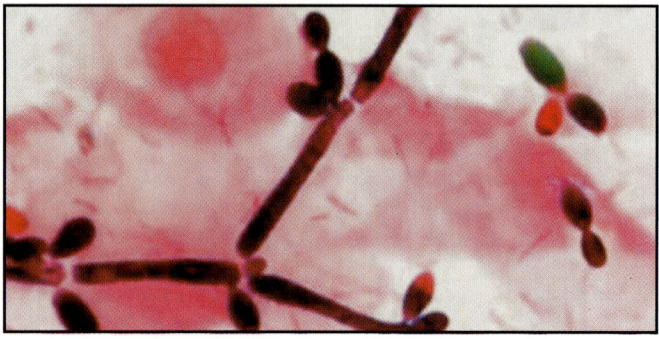

Fig. 47. Vaginal smear showing budding yeast cells, true hyphae and epithelial cells (PAS stain, ×400).

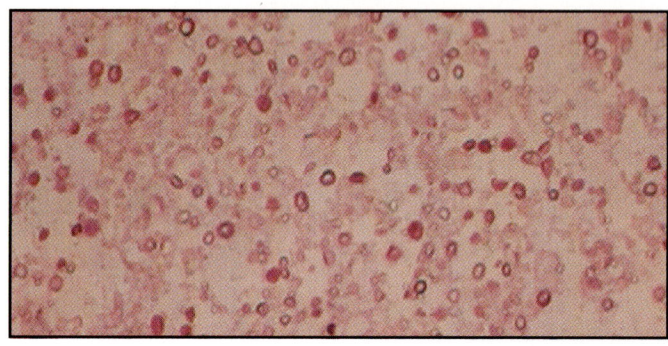

Fig. 48. Cryptococci stained with Mayer's mucicarmine stain (×400) The capsule is stained bright carmine red in colour.

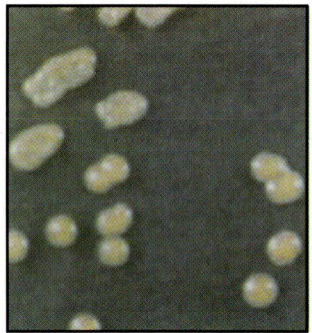 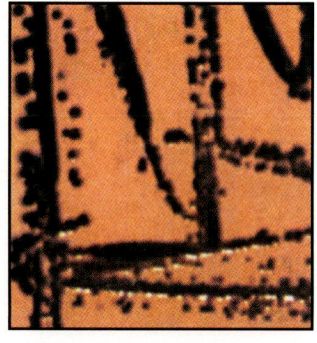

Fig. 49. *Cryptococcus neoformans* growing on SDA (left), and showing black colonies on niger seed agar (right).

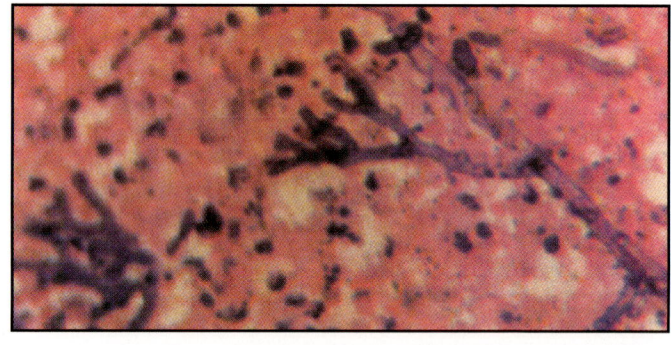

Fig. 50. *Aspergillus* showing septate hyphae with characteristic dichotomous branching.

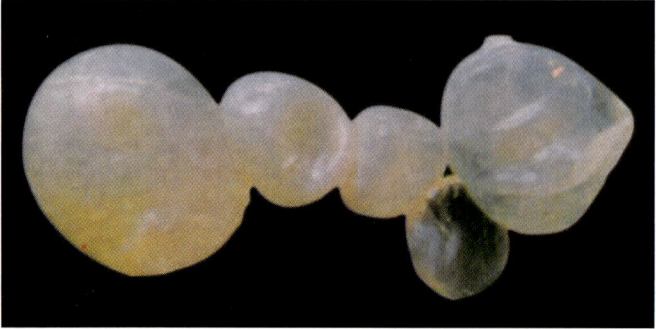

Fig. 51. Hydatid cysts.

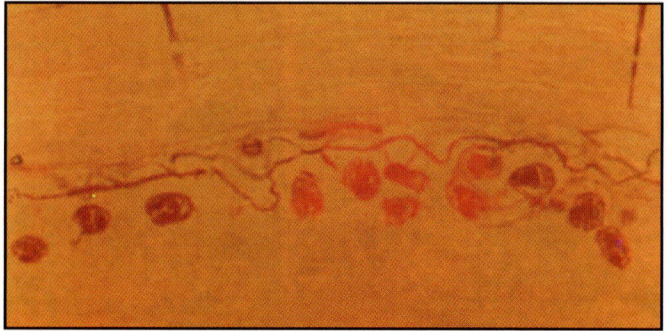

Fig. 52. Hydatid cyst showing laminated hyaline ectocyst, endocyst and scolices.

Section 1

General Bacteriology

- The compound microscope
- Gram staining
- Ziehl-Neelsen staining
- Albert's staining
- Spore staining
- Capsule staining
- Motility of bacteria
- Sterilization
- Liquid culture media
- Solid culture media
- Collection and transportation of specimen
- Cultivation of bacteria
- Identification of bacteria (biochemical reactions)
- Antimicrobial susceptibility testing

The Compound Microscope

Instructions while Using Microscope

- Keep the microscope on a table that is free from vibration.
- Do not place it in front of a window where bright day light causes unwanted glare. Use artificial light for the microscope.
- Always adopt a comfortable posture.
- Identify all the essential parts of microscope (Fig. 1.1).
- If wearing spectacles, take care to avoid contact between the eyepiece and the spectacles.
- Before using a microscope, first clean the eyepieces, objectives, condenser lens and stage.

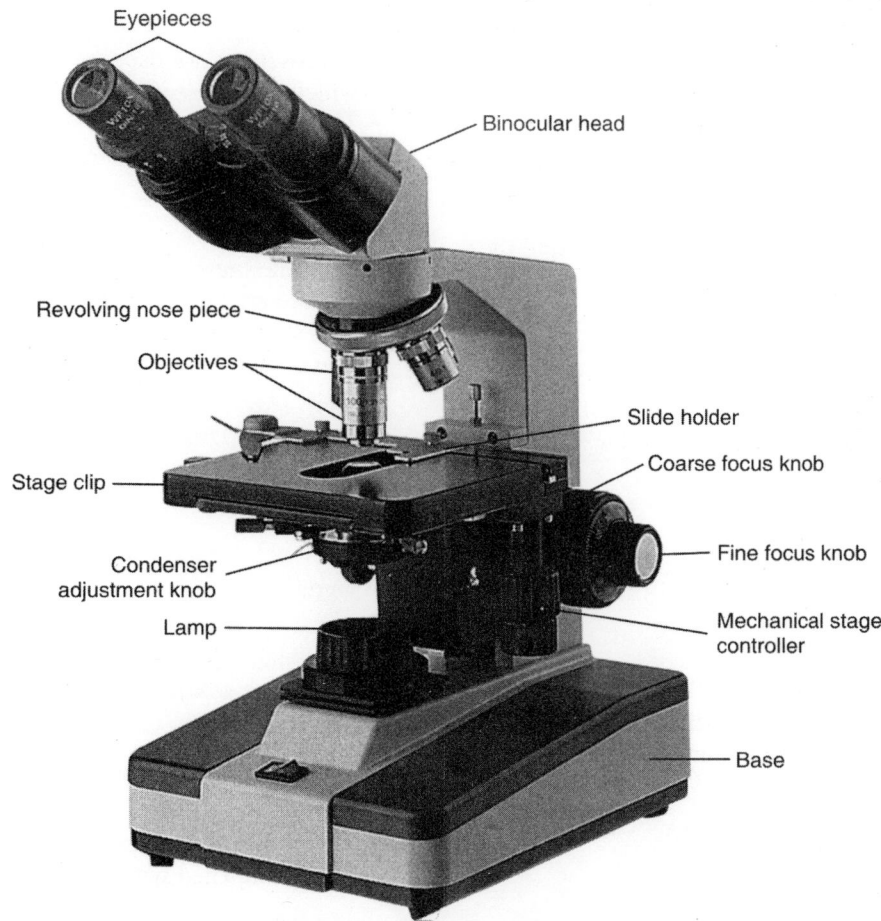

Fig. 1.1. Binocular microscope.

- Make sure the underside of the slide and surface of the stage are completely dry and clean.
- Use plane side of the mirror.
- Raise the condenser to within 1 mm of its topmost position and open the iris.
- Adjust the light by moving up and down the condenser and also by closing or opening the iris diaphragm.
- Obtain the best possible image by adjusting the condenser iris:
  - for the 10× objective, close the iris about two-thirds.
  - for the 40× objective, open the iris more.
  - for the 100× objective, open the iris fully and use 7× eyepiece with this objective.
- Always focus the slide first with the 10× objective followed by 40× or 100× as required. While changing the objective from one power to another, always hear the click sound otherwise objective may not be in place for proper illumination.
- Move the objective carefully downwards using the coarse focusing knob until the lens is near the slide. Then looking through the eyepiece, move the objective slowly upwards with the coarse adjustment knob until the image comes into the view. Then adjust with the fine adjustment knob until image is clear.
- Focus continuously to avoid organisms and structures in different planes being missed or misidentified.
- Use a coverslip when examining the specimen with the 10× or 40× objective.
- Put a drop of oil on the dried slide, when using 100× objective. Always check that the oil has been added to the smear side of the slide. Mark the smear side of the slide with glass marker.
- The oil-immersion objective must be cleaned after use with a tissue paper. Use xylene to remove the dried oil.
- Always move the 100× objective to one side when inserting and removing slide to prevent scratching of the front lens of the objective.
- Keep the microscope under a plastic cover after the work is over. If the microscope is to be moved, do not hold it by the body limb. It should be lifted by the upright limb.

Discussion

1. **Define resolving power of microscope.**

   This is defined as the ability to distinguish clearly two points that are close together within the structure of a particular object.

2. **How do you calculate the resolving power?**

   Resolving power is calculated as:

   $$r = \frac{0.6 \times \lambda}{NA}$$

   where λ = wavelength of light; NA = numerical aperture of objective.

3. **Define numerical aperture (NA).**

   This is defined as the ratio of diameter of the lens to its focal length.

4. **What is magnification?**

   The degree of enlargement of the object is known as magnification.

5. **How do you calculate the magnification?**

   This is calculated by multiplying the magnification of the objective lens with that of the eyepiece lens.

6. **What is the limit of resolution of naked eye, light microscope and electron microscope?**

   These are 200 μm, 0.2 μm and 0.3 nm for naked eye, light microscope and electron microscope, respectively.

7. **Enumerate various compound microscopes.**

   - Light microscope
   - Phase-contrast microscope
   - Dark-ground (dark-field) microscope
   - Fluorescence microscope
   - Electron microscope

8. **What are the major advantages of microscopes?**

   - Microscopes are used to visualize very small objects which are not seen clearly with naked eye.
   - They are used for diagnosing many diseases especially those caused by parasites.

9. **Why oil is used while examining the object under oil-immersion lens?**

   Oil has the same refractive index as that of glass. Due to the presence of oil, light is not refracted outwards but passes straight into the objective and helps in visualization of the object (organisms).

10. **Which side of mirror is used for reflecting light up through the condenser?**

    Plane mirror.

11. **Which agent should be used to clean the oil-immersion objective?**

    Xylene.

12. **Why alcohol should not be used for cleaning the oil-immersion objective?**

    Because alcohol will dissolve the cement holding the lens in its mount.

13. **How do you decontaminate the stage of the microscope?**

    Stage of the microscope can be decontaminated by using a linen dampened with 70% ethanol.

14. **How do you differentiate, whether dirt seen in the image is from the objective or eyepiece?**

    Rotate one of the eyepieces, if the dirt also rotates it is in the eyepiece.

15. What do you suspect, if blurred image is seen with 40× objective lens?

The objective lens may become contaminated from a wet preparation or may have oil.

16. What is the correct use of a binocular head?

The distance between the user's eyes (interpupillary distance) should be matched with the distance between the eyepieces of the binocular head.

17. What is advantage of trinocular head?

In trinocular head, an additional tube is used for holding a camera for photomicrography work.

18. Why monocular microscopes should be avoided wherever there is heavy use of microscopes?

Because eye strain is associated with the use of monocular microscope.

19. How glare is minimized while using microscope?

- Adjust the iris diaphragm according to the objective in use.
- Avoid using a large source of illumination than is necessary.
- Do not position a microscope in front of sunlight.

20. What are the uses of filters in microscopy?

- To reduce the intensity of light, when required.
- To transmit light of a selected wavelength, e.g., an exciter filter is used in fluorescence microscope.
- To increase contrast and resolution.
- To protect eye from injury caused by ultraviolet light, e.g., barrier filter is used in fluorescence microscope.

21. What are the uses of dark-field microscopy?

Dark-field microscopy is useful for detecting spirochaetes such as:

- *Treponema pallidum* in the lesions.
- Borreliae in blood.
- Leptospires in urine.

22. Which light is used in fluorescence microscope?

Ultraviolet light.

23. What are the applications of fluorescence microscopy?

- Examination of auramine-phenol stained sputum and cerebrospinal fluid for acid-fast bacilli.
- Immunodiagnosis by indirect and direct fluorescent antibody test.
- Examination of acridine orange stained blood films for detection of malaria parasites, microfilariae and trypanosomes.

24. What do you mean by micrometry?

The measurement of size of microorganisms using a calibrated eyepiece scale is called micrometry.

25. How do the organisms appear in dark-field microscopy?

Organisms appear as bright objects against a dark background.

26. What is the main use of phase-contrast microscopy?

It is used to study the internal structures of microorganisms.

Gram Staining

Introduction

The Gram stain was introduced by Hans Christian Gram, a Danish physician in 1884. This is the most frequently used differential stain that divides bacteria into two major groups: (1) Gram-positive, and (2) Gram-negative. Gram staining reaction depends on whether or not the organism resists decolourization with acetone or alcohol after staining with pararosaniline dye and further treatment with mordant (Gram's iodine). Bacteria which resist decolourization and remain dark purple after counterstaining are called Gram-positive bacteria while bacteria which get decolourized and take the light pink colour after counterstaining with safranin, neutral red or dilute carbol fuchsin are called Gram-negative bacteria.

Principle

The exact mechanism of Gram reaction is not known. It may, however, be attributed to:

- Gram-positive bacteria have more acidic protoplasm, which may account for their retaining the basic primary dye more strongly than Gram-negative bacteria.
- The violet basic dye and the iodine forms a dye–iodine complex inside both Gram-positive and Gram-negative bacteria, but during decolourization, cell membranes are dissolved (outer membrane of cell wall and cytoplasmic membrane). However, dye–iodine complex is retained in Gram-positive cells by the thick peptidoglycan mesh, whereas, it is readily washed out through the very thin peptidoglycan layer remaining in Gram-negative cells after both membranes have been dissolved.

Requirements

- Slides
- Spirit lamp
- Nichrome loop
- Glass marker
- Distilled water
- Cedar-wood oil
- Gauge piece
- Light microscope

Reagents

- Crystal violet (2%) or methyl violet (0.5%) or gentian violet (1%).
- Gram's iodine:
  - Iodine crystal   1 g
  - Potassium iodide   2 g
  - Distilled water   100 ml

  Dissolve 2 g potassium iodide in 25 ml water, and then add 1 g iodine. When iodine is dissolved, make up to 100 ml with water.
- Acetone or alcohol.
- Safranin (0.1%) or dilute carbol fuchsin (1:10).

Procedure

Smear preparation

1. Take a grease-free clean slide and make an oval-shaped mark at the centre by using a glass marker.
2. Transfer a loopful of liquid culture with a sterile nichrome loop and make a smear in the premarked area on the slide (for solid culture, take a loopful of saline on the slide and emulsify the organisms in an area of 1 cm^2).
3. Allow the smear to air dry.
4. Fix the dry smear by passing the slide 3 to 4 times over the flame quickly with smear side facing-up. The smear is said to be fixed when it is just tolerable on the dorsum of hand. Overheating chars the smear.

Staining

1. Place the slide on the staining glass rods.
2. Cover the smear with 2% crystal violet and leave for 1 minute.

3. Wash the slide with Gram's iodine.
4. Cover the smear with Gram's iodine and allow it to act for 1 minute.
5. Drain off the iodine.
6. Decolourize with alcohol or acetone. Acetone is the fastest decolourizer. It is applied to smears for only 2–3 seconds. While alcohol acts more slowly than acetone and should be applied and re-applied for about 1 minute until on tilting the slide from side-to-side and viewing against a white background, colour is no longer seen to flow out of the preparation.
7. Wash under tap water.
8. Counterstain the smear with dilute carbol fuchsin or 1% safranin for 30 seconds.
9. Wash with water and allow the stained smear to dry in air (or dry with blotting paper).
10. Put a drop of cedar-wood oil on the stained smear and observe under oil-immersion lens (100×) of microscope.

Result

- Gram-positive bacteria (Colour Plate I, Fig. 1) Dark purple
- Gram-negative bacteria (Colour Plate I, Fig. 2) Light pink or red
- Yeast cells Dark purple
- Tissue cells Pink
- Red blood cells Pink
- White blood cells Pink
- Nuclei of pus cells Pink to red
- Epithelial cells Pale red

Uses

1. It helps to differentiate bacteria into two groups, i.e. Gram-positive and Gram-negative.
2. This differentiation is helpful in determining the use of subsequent culture media and biochemical tests.
3. On the basis of the shape, we can differentiate between cocci and bacilli.
4. It helps in identification of organisms on the basis of arrangement, e.g., Gram-positive cocci in chains (streptococci), and Gram-positive bacilli with Chinese letter arrangement (*Corynebacterium diphtheriae*).
5. Presence of spore (unstained area) and its position can be determined.
6. It helps in starting antibacterial treatment, e.g., cell wall acting antibiotics in case of Gram-positive cocci and broad spectrum antibiotics in case of Gram-negative bacilli.
7. It helps to identify host cells. Presence of host cells such as squamous epithelial cells in respiratory specimen indicates contamination with organisms and cells from the mouth.
8. Presence of inflammatory cells (e.g., phagocytes) is key indicator of an infectious process.

9. It can identify non-bacterial forms such as trichomonads, *Strongyloides* larvae and *Pneumocystis jirovecii* cysts, although, it is not as sensitive as other special stains used for their visualization.

Gram-positive organisms that have lost cell wall integrity because of antibiotic treatment, old age, or action of autolytic enzymes may allow crystal violet to wash out with the decolourizing step and may appear Gram-variable, with some cells staining pink and others staining violet. However, for identification purposes, these organisms are considered Gram-positive. On the other hand, Gram-negative bacteria rarely, if ever, retain crystal violet, if staining procedure has been properly performed.

Not all bacteria can be seen in the Gram stain. Table 2.1 lists the medically important bacteria that cannot be seen in Gram stain and describes the reason why. The alternative microscopic approach to Gram stain is also given.

Table 2.1. Medically important bacteria that cannot be seen by Gram staining

Microorganism	Reason	Alternative microscopic approach
Mycobacteria including *M. tuberculosis*	Too much lipid in cell wall so dye cannot penetrate	Acid-fast stain
Treponema pallidum	Too thin to see	Dark-field microscopy, silver impregnation method or fluorescent-antibody staining
Mycoplasma pneumoniae	No cell wall; very small	Giemsa
Legionella pneumophila	Poor uptake of red counterstain	Prolong time of counter-stain
Chlamydiae including *C. trachomatis*	Intracellular; very small	Giemsa
Rickettsiae	Intracellular; very small	Giemsa or other tissue stains

Modifications of Gram staining

These are given in Table 2.2.

Table 2.2. Modifications of Gram staining

Method	Decolourizing agent	Counterstain
Kopeloff and Beerman's method	Acetone	Basic fuchsin
Burke's modification	Acetone	Safranin
Jensen's modification	Alcohol	Neutral red
Preston and Morrell's method	Iodine-acetone	Dilute carbol fuchsin
Weigert's modification	Aniline-xylol	Carmalum solution

Discussion

1. What are mordants?

Mordants are substances used in staining treatment which penetrate into a bacterial cell and which help to retain the original dye within the cell (by forming a link between organism and stain).

2. Can Gram-positive organisms appear as Gram-negative?

Yes, under following situations, it can be so:
- Overdecolourization of the smear.
- Smear prepared from old cultures.
- Use of iodine solution which is too old (yellow instead of brown).
- Cell wall damage due to excessive heat fixation of the smear, antibiotic therapy or action of autolytic enzymes.

3. Name Gram-positive bacilli.
- *Corynebacterium*
- *Clostridium*
- *Bacillus*
- *Actinomyces*
- *Nocardia*
- *Streptomyces*
- *Listeria*
- *Erysipelothrix*

4. Name various agents to which Gram-positive organisms are more susceptible as compared to Gram-negative.

Gram-positive organisms are more susceptible to antibacterial action of penicillin, acids, iodine, basic dyes, detergents and lysozyme and less susceptible to alkali, azide, tellurite, proteolytic enzymes, lysis by antibody, complement and plasmolysis in solutes of high osmotic pressure.

5. Name Gram-negative cocci.
- Meningococci
- Gonococci
- *Veillonella*

6. Differentiate between cell walls of Gram-positive and Gram-negative organisms.

Differences between cell walls of Gram-positive and Gram-negative organisms are given in Table 2.3.

7. Name organisms which lack cell wall.
- *Mycoplasma*
- *Ureaplasma*
- *Spiroplasma*
- *Anaeroplasma*

8. Mention coccobacilli.
- *Kingella*

Table 2.3. Differences between cell walls of Gram-positive and Gram-negative organisms

	Gram-positive	Gram-negative
Thickness	Thicker	Thinner
Teichoic acid	Present	Absent
Lipids	Absent/scanty	Present
Aromatic and sulphur-containing amino acids	Absent	Present
Peptidoglycan	50–90% of the dry weight of the cell wall	5–10% of the dry weight of the cell wall

- *Acinetobacter*
- *Klebsiella granulomatis*

9. Mention any organism which occurs in octad pattern.

Sporosarcina

10. Which is the fastest and most specific decolourizing agent?

Acetone.

11. Name various decolourizing agents.

Acetone, absolute alcohol, acetone-alcohol and iodine-acetone.

12. Which is the strongest counterstain?

Dilute carbol fuchsin.

13. What is the disadvantage of dilute carbol fuchsin?

This counterstain when applied for 10–30 seconds gives the strongest red staining. The colouration may be so dark that some Gram-negative bacteria may be difficult to distinguish from Gram-positive ones.

14. Name any slowly acting decolourizing agent?

Iodine-acetone (Addition of small concentration of iodine to acetone slows its rate of decolourization without reducing its specificity.)

15. Which two dyes constitute gentian violet?

Crystal violet and methyl violet.

16. Who invented Gram staining?

Hans Christian Gram.

17. Name other stains which can be used in place of crystal violet in Gram staining?

Methyl violet or gentian violet may be used.

18. What do you mean by Gram-positive or Gram-negative organisms?

Gram-positive bacteria resist decolourization and retain the colour of primary stain, i.e., violet colour. Gram-negative bacteria are decolourized by acetone and, therefore, take the colour of the counterstain (dilute carbol fuchsin or safranin), i.e. light pink or red.

Ziehl-Neelsen Staining

Introduction

Ziehl-Neelsen staining method is used for staining of acid-fast bacilli (AFB). Acid-fastness has been attributed to the high content of lipids, fatty acids and higher alcohols found in acid-fast bacteria. Of the lipids, mycolic acid, a high molecular weight hydroxy acid wax containing carboxyl groups, is the most important because it is acid-fast even in free state. Because of these lipids, ordinary aniline dye solutions do not penetrate the cell wall. The staining solution used to stain acid-fast bacilli is prepared by using a strong mordant dye like basic fuchsin with phenol. For penetration of the dye into the bacillus, heating of the stain is necessary.

Principle

Basic fuchsin in combination with phenol penetrates the cell wall and stains the bacilli bright red. Once stained, they resist decolourization with strong acid. The basic dye in combination with mineral acid forms a yellowish-brown compound which easily comes out of the non-acid-fast bacilli after decolourization but not out of the acid-fast bacilli. Counter-staining with methylene blue is done to form a contrast to red-coloured acid-fast bacilli.

Reagents

- Ziehl-Neelsen carbol fuchsin
  - Basic fuchsin (powder)   5 g
  - Phenol (crystalline)   25 g
  - Absolute alcohol (ethanol)   50 ml
  - Distilled water   500 ml
- Sulphuric acid   20%
- Loeffler's methylene blue   0.5%

Requirements

Same as in Practical 2.

Procedure

Smear preparation

1. Take a new, unscratched slide and make an oval-shaped mark at the centre by using a glass marker.
2. Make a smear from blood tinged or yellow purulent portion of the sputum using a stick in the premarked area.
3. Allow the smear to air dry for 15–30 minutes.
4. Fix the smear by passing the slide over the flame quickly 3–4 times with smear side facing up.

Staining

1. Place the slide on the staining glass rods with the smeared side facing upwards.
2. Pour filtered carbol fuchsin over the slide so as to cover the entire slide.
3. Heat the slide underneath until vapours start rising. Do not allow carbol fuchsin to boil or the slide to dry. Continue the process for five minutes.
4. Wash both sides of the slide with tap water.
5. Cover the slide with 20% sulphuric acid. The red colour of the preparation is changed to yellowish-brown. After about a minute in the acid, wash the slide with water, and pour on more acid. Repeat this process several times. The object of the washing is to remove the compound of acid with stain and allow fresh acid to gain access to the preparation. The decolourization is finished when, after washing, the film is only faintly pink. Decolourization generally requires contact with sulphuric acid for a total of at least 10 minutes.
6. Counterstain with Loeffler's methylene blue for 15–20 seconds.
7. Wash with water.
8. Place the slide in slide tray and allow it to dry.
9. Put a drop of oil on the stained area and observe under oil-immersion (100×) magnification.

General Bacteriology

1

Result

- Acid-fast bacilli   Bright red bacilli against blue
  (Colour Plate I, Fig. 3)   background
- Pus cells   Blue
- Squamous epithelial cells   Blue
- Elastic fibres   Blue

Uses

1. Ziehl-Neelsen method of staining is useful in detection of acid-fast organisms.
2. Number of bacilli in the smear may be counted and correlated with infectiousness of the person. Ziehl-Neelsen smear grading as per RNTCP recommendations (Table 3.1).

Table 3.1. Ziehl-Neelsen smear grading as per RNTCP recommendations

If the slide has	Result	Grading	No. of fields to be examined
More than 10 AFB per oil-immersion field	Positive	3+	20
1–10 AFB per oil-immersion field	Positive	2+	50
10–99 AFB per 100 oil-immersion fields	Positive	1+	100
1–9 AFB per 100 oil-immersion fields	Positive	Scanty	100
No AFB in 100 oil-immersion fields	Negative	—	100

3. This is useful in following a patient's response to treatment.
4. To know the drug resistance. If organisms fail to decrease after therapy in the smear, the possibility of drug resistance must be considered.

How to prevent false positive sputum results?

- Ask the patient to rinse the mouth with water before collecting sputum sample.
- There should not be any food particle or fibre in the sputum sample.
- Use only new, unscratched slides.
- Always use filtered carbol fuchsin.
- Do not allow the carbol fuchsin to boil during staining.
- Decolourize adequately with sulphuric acid.
- Never touch the oil-immersion applicator to the slide.
- Always clean the oil-immersion lens after screening each smear.

How to prevent false negative sputum results?

- Make sure that sample contains sputum and not just saliva.
- There should be enough sputum (at least 2 ml).
- Select blood-tinged or purulent portions to make the smear.
- Fix the smear with correct length of time.
- Prepare smear with adequate material.
- Stain with carbol fuchsin for 5–7 minutes.
- Do not decolourize with sulphuric acid too intensively.
- Examine every smear for at least five minutes observing at least 100 fields before recording as negative.

Discussion

1. **What do you mean by acid-fastness?**

   Acid-fast bacteria do not stain readily with dilute solutions of dyes. But when stained with hot concentrated carbol fuchsin, subsequently resist decolourization by mineral acid.

2. **Name various acid-fast organisms.**

   Tubercle bacilli, lepra bacilli, nontuberculous myco-bacteria, *Nocardia* spp., *Legionella micadadei*, *Rhodococcus* spp., bacterial spores, and oocysts of *Cryptosporidium parvum*, *Isospora belli* and *Cyclospora cayetanensis*.

3. **What are the factors which affect acid-fastness of an organism?**
   - Age of colonies
   - Medium on which growth occurs
   - Ultraviolet light
   - Lipid content and integrity of the cell wall of the organism

4. **Why tubercle bacilli are acid-fast?**

   Due to presence of mycolic acid in their cell wall.

5. **Why heating of carbol fuchsin is necessary in Ziehl-Neelsen staining?**

   Heating helps in penetration of dye (carbol fuchsin) through waxy coat surrounding the cell wall of myco-bacteria.

6. **What are the other methods of acid-fast staining?**
   - Kinyoun acid-fast stain
   - Fluorochrome stain.

7. **Why Kinyoun acid-fast stain method is known as cold method?**

   The Kinyoun stain is known as "cold stain" because the high concentration of phenol in the reagent serves to 'dissolve' the lipid material in the cell wall, allowing penetration of the carbol fuchsin dye without the use of heat.

8. **Which method of staining is most useful screening procedure?**

   Fluorescent dye staining.

9. **What are the advantages of fluorescent staining over Ziehl-Neelsen staining?**

Fluorescent staining is:

- More sensitive.
- No heating is required.
- Slide is scanned under low power and hence scanning is quick.
- Positive fluorescent smear may be restained by Ziehl-Neelsen or Kinyoun procedure, thereby saving the time needed to make a fresh smear.
- Mycobacteria appear as bright luminous yellow rods against a dark background.

10. What are the drawbacks of fluorochrome staining?

- Many rapid growers (e.g., *Mycobacterium chelonae* and *M. fortuitum*) may not appear fluorescent with these reagents.
- Fluorescence microscope and reagents are expensive.
- Expert hands are required to distinguish between positive bacilli and artifacts.

11. What are the limitations of acid-fast staining?

- Organisms other than mycobacteria may demonstrate various degree of acid-fastness.
- Rapidly growing mycobacteria may stain poorly or acid-fast variable.

12. What is the number of bacilli which must be present in the sputum for detection by direct microscopy?

Fifty thousand to 100,000 bacilli per ml.

13. What is the minimum number of bacilli which must be present in the sputum for detection by direct microscopy while using standard concentration technique?

Ten thousand/ml.

14. Can we use counterstain other than methylene blue?

Yes, malachite green may be used.

15. What is the disadvantage of malachite green?

This is a strong counterstain and may mask the presence of AFB.

16. Can we decolourize the smear with acids other than sulphuric acid?

Yes, nitric acid or hydrochloric acid may be used.

17. What is the role of phenol in carbol fuchsin?

It acts as mordant. It also makes the cell surface easily penetrable for basic fuchsin by dissolving fats.

18. Which method is more sensitive (Ziehl-Neelsen or Kinyoun)?

Ziehl-Neelsen is more sensitive. Weak acid-fast strains of rapidly growing species may stain better with Ziehl-Neelsen than Kinyoun.

19. What is the concentration of sulphuric acid used for decolourization of various acid-fast organisms?

Concentration of sulphuric acid used for decolourization of various acid-fast organisms is given in Table 3.2.

Table 3.2. Concentration of sulphuric acid used for decolourization of various acid-fast organisms

Microorganisms	% concentration of sulphuric acid
Mycobacterium tuberculosis	20
Nontuberculous mycobacteria	20
M. leprae	5
Cryptosporidium	1–5
Nocardia spp.	1
Bacterial spores	0.25–0.5

20. How can you differentiate smegma bacilli present in the urine from *Mycobacterium tuberculosis*?

M. tuberculosis is acid- and alcohol-fast while smegma bacilli (commensal) are only acid-fast.

21. Describe the morphology of *M. leprae* on Ziehl-Neelsen staining.

M. leprae is acid-fast, slender, slightly curved or straight bacillus. The bacilli are seen singly and in groups, intracellularly or lying free outside the cell. Inside the cells, they are usually present in parallel bundles of 50 or more organisms bound together by a lipid-like substance, the **glia**. These masses of bacteria are known as **globi** which are seen inside the histiocytes which have a foamy appearance. These are known as **lepra cells**.

22. How do you differentiate live and dead lepra bacilli in smear stained with Ziehl-Neelsen staining?

The live bacilli stain uniformly and appear solid, whereas the dead bacilli are fragmented and granular. This helps to monitor the efficacy of treatment in leprosy patients.

23. Define morphological index (MI).

It is defined as the percentage of uniformly stained bacilli out of the total number of bacilli counted. A continuing fall in the MI is encouraging and a fall succeeded by a rise indicates development of drug resistance in the bacteria.

24. What is bacteriological index (BI)?

Bacteriological index of a smear is the total number of acid-fast bacilli in an oil-immersion field. It is expressed from 1+ to 6+ by Ridley's scale (Table 3.3).

Table 3.3. Bacteriological index (Ridley scale)

Bacteriological index	Number of acid-fast bacilli
6+	More than 1000 per oil-immersion field
5+	100–1000 per oil-immersion field
4+	10–100 per oil-immersion field
3+	1–10 per oil-immersion field
2+	1–10 per 10 oil-immersion fields
1+	1–10 per 100 oil-immersion fields

Albert's Staining

Introduction

Albert's staining method is commonly used for staining and demonstration of *Corynebacterium diphtheriae*, the causative agent of diphtheria. They are thin, Gram-positive bacilli of varying length with an average size of 3×0.3 μm. They frequently possess club-shaped swellings at one or both ends, a characteristic feature, which is responsible for the name of the genus. When dividing, the bacilli snap and bend abruptly and appear as angled pairs or parallel rows of 3 to 4 bacilli (palisades) which resemble Chinese letters (Chinese letter arrangement).

Principle

The granules consist of long-chain inorganic polyphosphates and because of their characteristic reaction, they are termed as **metachromatic granules** or **volutin granules** or **Babes-Ernst bodies**. In unstained wet preparation, they appear as round refractile bodies within the bacterial cytoplasm. Most cells contain 2 or 3 of these, and they tend to be on poles. Their presence in thin slender bacilli helps to distinguish *C. diphtheriae* from short, thick plumpy, nonpathogenic diphtheroids which lack them. With Albert's stain, the granules stain bluish-black and cytoplasm green.

Requirements

Same as in Practical 2.

Reagents

Albert's stain

• Toluidine blue	0.15 g
• Malachite green	0.20 g
• Glacial acetic acid	1 ml
• Alcohol (95%)	2 ml
• Distilled water	100 ml

   Dissolve the dyes in the alcohol and add to the water and glacial acetic acid. Allow to stand for one day and then filter.

Albert's iodine

• Iodine	2 g
• Potassium iodide	3 g
• Distilled water	300 ml

Procedure

1. Make film, dry in air, and fix by heat.
2. Place the slide on the staining glass rods.
3. Cover the smear with Albert's stain and allow to act for 3–5 minutes.
4. Drain the staining solution, but do not wash.
5. Cover the smear with Albert's iodine and allow to act for 1 minute.
6. Wash with water.
7. Dry with blotting paper and observe under 100× magnification of microscope.

Result

• Metachromatic granules (Colour Plate I, Fig. 4)	Bluish-black
• Bacillary body or protoplasm	Green

Uses

1. Albert's staining is useful in the demonstration of metachromatic granules.
2. Presence of metachromatic granules help to distinguish *C. diphtheriae* from diphtheroids which lack them.
3. Differentiation of three biotypes of *C. diphtheriae* can be done on the basis of granules.

Discussion

1. What is the chemical nature of metachromatic granules?

The granules consist of long-chain inorganic polyphosphates. It appears that they represent storage depots for materials needed to form high-energy phosphate bonds.

2. **What are the other names of metachromatic granules?**

   Babes-Ernst granules, volutin granules and polar bodies.

3. **On which medium granule formation is best seen?**

   Loeffler's serum slope.

4. **How can you differentiate *C. diphtheriae* from diphtheroids on the basis of granules?**

   Diphtheroid bacilli do not exhibit metachromatic granules.

5. **In which biotype of *C. diphtheriae* prominent granulation is seen?**

   Mitis.

6. **In which biotype of *C. diphtheriae* few or no granules are present?**

   Gravis.

7. **How can you differentiate diphtheroids from biotype gravis?**

   Diphtheroids are arranged in V forms or palisades rather than Chinese letter arrangement. They can also be differentiated on the basis of toxigenicity test and fermentation of starch and glycogen, which are shown by biotype gravis.

8. **What is the maximum number of these granules in a single bacillus?**

   Six

9. **Why are they called corynebacteria?**

   They frequently show club-shaped swellings and hence the name corynebacteria (*coryne* meaning club).

10. **What is the other name of *C. diphtheriae*?**

    Klebs-Loeffler bacillus.

11. **In which other organism volutin granules are found?**

    Lactobacillus spp.

Spore Staining

Introduction

Spores are highly resistant resting forms which occur after a period of vegetative growth. Members of several bacterial genera are capable of forming spores. The two most common are Gram-positive rods—the aerobic genus *Bacillus* and the anaerobic genus *Clostridium*. The other bacteria known to form spores are the Gram-positive coccus *Sporosarcina* and possibly the rickettsial agent of Q fever and *Coxiella burnetti*.

Principle

Spores are most simply observed as intracellular refractile bodies in unstained cell suspension or as unstained bodies in Gram stain (Colour Plate I, Fig. 5). The spore wall is relatively impermeable, but dyes can be made to penetrate it by heating the preparation. The same impermeability then serves to prevent decolourization of the spore by a period of alcohol treatment sufficient to decolourize vegetative cells. The latter can finally be counterstained. They are commonly stained with malachite green or modified Ziehl-Neelsen staining (0.25% sulphuric acid as decolourizer).

MALACHITE GREEN STAIN FOR SPORES (SCHAEFFER AND FULTON METHOD)

Requirements

Same as in practicals 2–4.

Reagents

- Malachite green 5%
- Safranin (0.5%) or basic fuchsin (0.05%)

Procedure

1. Prepare a smear on a clean glass slide, dry it in air and fix it by heat.
2. Place the slide over a beaker of boiling water, resting it on the rim with the bacterial film uppermost.
3. When, within several seconds, large droplets have condensed on the underside of the slide, flood it with 5% acqueous solution of malachite green and leave it to act for 1 minute while the water continues to boil.
4. Wash under running tap water.
5. Cover the smear with 0.5% safranin or 0.05% basic fuchsin for 30 seconds.
6. Wash and dry.
7. Observe under oil-immersion lens.

Result (Colour Plate I, Fig. 6)

- Spore   Green
- Vegetative bacilli   Red
- Lipid granules   Unstained

Other methods of spore staining are given in Table 5.1.

Table 5.1. Other methods of spore staining			
Method	**Primary stain**	**Decolourization with**	**Counterstain**
Fleming's method	Carbol fuchsin	5% Sodium sulphate	10% Nigrosin
Mueller's method	Carbol fuchsin	Alcohol	Loeffler's methylene blue

Uses

1. It helps in identification of spore-bearing organisms.
2. Position of spores can be determined (i.e. central, terminal or subterminal).
3. Morphology of spores can be determined (bulging, non-bulging, spherical or oval).

Discussion

1. **Mention any coccus exhibiting the presence of spore.**
   Sporosarcina.

2. **What is the concentration of sulphuric acid used for decolourization of bacterial spores?**
   0.25%.

3. **What is the advantage of malachite green stain over modified Ziehl-Neelsen stain for staining bacterial spores?**
   In malachite green stain, spores are green and lipid granules are unstained, while in modified Ziehl-Neelsen stain, both spores and lipid granules are stained red.

4. **What are the uses of bacterial spores?**
   Bacterial spores are used as biological control to check the efficiency of sterilization methods (Table 5.2).

Table 5.2. Biological controls of hot air oven and autoclave

Method of sterilization	Biological control
Hot air oven	*Bacillus subtilis* subsp. *niger*
Autoclave	*Bacillus stearothermophilus*

5. **Why spores of *B. anthracis* are known as perfect germs for bioterrorism?**
   They are called perfect germs for bioterrorism because of the following reasons:
   - Production of spores of *B. anthracis* is easy and cheap.
   - These are extremely stable and can be stored almost indefinitely as dry powder.
   - These can be loaded in a freeze-dried condition and disseminated as an aerosol with crude sprayer.
   - A millionth of a gram of anthrax spores constitutes a lethal inhalation dose.

6. **By which method spores of all medically important species are destroyed?**
   Autoclaving at 121°C for 10–20 minutes.

7. **Compare bacterial spores with fungal spore.**
   Comparison of bacterial spores and fungal spores is given in Table 5.3.

Table 5.3. Comparison of bacterial and fungal spores

Bacterial spores	Fungal spores
Method of preservation	Method of reproduction
Highly resistant	Delicate

Capsule Staining

Introduction

Cell wall in many bacteria is enclosed by a protective gelatinous covering layer. If it is easily washed off and does not appear to be associated with the cell, in any definite fashion, it is referred to as a slime layer, on the other hand, if it appears as discrete, thickened gel around each cell, it is known as capsule. Capsule cannot be stained with ordinary stains like Gram staining. They are demonstrated by negative staining methods, either by the wet-film India ink preparation or by dry-film India ink or nigrosin preparation.

Wet India Ink Film

This is the simplest and most widely applicable method. In this method, capsules are not shrunken, as they are not dried or fixed and hence demonstrated clearly.

Requirements and Reagents

- Bacterial culture
- Glass slide
- Coverslip
- Inoculating loop
- Spirit lamp
- India ink

Procedure

1. Place one loopful of India ink on a perfectly clean glass slide.
2. Emulsify a small portion of bacterial culture in the drop of India ink with the help of a sterile loop.
3. Place a clean coverslip on drop of India ink without introducing air bubbles.
4. Press down the coverslip through a sheet of blotting paper so as to get thin film.
5. Observe under oil-immersion objective (100× magnification).

Result

On microscopical examination with the oil-immersion objective, the highly refractile outline of the bacterium is seen. Between the refractile surface-membrane and the dark background of ink particles, there is a clear space which represents the capsule (Colour Plate I, Fig. 7). Non-capsulated bacteria do not show this clear zone. The ink particles directly abut the refractile wall and in consequence, these bacteria are not easily seen.

Uses

This method is useful in identification of capsulated organisms.

Discussion

1. **Name capsulated organisms?**
   - *Streptococcus pneumoniae*
   - *Neisseria meningitidis*
   - *Klebsiella pneumoniae*
   - *Haemophilus influenzae*
   - *Yersinia pestis*
   - *Bacillus anthracis*
   - *Cryptococcus neoformans*

2. **What is the chemical nature of capsule?**

   In most species, it is made-up of complex polysaccharide, though in some species, its main constituent is polypeptide or protein (*Bacillus anthracis*).

3. **Why wet-film India ink method is better than dry-film method?**

   Dry-film negative staining method is less reliable since occasionally shrinkage space gives the appearance of capsule around bacteria that are non-capsulated and occasionally, especially in thick films, capsules may be shrunken or obscured to the point that they are rendered invisible. In wet-film, capsules do not become shrunken, since they are not dried or fixed.

4. **For what purpose dry-film India ink method is used?**

   If a permanent preparation is required for demonstration of bacterial capsules, it is necessary to use a dry-film method.

5. **What are common errors when preparing wet-film India ink?**

   • Use of diluted ink.
   • Making the films too thick (capsule is obscured by overlying ink).

6. **What are the characteristics of India ink used for capsule staining?**

   It must be:

   • Dense and homogeneous
   • Very finely granular
   • Free from contamination with capsulate or non-capsulate bacteria

7. **What are the functions of capsule?**

• Capsule protects the bacteria from antibacterial agents.
• It inhibits phagocytosis, thus, contributing to the virulence of bacteria.

8. **Mention any organism where capsule is polypeptide in nature?**

   Bacillus anthracis.

9. **Mention organisms in which both capsule and slime layer are present?**

   Klebsiella spp. and *Streptococcus salivarius.*

10. **Which serological method is used to demonstrate capsule?**

    Quellung reaction or capsule swelling.

11. **Briefly describe Quellung reaction?**

    Capsular material is antigenic. So, when a suspension of a capsulated bacterium is mixed with its specific anticapsular serum and examined under the microscope, the capsule becomes very prominent and appears 'swollen' due to an increase in its refractivity. This is known as Quellung reaction and employed for the identification of capsular serotypes.

Motility of Bacteria

Method

Hanging drop method.

Introduction

Bacteria are motile with the help of flagella. On microscopic examination of wet-films, motile bacteria are seen swimming in different directions across the field. True motility should be differentiated from passive drifting and Brownian movement.

True Motility

The organisms move in different directions and change their position in the field.

Passive Drifting

Organisms move in the same direction in a convectional current in the fluid.

Brownian Movement

This is a rapid oscillation of bacterium within a very limited area due to bombardment by the water molecules.

Requirements

- Glass slide
- Plasticine ring
- Coverslip
- Nichrome loop
- Spirit lamp
- Light microscope
- Bacterial culture (suspension)

Procedure

1. Place a small ring of plasticine over a clean glass slide. Alternatively, a slide with concavity may be used.
2. Put a drop of bacterial suspension on a coverslip.

3. Invert the glass slide over the coverslip, allowing coverslip to adhere to the slide.
4. Now, turn around the slide so that coverslip is on the top and drop of bacterial suspension hangs in the centre of plasticine ring from the under surface of coverslip (Fig. 7.1).

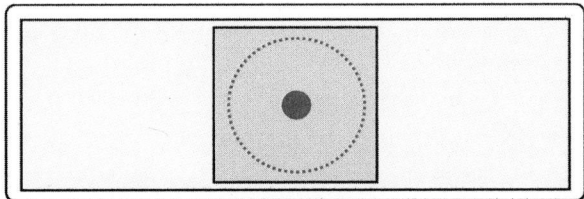

Fig. 7.1. Hanging drop preparation.

5. Examine under the microscope with condenser lying low. Focus the margin of hanging drop with low power and then swing the objectives to the high power lens (40× magnification) (Fig. 7.2).

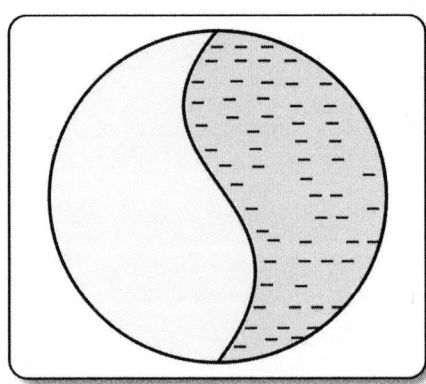

Fig. 7.2. Hanging drop examination under 40× magnification.

6. Observe for motility of bacteria.

Result

- Motile organisms: Detected by the presence of directional motion.
- Non-motile organisms: No movement.

Uses

1. Detection of motility of organisms.
2. Shape, approximate size and general structure can be observed.
3. Type of motility can be observed, e.g., darting motility is shown by *Vibrio cholerae*.

Discussion

1. **Name motile Gram-positive cocci.**
   - Planococci
   - *Sporosarcina*

2. **Enumerate various types of motility giving examples.**
   Various types of motility along with examples are given in Table 7.1.

   Table 7.1. Types of motility with examples

Type of motility	Example
Darting motility	*Vibrio cholerae*
Very actively motile	*Proteus* spp.
Actively motile	*Escherichia coli*
Tumbling motility	*Listeria monocytogenes*
Gliding motility	*Mycoplasma pneumoniae*
Corkscrew motility	*Campylobacter* spp. and spirochaetes

3. **Name the organelles of motility.**
   Flagella.

4. **Name any organism which is motile by fimbriae.**
   Eikenella corrodens. It lacks flagella and shows jerking or twitching motility which is due to its possession of contractile fimbria-like filamentous appendages.

5. **Name the organelles of locomotion in spirochaetes.**
   The motility in spirochaetes is due to one or more pairs of axial filaments which run between outer membrane and peptidoglycan layer and are anchored by knobs at both poles.

6. **Name non-motile Gram-positive bacilli.**
   - *Clostridium perfringens*
   - *Bacillus anthracis*

7. **Name other methods of determining motility of bacteria.**
   - Cragie's tube technique
   - Mannitol motility medium
   - Swarming on solid medium

8. **How do you interpret motility in mannitol motility medium?**
   This medium has agar concentration of 0.4% or less to allow free spread of organisms. Inoculation is done by a single stab into the medium. After overnight incubation, movement away from the stab line or a hazy appearance throughout the medium indicates a motile organism.

9. **What are the other features observed in mannitol motility medium?**
   - Fermentation of mannitol
   - Gas production (aerogenic organisms)

10. **How motile organisms are converted into non-motile?**
    - Temporary phenotypic change
    - Mutation

11. **Why edge of hanging drop is preferred for examination?**
    Because due to surface tension, number of bacteria present are more near the edge of the drop.

Sterilization

Introduction

Sterilization is defined as the process by which an article, a surface or a medium is freed of all microorganisms including viruses, bacteria, their spores and fungi, both pathogenic and nonpathogenic. The process of sterilization is used in microbiology for prevention of contamination of culture media from bacteria in air, dust, etc. Heat is the most reliable, certain and rapid method of sterilization. There are two types of heat: dry heat and moist heat (Tables 8.1 and 8.2). Dry heat is believed to kill microorganisms by causing destructive oxidation of essential cell constituents. The moist heat causes denaturation and coagulation of proteins.

HOT AIR OVEN

It is a method of choice for sterilization of glassware such as test tubes, petri dishes, pipettes and flasks; metal instruments such as forceps, scissors and scalpel; materials such as oils, jellies and powders which are impervious to steam and swab sticks packed in test tubes. It is not suitable for materials like fabrics which may be damaged by heat. Hot air oven is electrically heated and is fitted with a thermostat that maintains the chamber air at a chosen temperature and a fan that distributes hot air in the chamber (Fig. 8.1). It must not be overloaded and spaces must be left for circulation of air through the load. Holding time for sterilization in hot air oven is one hour at 160°C for one hour or 20 minutes at 180°C. It is timed as beginning when the thermometer first shows 160°C or 180°C, respectively.

Sterilization Controls

Two types of controls are available.

Chemical control

A Browne's tube containing red solution is placed within the

Table 8.1. Sterilization by dry heat

Mode of sterilization	Instrument	Temperature and time	Sterilization of
Red heat	Bunsen burner	Till red hot	Inoculating wire loops and forceps
Flaming	Bunsen burner	Waving through the flame	Scalpel blades, glass slides, mouth of culture tubes and bottles
Hot air	Hot air oven	160°C for 1 hour or 180°C for 20 minutes	Glassware, metal instruments, sealed materials such as oils, greases, dry powder, swab sticks packed in test tubes, etc.

Table 8.2. Sterilization by moist heat

Mode of sterilization	Instrument	Temperature and time	Sterilization of
Below 100°C	Water bath	56°C for 1 hour	Serum
At 100°C	Boiling water bath	100°C for 10–20 minutes	Glass, metal and rubber items
Steaming at 100°C	Arnold steamer	100°C for 20 minutes on 3 successive days	Culture media containing sugar and gelatin
Steaming above 100°C	Autoclave	121°C for 15–20 minutes	Culture media and aqueous solutions, dressing material, linen, gloves, etc.

General Bacteriology

1

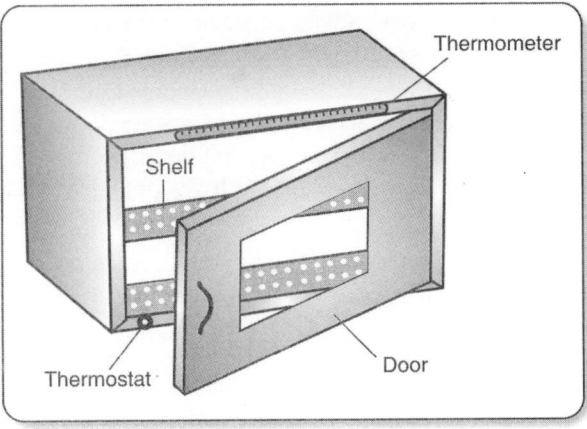

Fig. 8.1. Hot air oven.

load. A change of colour of the solution to green indicates proper sterilization.

Biological control

An envelope containing a filter paper strip impregnated with 10^6 spores of *Bacillus subtilis* subsp. *niger* is placed within the load. After sterilization is over, the strip is removed and inoculated into tryptone soy broth and incubated aerobically at 37°C for five days. No growth of *B. subtilis* subsp. *niger* indicates proper sterilization.

AUTOCLAVE

Sterilization by steam under pressure (autoclaving) is suitable for culture media and aqueous solutions, dressing materials, linen, gloves, etc. Satisfactory sterilization can be achieved at 15 pounds per square inch (psi) pressure equivalent to 121°C in 15–20 minutes. The laboratory autoclave (Fig. 8.2) consists of a vertical or horizontal cylinder of gun metal or stainless steel in a supporting frame.

The lid is fastened by screw clamps and rendered air tight by asbestos gasket. Lid bears a pressure gauge and a steam release valve or safety valve. The latter opens and closes when the steam pressure rises or falls the desired level, respectively. On its upper part of the side, the autoclave has a discharge tap for air and steam, and an air and steam release knob. Heating is done by electricity. Water is added on the bottom of the autoclave. Above this is a perforated shelf on which articles to be sterilized are placed. The lid is closed, discharge tap is opened and safety valve is adjusted to the required pressure. As heating continues, the steam and air mixture escapes. When all the air from inside the autoclave has been removed then the discharge tap is closed. Steam pressure rises inside and when it reaches the desired set level (15 psi) the safety valve opens and excess steam escapes. From this point, the holding time (15 minutes) is counted. When the holding time is over, the heating is stopped and autoclave allowed to cool till pressure gauze indicates that inside pressure has reached to the atmospheric pressure. The discharge tap is now

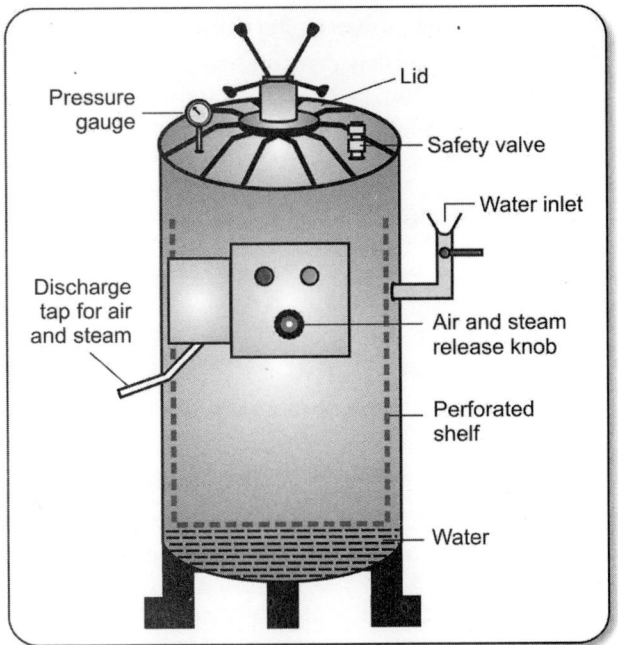

Fig. 8.2. Autoclave.

opened and air allowed to enter the autoclave. The lid is now opened and the sterilized articles removed.

Biological control

Bacillus stearothermophilus. It is processed as in case of hot air oven. However, incubation is done at 56°C.

Chemical control

A Browne's tube containing red solution as in case of hot air oven.

Discussion

1. **Define the term sterilization.**
   Sterilization is defined as the process by which an article, a surface or a medium is freed of all microorganisms including viruses, bacteria, their spores and fungi, both pathogenic and nonpathogenic.

2. **Define the term disinfection.**
   Disinfection is a process of destruction or removal of organisms capable of giving rise to infection. Disinfectants are capable of killing vegetative bacteria, fungi, viruses and rarely bacterial spores.

3. **What do you mean by antiseptic?**
   A disinfectant that is applied to living tissue is referred to as an antiseptic.

4. **What is the mechanism of sterilization by dry heat?**
   Dry heat is believed to kill microorganisms by causing destructive oxidation of essential cell constituents.

5. **What is the mechanism of sterilization by moist heat?**

   The moist heat causes denaturation and coagulation of proteins. When steam condenses on cooler surface, it releases its latent heat and raises the temperature of its surface. If spores are present, steam condenses on them and increases their water content leading to hydrolysis and breakdown of bacterial proteins.

6. **What is the holding time for sterilization in hot air oven?**

   Holding time for sterilization in hot air oven is one hour at 160°C or 20 minutes at 180°C.

7. **Name biological control to check the efficacy of hot air oven.**

   Bacillus subtilis subsp. *niger* (NCTC 10075 or ATCC 9372).

8. **What do you mean by low temperature steam-formaldehyde (LTSF) sterilization?**

   Items which cannot withstand heat at 100°C may be disinfected by steam at sub-atmospheric pressure at a temperature of 75°C with formaldehyde vapour. This is known as LTSF sterilization.

9. **How many methods of pasteurization are there?**

   • *Holder method:* The temperature employed is 63°C for 30 minutes.
   • *Flash method:* 72°C for 20 seconds followed by rapid cooling to 13°C or lower.

10. **Which organism may survive pasteurization by Holder methods?**

    Coxiella burnetti, causative agent of Q fever.

11. **What do you mean by tyndallization or intermittent sterilization?**

    One single exposure to free steam at 100°C for 90 minutes ensures complete sterilization but for culture media containing sugar and gelatin, which may get decomposed on long heating, an exposure of 100°C for 20 minutes on three consecutive days is employed. This is known as tyndallization.

12. **Why an exposure of three consecutive days is required in tyndallization?**

    First exposure to steam kills vegetative bacteria and any spores present, being in a favourable medium, will germinate and will be killed on the subsequent occasions.

13. **Enumerate items which can be sterilized in hot air oven.**

    • Glassware
    • Metal instruments
    • Liquid paraffin
    • Jellies
    • Powders
    • Swab sticks packed in test tubes

14. **Why steam above 100°C or saturated steam is more efficient sterilizing agent than hot air?**

    • It provides greater lethal action of moist heat.
    • It is quicker in heating-up the exposed articles.
    • It can penetrate easily porous materials such as cotton-wool stoppers, paper and cloth wrappers, bundles of surgical linen, and hollow apparatus.

15. **Enumerate articles which are sterilized in autoclave.**

    • Culture media
    • Aqueous solutions
    • Dressing material
    • Linen
    • Gloves

16. **What temperature and pressure are required for sterilization by autoclaving?**

    Sterilization can be achieved at 15 pounds per square inch (psi) pressure equivalent to 121°C in 15–20 minutes.

17. **Name biological control to check the efficacy of autoclave.**

    Bacillus stearothermophilus (NCTC 10003 or ATCC 7953).

18. **Enumerate physical agents of sterilization.**

    • Sunlight
    • Drying
    • Heat
    • Filtration
    • Radiation

19. **Which method of sterilization can kill all bacterial spores?**

    Autoclaving at 121°C for 15–20 minutes.

20. **Name one steam sterilizer.**

    Koch or Arnold steam sterilizer.

21. **What do you mean by 'thermal death time'?**

    Thermal death time is the minimum time required to kill a suspension of organisms at a pre-determined temperature in a specified environment.

22. **Enumerate factors influencing 'sterilization by heat'.**

    • Number of microorganisms.
    • Presence or absence of spores.
    • Species, strain and spore-forming ability of the microorganisms.
    • Nature of the material in which microorganisms are heated.

23. **Enumerate media which are sterilized in an inspissator.**

    Lowenstein-Jensen medium and Loeffler's serum slope.

24. **What temperature and time are required for sterilization in an inspissator?**

    80–85°C for half an hour on three successive days.

25. **Which rubber can withstand temperature of hot air oven?**

Silicon rubber.

26. **Why hot air oven is allowed to cool after sterilization process?**

It is allowed to cool for about two hours before the door is opened, since the glassware may crack due to sudden or uneven cooling.

27. **How do you sterilize inoculating loop or wire?**

It is sterilized by holding it vertical in a Bunsen burner flame until red hot.

28. **What is the method of sterilization of serum?**

Serum can be sterilized by heating for one hour at 56°C in a water bath.

29. **Define cold sterilization.**

Sterilization of disposable items by ionizing radiations or ethylene oxide is known as cold sterilization.

Liquid Culture Media

Introduction

Culture media are essential for isolation and identification of microorganisms which help in diagnosis and treatment of infectious diseases.

Classification of Media

Culture media have been classified as under:

1. Solid, semisolid and liquid media.
2. Simple (basal), complex, synthetic, defined, semidefined, and special media. Special media are further divided into enriched, selective, enrichment, indicator or differential, sugar media and transport media.
3. Aerobic media and anaerobic media.

Commonly Used Liquid Culture Media

1. Peptone water
2. Nutrient broth
3. Sugar media
4. Bile broth and glucose broth
5. Cooked meat broth (CMB)
6. Hiss serum sugar media
7. Buffered glycerol saline
8. Tetrathionate broth
9. Selenite-F broth
10. Venkatraman-Ramakrishnan medium (VR medium)

1. Peptone Water

This is a sugar-free basal medium. It contains peptone (10 g), sodium chloride (5 g) and distilled water (1000 ml). It is a watery colourless solution with pH 7.4–7.6 (Colour Plate II, Fig. 8A).

Uses

- It is a liquid basal medium used for preparation of sugar media.

- It is mainly used for culturing a large number of non-fastidious organisms.
- Peptone water is used for testing indole production.
- It is also used for studying the motility of organisms.
- It is used for cultivation and as an enrichment medium for *Vibrio cholerae* by raising the pH to 8.4 (alkaline peptone water).

2. Nutrient Broth

This is a basal medium for the preparation of other media. It contains meat extract (10 g), peptone (10 g), sodium chloride (5 g) and distilled water (1000 ml). It is a clear, straw-coloured transparent fluid with pH 7.4–7.6 (Colour Plate II, Fig. 8B).

Uses

- It is more nutritious than peptone water and may be used for growth of fastidious organisms.
- This medium is routinely used for culture of common bacteria.
- It is used as a basal medium for preparation of cooked meat broth employed for cultivation of anaerobes.
- It is used for preparation of bile broth and glucose broth.
- It is used for testing of disinfectants.

3. Sugar Media

A large variety of carbohydrates are used for identification of organisms. The basal medium for sugars is peptone water. It contains 1% sugar (glucose, lactose, mannitol, sucrose, etc.) in a sterilized peptone water (pH 7.2–7.4). It also contains 1% Andrade's indicator. Various other indicators having a pH range between 6 and 8, such as bromothymol blue and neutral red, can also be used. Sugar media are dispensed in tubes containing inverted Durham's tube (Colour Plate II, Fig. 8C). Various sugar media in tubes can be identified by incorporating cotton-wool stoppers of different colours.

Uses

- Sugar media are used for testing the sugar fermentation reactions for identification of various organisms. (Fermentation is indicated by development of red colour due to the production of acid.)
- Gas producing bacteria can be identified by observing air in Durham's tube.

4. Bile Broth and Glucose Broth

These are primary culture media for blood culture. These contain nutrient broth (100 ml), glucose/bile (1 g) and sodium citrate (0.2 g) (Colour Plate II, Fig. 8D and E). In most of the patients with septicaemia and pyrexia of unknown origin, the organisms present in the blood are very few, so large amount of blood (5–10 ml) is required. Blood itself contains antibacterial substances. Hence, for diluting these antibacterial substances, 10-fold dilution of the blood in the medium (50–100 ml) is required. The addition of liquoid (sodium polyanetholsulphonate) counteracts the bactericidal action of blood.

Uses

- Bile broth is used for isolation of *Salmonella* spp. from blood of the patients suffering from enteric fever.
- Glucose broth is used for isolation of pyogenic organisms from blood, e.g., streptococci from cases of bacterial endocarditis.

5. Cooked Meat Broth (CMB)

This medium is used for the isolation of anaerobic organisms. It contains meat cooked in sodium hydroxide and then filtered and squeezed. The meat particles in the medium act as a reducing agent and provide anaerobic atmosphere. The meat particles are dispensed in sterile test tube to give a tall column (approximately 2.5 cm). Sterile nutrient broth is added to give a column of 5 cm above the meat particles. A tall column of meat is essential because the conditions are anaerobic only when the column of meat is sufficiently high. Addition of paraffin on the top of nutrient broth further seals off the atmospheric oxygen (Colour Plate II, Fig. 8F).

Uses

It is used:

- For isolation of anaerobic organisms.
- As a transport medium for anaerobic organisms.
- To distinguish proteolytic clostridia from saccharolytic. In CMB, saccharolytic clostridia produce acid and gas but they do not digest the meat. The culture may have a slightly sour smell and the meat is often reddened. On the other hand, proteolytic clostridia produce blackening of meat, decompose it and reduce it in volume with the formation of foul-smelling products.

- For preservation of stock cultures of aerobic organisms, e.g., streptococci.

6. Hiss Serum Sugar Medium

It consists of 1 part of ox serum and 3 parts of peptone water.

Uses

It is used for biochemical reactions of organisms requiring serum for growth, e.g., neisseriae, corynebacteria, etc.

7. Buffered Glycerol Saline

It contains disodium hydrogen phosphate (10 g), glycerol (300 ml), sodium chloride (4.2 g), phenol red (15 ml) and distilled water (700 ml). This medium is purple-pink in colour (Colour Plate II, Fig. 8G) and dispensed in 6 ml amount in universal container.

8. Tetrathionate Broth

It contains thiosulphate solution, iodine solution, phenol red, calcium carbonate and nutrient broth. This medium should be used within 24 hours of preparation.

Uses

- This medium is used as an enrichment medium for *Salmonella* and *Shigella*.
- **Brilliant green tetrathionate broth:** This broth can be prepared by addition of 0.001% brilliant green to this medium (Colour Plate II, Fig. 8H).

9. Selenite-F Broth

It contains sodium hydrogen selenite (4 g), peptone (5 g), lactose (4 g), disodium hydrogen phosphate (9.5 g), sodium dihydrogen phosphate (0.5 g) and distilled water (100 ml) (Colour Plate II, Fig. 8I). This medium is sterilized by steaming at 100°C for 30 minutes.

Uses

This is an enrichment medium for the isolation of *Salmonella* and *Shigella*.

10. Venkatraman-Ramakrishnan Medium (VR Medium)

This medium contains crude sea salt (20 g), peptone (5 g) and distilled water (100 ml). It is dispensed in screw-capped bottles in 10–15 ml amounts. About 1–3 ml stool is to be added to each bottle.

Uses

This is used as transport or holding medium for *Vibrio cholerae*. In this medium, vibrios do not multiply but remain viable for several weeks.

Discussion

1. **What are the advantages of liquid media?**

   In liquid media, rapid growth of organism is obtained. These are used for:

   - Biochemical tests,
   - Antibiotic sensitivity tests,
   - Studying motility of bacteria, and
   - For bulk cultures for the preparation of antigens and vaccines.

2. **What are the disadvantages of liquid media?**

   - The growth of organisms does not exhibit characteristic appearances. However, pigment production, as in case of *Pseudomonas aeruginosa*, can be easily detected.
   - Individual organisms cannot be identified from a mixture containing different organisms.

3. **What is peptone?**

   Peptone consists of water-soluble products obtained from lean meat or other protein materials, such as heart muscle, casein, fibrin or soya fluor, by digestion with the proteolytic enzymes, pepsin, trypsin or papain. The important constituents are peptones, proteoses, amino acids, a variety of inorganic salts (phosphates, potassium and magnesium), and certain accessory growth factors such as nicotinic acid and riboflavin.

4. **What are the essential requirements of a good peptone?**

   - Able to support the growth of moderately exacting bacteria from small inocula.
   - Absence of fermentable carbohydrates.
   - A very low content of copper.

5. **What do you mean by term 'Sugar'?**

The term 'sugar' in microbiology denotes any fermentable substance. They may be monosaccharides (pentoses, hexoses), disaccharides (lactose), trisaccharides (raffinose), polysaccharides (starch, inulin), alcohols (glycerol, sorbitol), glucosides (salicin, aesculin) and non-carbohydrate substances (inositol).

6. **What is the reducing agent in cooked meat broth?**

   Meat particles act as reducing agent.

7. **Name various reducing agents used in culture media.**

   Glucose (0.5–1%), ascorbic acid (0.1%), cysteine (0.1%) and sodium thioglycolate (0.1%).

8. **What are the essential requirements of a culture medium?**

   The culture medium should provide energy source, nitrogen source, carbon source, salts (phosphates, sodium, potassium, calcium and magnesium), satisfactory oxidation-reduction potential, certain growth factors and pH corresponding to the pH of body cells.

9. **What is the disadvantage of copper-distilled water for preparation of culture media?**

   Copper-distilled water should not be used as even traces of copper are inhibitory for bacterial growth. Demineralized glass-distilled water is preferred.

10. **Define enrichment media.**

    When a substance is added to a liquid medium which inhibits the growth of unwanted bacteria and favours the growth of wanted bacteria, it is known as enrichment medium.

11. **Name enrichment media.**

    Tetrathionate broth and selenite broth for *Salmonella* and *Shigella*, and alkaline peptone water for *Vibrio cholerae*.

Solid Culture Media

Introduction

Robert Koch described means of cultivating bacteria on solid media. Most solid media are solidified by adding agar (a long-chain polysaccharide gelling agent obtained from certain seaweeds). A concentration of 1–2% usually yields a suitable gel. The melting and solidifying points of agar are not the same. At the concentration, normally used, most bacteriological agars melt at about 95°C and solidify only when cooled to about 42°C. It does not melt at 37°C (incubation temperature of most pathogenic bacteria)—a property that makes it a suitable solidifying agent for culture media. Most of the culture media are sterilized by autoclaving at 121°C for 15 minutes. Nutrients that are damaged by autoclaving are sterilized separately by filtration, etc. The sterilized agar base is then melted in the steamer and cooled to about 45–50°C followed by addition of heat-labile ingredients, but once these are added, the medium must at once be poured into petri dishes because it cannot be remelted without damaging the heat-sensitive ingredients. Solid media are used to obtain isolated colonies of organisms.

Commonly Used Solid Media

1. Nutrient agar
2. Blood agar
3. Chocolate agar
4. MacConkey agar
5. Loeffler's serum slope
6. Lowenstein-Jensen medium
7. Sabouraud dextrose agar
8. Mueller-Hinton agar
9. Triple sugar iron agar

1. Nutrient Agar

It is a solid basal medium for routine use. It contains peptone (10 g), sodium chloride (5 g), meat extract (10 g), agar (20 g) and distilled water (1000 ml). It is pale yellowish (Colour Plate II, Fig. 9A) dispensed in petri dishes and test tubes.

Uses

- It is used for growth of common pathogenic organisms.
- It acts as basal medium for the preparation of other media, e.g., blood agar, milk agar, salt agar, etc.
- It is used for antibiotic sensitivity testing.
- It is used for demonstration of pigment production in staphylococci and *Pseudomonas*.
- Semisolid nutrient agar (0.2–0.5% agar) is used for demonstrating motility (Craigie's tube method).
- Concentrated nutrient agar (4–6%) is used for inhibiting the swarming of *Proteus* species.
- Slopes of nutrient agar are used for maintenance of stock cultures.
- It is used as a transport medium for bacterial cultures.

2. Blood Agar

It contains 5–10% sheep blood in nutrient agar. It is red-coloured opaque medium contained in petri dishes (Colour Plate II, Fig. 9B). It is a widely used enriched medium in bacteriology.

Uses

- It is used for demonstrating haemolytic property (α, β and γ) of organisms.
- It is useful for growth of most of the pathogens.
- It is used for testing the drug sensitivity of *Haemophilus influenzae* and *Neisseria* species.
- It is used for preparation of chocolate agar.
- It may become selective medium by addition of certain chemicals, e.g., potassium tellurite, neomycin, crystal violet, etc.

General Bacteriology

1

3. Chocolate Agar (Heated Blood Agar)

This medium is more enriched medium than blood agar. It is prepared by heating 10% of sterile blood in sterile nutrient agar. Melt the agar, cool it in a water bath at 75°C, add the blood and allow the medium to remain at 75°C, mixing the blood and agar by gentle agitation from time to time until the blood becomes chocolate-brown in colour, within about 10 minutes. Then pour in petri dishes. Alternatively, it can also be prepared by simply heating the blood agar plates at 55°C by placing in an incubator for 1–2 hours. It is identified by its typical chocolate colour (Colour Plate II, Fig. 9C).

Uses

This medium is used for the culture of *Neisseria*, pneumococci, *Haemophilus influenzae*, etc.

4. MacConkey Agar

MacConkey agar is a differential or indicator medium used for the culture of the organisms of the family Enterobacteriaceae. It contains peptone (20 g), sodium taurocholate (5 g), lactose (1%) neutral red solution, 2% in 50% ethanol (3.5 ml), agar (20 g) and distilled water (1000 ml). It is transparent, pink red in colour and is dispensed in petri dishes (Colour Plate II, Fig. 9D). Presence of bile salts in the medium inhibits the growth of non-intestinal organisms. Lactose with an indicator neutral red distinguishes the lactose-fermenting coliforms from non-lactose-fermenting organisms. Fermentation of lactose by organisms results in acid production, which is indicated as pink colour colonies when the indicator is neutral red.

Uses

- It is a useful medium for the culture of the organisms of the family Enterobacteriaceae.
- It differentiates lactose-fermenting organisms from non-lactose-fermenting organisms.
- It can be used as a selective medium for *Salmonella* spp. by the addition of brilliant green.
- It can be made differential for *Escherichia coli* 0157: H7 by addition of sorbitol and omission of lactose. It produces colourless colonies on this medium, as it does not ferment sorbitol. Other strains of *E. coli* produce pink colonies on this medium.

5. Loeffler's Serum Slope (LSS)

It contains 3 parts of ox, sheep or horse serum and 1 part sterile glucose broth (1%). It is white opaque medium with small amount of water of condensation. It is dispensed in McCartney's bottle as a slope (Colour Plate II, Fig. 9E).

Uses

- This is used for the cultivation of *Corynebacterium diphtheriae*.

- Growth of *C. diphtheriae* on this medium is rapid (6–8 hours).
- Metachromatic granules of *C. diphtheriae* are well formed in this medium.
- The water of condensation is used for testing the toxigenicity in guinea pig.

6. Lowenstein-Jensen Medium

It contains whole egg, malachite green, mineral salt solution (asparagine, glycerol, magnesium sulphate, magnesium citrate, distilled water and potassium dihydrogen phosphate). It is green opaque slope dispensed in McCartney bottle (Colour Plate II, Fig. 9F). 0.75% glycerol enhances the growth of human tubercle bacillus, but glycerol at this concentration is inhibitory to *Mycobacterium bovis*, so it fails to grow on this medium. However, when the concentration of the glycerol is reduced to 0.5%, it still improves the growth of *M. tuberculosis* but generally does not inhibit the growth of *M. bovis*. Malachite green inhibits the growth of organisms other than mycobacteria and provides a colour contrast while egg serves both as enrichment and solidifying agent.

Uses

- It is used for cultivation of mycobacteria including *Mycobacterium tuberculosis* and nontuberculous mycobacteria.
- It is used for differentiation between human and bovine types of tubercle bacilli.
- It is used for drug sensitivity testing of tubercle bacilli.

7. Sabouraud Dextrose Agar

This is a selective medium for the cultivation of fungi. It contains glucose (40 g), peptone (10 g), agar (20 g) and distilled water (1000 ml). It is pale, semitransparent slope dispensed in large test tubes with pH 5.4 (Colour Plate II, Fig. 9G). Its low pH, high sugar content and incorporation of penicillin and streptomycin prevents the growth of bacteria, and cycloheximide inhibits the growth of contaminating fungi.

Uses

- It is used for cultivation of fungi.
- Sensitivity to antimycotic drugs may be determined in this medium.

8. Mueller-Hinton Agar

It contains beef infusion (300 ml), casein hydrolysate (17.5 g), starch (1.5 g), agar (20 g) and distilled water (1000 ml). Presence of starch in the medium acts as a colloidal agent against the toxic substances produced during the growth.

Uses

- This medium is used for antibiotic sensitivity testing of most pathogens.

- It is also used for the isolation of pathogenic *Neisseria* species.

9. Triple Sugar Iron (TSI) Agar

It contains 3 sugars (glucose, lactose and sucrose), sodium thiosulphate, yeast extract, sodium chloride, peptone, ferric citrate, phenol red, peptone, agar and distilled water. It is a red-coloured slope dispensed in a tube (Colour Plate II, Fig. 9H). It is advisable to inoculate both slant and the butt for demonstrating the varying patterns of fermentation in TSI medium.

Uses

This is used for differentiation of the members of the family Enterobacteriaceae according to their ability to ferment lactose, sucrose, glucose and production of hydrogen sulphide (H_2S) gas (Table 10.1).

Table 10.1. Interpretation of reactions seen on triple sugar iron agar

Appearance of medium	Interpretation of reaction
Orange red colour	Control (uninoculated)
Alkaline slant and alkaline butt (deep red)	No sugar fermented
Acid slant and acid butt (yellow)	Lactose and sucrose fermented along with glucose
Acid butt, alkaline slant (yellow butt, red slant)	Only glucose is fermented
Bubbles in butt or slant	Formation of gas during fermentation
Blackening in butt or at the junction of butt and slant	H_2S production

Discussion

1. **What are the advantages of solid media?**
   - Bacteria produce discrete visible growth (colonies) with distinct colonial morphology.
   - Different organisms form well-separated colonies from a mixed culture.
   - They exhibit many other characteristic features such as pigment production or haemolysis.

2. **What do you understand by the term enriched media?**
   In these media, substances like blood, serum and egg are added to basal medium to increase the nutritious value, e.g., blood agar, chocolate agar, Loeffler's serum slope, etc.

3. **Define indicator medium or differential medium.**
   When a substance is added into a medium which would produce a visible change in the medium following the growth of a particular organism, it is designated as indicator or differential medium, e.g., MacConkey agar.

4. **Define selective medium.**
   When a substance is added to a solid medium which inhibits the growth of unwanted bacteria but permits the growth of wanted bacteria it is known as selective medium, e.g., Lowenstein-Jensen medium for the isolation of *Mycobacterium tuberculosis*.

5. **What are the advantages of agar?**
   - Agar does not add to the nutritive properties of the medium and is not affected by the growth of bacteria.
   - The melting (95°C) and solidifying (42°C) points of agar are not the same, therefore, heat-labile ingredients can be added to sterilized agar base at 45–50°C.
   - Agar does not alter the pH of the medium.
   - Agar can be added to any nutrient liquid medium, if the advantages of a solid medium are desired.

6. **What is the advantage of low pH and high sugar content in Sabouraud dextrose agar?**
   It prevents bacterial contamination.

7. **What do you mean by the term "hard agar"?**
   To prepare a solid medium, usually 1–2% agar is used, if the concentration is raised to 6%, it is called hard agar.

8. **What is the concentration of agar in semisolid agar?**
   0.2–0.5%.

9. **Which blood is preferred for preparing blood agar plates?**
   Sheep blood is preferred because the haemolysis is better visualised, and moreover it does not have any toxic substances which can suppress the growth of bacteria.

10. **Name any medium containing serum.**
    Loeffler's serum slope.

11. **Name media containing egg.**
    - Dorset egg medium.
    - Lowenstein-Jensen medium.
    - NIH medium.

12. **How much medium should be poured in a 100 mm petri dish?**
    Medium should be poured to a depth of 4 mm (25 ml).

Collection and Transportation of Specimen

Introduction

The laboratory diagnosis of an infectious disease begins with the collection of a clinical specimen. Proper collection of an appropriate clinical specimen is the first step in obtaining an accurate laboratory diagnosis of an infectious disease. A poorly collected specimen not only may result in failure to recover important microorganisms, but may also lead to incorrect or even harmful therapy, if treatment is directed towards a commensal or contaminant.

General Rules for Collection and Transportation of Specimen

* Apply strict aseptic techniques throughout the procedure.
* Wash hands before and after the collection.
* Collect the specimen before the administration of anti-microbial agents.
* Prevent contamination of the specimen with externally present organisms or normal flora of the body.
* Collect the specimen at the appropriate phase of disease.
* Collect the specimen from the actual infection site.
* Collect adequate quantity for the desired tests.
* Collect the specimen aseptically in a sterile and appropriate container.
* Close the container tightly so that its contents do not leak during transportation.
* Ensure that the outside of the specimen container is clean and uncontaminated.
* Label the container appropriately and complete the requisition form.
* Immediately transport the specimen to the laboratory.

Criteria for Rejection of Specimens

* Missing or inadequate identification.
* Leaking container or blood-stained containers.
* Specimen collected in an inappropriate container.
* Insufficient quantity.
* Contamination suspected.
* Incomplete forms.
* Haemolysed blood sample.
* Inappropriate transport or storage.

Collection and Transportation of Specimens

Blood for culture

* Should be drawn under aseptic conditions.
* Disinfect the skin over the vein with tincture iodine and spirit and wait for a minute.
* Draw out 5–10 ml of blood for one blood culture bottle containing 50–100 ml of medium. For paediatric age group, 1 ml blood in 10 ml of medium in McCartney bottle (Fig. 11.1A) may be added.

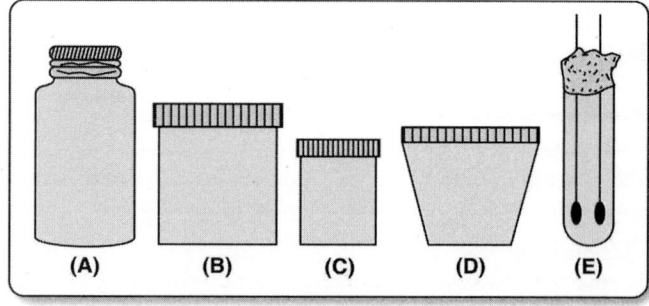

Fig. 11.1. (A) McCartney bottle, (B) Urine/stool container, (C) CSF container, (D) Sputum container, (E) Throat swabs.

* Collect blood during early stages of disease since the number of bacteria is higher in acute and early stages of disease.
* Collect blood during paroxysm of fever since the number of bacteria is higher during high temperature in patients with fever.

- In the absence of antibiotic administration, 99% culture positivity can be seen with three blood cultures.
- Transport the specimen to the laboratory. If not possible keep in incubator or at room temperature. Do not refrigerate.

Urine

- Mid-stream urine sample is collected after giving proper instructions to the patient.
  - *Clean the genitalia properly (in case of male, retract the prepuce, clean it with sterile normal saline. In case of female, wash perineum and periurethral area with soap and water).*
  - *Collect a "clean-catch" mid-stream urine sample in a sterile bottle (Fig. 11.1B).*
- Transport immediately to the laboratory. If a delay of more than 1–2 hours is unavoidable, refrigerate at 4°C.
- In catheterized patients, do not collect urine from collection bag or after opening the closed drainage. Clean the area over the collecting tube and puncture with the help of a sterile needle and syringe and draw out the sample.
- Suprapubic aspiration under aseptic condition may be done in infants.

Cerebrospinal fluid (CSF)

- Collect CSF in a screw-capped sterile container (Fig. 11.1C) under aseptic conditions.
- Immediately transport to the laboratory and process.
- If delay in processing is inevitable, then store it at 37°C.
- Do not refrigerate.

Sputum

- Collect the sputum in a wide-mouthed container, which is preferably disposable, made-up of clear thin plastic, unbreakable and leak-proof container (Fig. 11.1D).
- Ask the patient to rinse the mouth with plain water and then inhale deeply 2–3 times, cough up deeply and spit in the sputum container by bringing it close to the mouth. If the patient has difficulty in coughing sputum, postural drainage and appropriate physiotherapy often cause exudate to move in the bronchi and stimulate productive coughing.
- Make sure the sputum sample is of good quality and not just the saliva. A good sputum sample is thick, purulent and sufficient in amount (2–3 ml).
- Sputum sample may be refrigerated up to 3–4 hours.

Throat swab

- Two swabs should be collected (Fig. 11.1E).
- Depress the tongue with a tongue blade.
- Swab the inflamed area of the throat, pharynx or tonsils with a sterile swab, taking care to collect the pus or piece of membrane, if formed.
- Transport in a sterile transport tube.

Pus and other discharge

- Do not apply antiseptic before collection.
- Clean with normal saline.
- In case of discharge, 1–2 ml of sample is collected in a sterile tube.
- If swabs are collected, 2 swabs in a sterile container should be collected (one for direct microscopic examination and the other for culture).

Bone marrow

- Decontaminate the skin overlying the site from where specimen is to be collected with tincture iodine and spirit.
- Aspirate 1 ml or more of bone marrow by sterile percutaneous aspiration.
- Collect in a sterile screw-cap tube.
- Immediately transport to the laboratory.

Stool

- Should be collected in early stage of disease and prior to treatment with antimicrobials.
- Do not collect the specimen from bed pan.
- Should not be contaminated with urine.
- Collect the sample in a wide-mouthed clean container (Fig. 11.1B).
- If mucus or flakes are present, these must be included.
- If possible, submit more than one specimen on different days.
- The fresh stool specimen must be processed within 1–2 hours of passage.
- If delay is unavoidable, then store it at 2–8°C.

Rectal swab

- Collect the swab only if stool collection is not possible.
- Insert swab at least 2.5 cm beyond the anal sphincter so that it enters the rectum.
- Rotate it once before withdrawing.
- Transport in Cary-Blair or other transport medium.

Catheters and tips

- Mark the junction of skin and catheter.
- Withdraw the catheter a little and cut it at about 1 cm distal to the mark.
- Send 5 cm length of the catheter in a sterile container.

Discussion

1. **Name transport media.**
   - Venkatraman-Ramakrishnan medium
   - Cary-Blair medium
   - Amies medium
   - Stuart's medium

2. **What is the advantage of transport media?**

They preserve the viability of bacteria (pathogen) during transport without allowing their multiplication.

3. **Why Dacron or polyester swabs are preferred for collection of fastidious organisms?**

Cotton swab may contain residual fatty acid, and calcium alginate may emit toxic products that may inhibit certain fastidious bacteria.

4. **Name the conditions in which urine shows pus cells but the routine culture is negative.**

- Patient on antibiotics.
- Infection with anaerobic bacteria or nutritionally exacting bacteria, that cannot grow on media, normally used for routine investigation.
- Genitourinary tuberculosis or gonococcal infection.

5. **Which is the most suitable sample for the diagnosis of urinary tuberculosis?**

Three early morning specimens of urine should be collected. Each specimen should consist of 50–100 ml.

6. **Which type of container is used for collection of stool sample?**

A 25 ml screw-capped, wide-mouthed glass or plastic bottle, preferably with a spoon projecting from the underside of the cap.

7. **How much CSF sample should be collected?**

Three to five ml of CSF should be collected and rate of collection should be slow, about 4–5 drops a second. Removal of a large volume may lead to headache.

8. **Why CSF sample should not be refrigerated?**

Refrigeration of CSF sample tends to kill *Haemophilus influenzae*.

9. **What is the best condition for storage of CSF?**

The specimen is best kept in an incubator at 37°C.

10. **How do you collect the vaginal swab and endocervical swab?**

- Vaginal swab is inserted into the upper part of vagina and rotated there before withdrawing it, so that exudate is collected from the upper as well as lower vaginal wall.
- An endocervical swab is collected for examination of gonococci. A vaginal speculum is used to provide a clear sight of the cervix and the swab is rubbed in and around the introitus of the cervix and withdrawn without contamination from the vaginal wall.

11. **Why do you collect two swabs?**

One swab is for making film and the other for seeding culture.

12. **What is the method of collection of throat swab?**

The swab should be rubbed with rotation over one tonsillar area, then arch of the soft palate and uvula, the other tonsillar area, and finally the posterior pharyngeal wall. Pseudomembrane, if formed, should be scraped with swab stick.

13. **How do you differentiate saliva from sputum sample on Gram staining?**

If a Gram-stained smear of a homogenized specimen shows less than 10 polymorphs to every squamous epithelial cell, and if the patient is not leucopenic, the material probably consists mainly of saliva.

14. **In which clinical situations, blood culture is requested?**

Blood culture is requested mainly in two clinical situations:

- Septicaemia or bacteraemia suggested by presence of fever, shock or other signs and symptoms occurring in association with a known or suspected local infection such as sepsis in surgical wound, puerperal sepsis, pneumonia, meningitis, osteomyelitis or endocarditis.
- Pyrexia of unknown origin (PUO).

15. **When do you collect nasal swabs?**

Nasal swabs are often taken to detect healthy carriers than to diagnose infection, deep nasal swabs being taken for *Streptococcus pyogenes* and diphtheria bacillus, and swabs from the skin of anterior nares for *Staphylococcus aureus*.

16. **In which clinical conditions, swabs are taken from external auditory meatus?**

Acute otitis media, chronic suppurative otitis media and otitis externa.

17. **How do you collect exudate from eye?**

The exudate from eye may be collected with:

- Sterile platinum loop.
- Smooth rounded tip of a thin glass or plastic rod.
- Serum-coated swab.

18. **Why cotton swabs are not used for the collection of exudates from eye?**

Cotton swabs are not used for the collection of exudate from eye because the volume of exudate obtainable is generally small, a dry cotton wool swab, which would absorb and retain most of the specimen, is unsuitable as a means of collection of exudate from eye.

19. **What is the advantage of homogenization of sputum sample?**

Most sputum samples are not homogeneous. If the specimen is homogenized, every drop and loopful of it will contain some of the pathogens present. Moreover, the homogenized material is suitable for quantitative examinations.

20. **Describe the characteristic features of pus due to different organisms?**

Characteristic features of pus due to different organisms are given in Table 11.1.

Table 11.1. Characteristic features of pus due to different organisms

Causative organisms	Characteristic features of pus
Staphylococcus aureus	Thick creamy
Streptococcus pyogenes	Watery and straw-coloured
Proteus spp.	Fishy smell
Pseudomonas spp.	Sweet, musty odour and often a blue pigmentation
Anaerobes	Offensive putrid smell
Actinomycetes	Sulphur granules
Fungi	Black or brown granules

Cultivation of Bacteria

Introduction

For the cultivation of bacteria, clinical specimens are inoculated onto various culture media. Inoculation is carried out with platinum or nichrome loops of different gauges. Nichrome has oxidizing properties and hence in some of the tests where this property of bacterium is to be tested (e.g., oxidase test), platinum loop, instead of nichrome should be used. The loop is sterilized by holding it vertically in the flame of burner, so that the whole length of wire becomes red hot. It is allowed to cool down before it touches any material suspected to be having bacteria to avoid the heat killing of the organisms.

Important Points about Inoculation of Culture Media

- Aseptic technique is important to avoid contamination of the material under process and to protect the worker from acquiring infection from the clinical specimen.
- Inoculate the media with clinical specimen as soon as possible.
- Open the caps and lids of the containers containing the specimen for the briefest period required.
- Do not keep the caps and lids on the workbench.
- Inoculating loops should be sterilized prior to introducing them into the specimen container.
- While working on the infectious material, keep the specimen away from the face.
- Avoid vigorous shaking of the specimen prior to opening. Open the caps slowly to minimize aerosol production.
- Loop should not contain fluid or large particle that may splatter when placed in flame.
- Keep all the specimens in racks to reduce the risk of accidental spillage.
- Prepare smears for staining after all media have been inoculated.

- When more than one medium is inoculated, follow a particular order. Inoculate media without inhibitors, followed by indicator and then selective media.
- While processing fluid specimen, inoculate liquid media first to reduce the chances of carrying over any possible contamination from solid media.
- Properly label the media to be inoculated.
- Minimize the aerosol production by opening the caps of liquid media slowly and avoid expulsion of the last drop from the pipette.
- Mop-up the workbench clean with a disinfectant at the start and close of work.
- Wash hands with soap and water before and after handling specimens.

Culture Methods

- Streak culture
- Lawn culture
- Stroke culture
- Stab culture
- Shake culture
- Pour-plate culture
- Liquid culture

Requirements

- Inoculation loop/wire
- Marker
- Peptone
- Nutrient agar medium
- Incubator
- Blood culture bottle
- Spirit lamp
- Light microscope
- Pipettes

Streak culture

This method is routinely employed for the isolation of bacteria in pure culture from clinical specimen. Owing to the high cost of platinum, loops for routine use are made of nichrome, No. 24 SWG with internal diameter 2–4 mm. One loopful of the specimen is smeared thoroughly over area A (Fig. 12.1), on the surface of a well dried plate, to give a well inoculum or 'well'. The loop is re-sterilized and drawn from the well in 2 or 3 parallel lines on the fresh surface of the medium (B). This process is repeated as shown (C, D and E), care being taken to sterilize the loop, and cool it on unseeded medium, between each sequence. On incubation, growth may be confluent at the site 'well', but becomes progressively thinner, and well separated colonies are obtained over the final series of streaks.

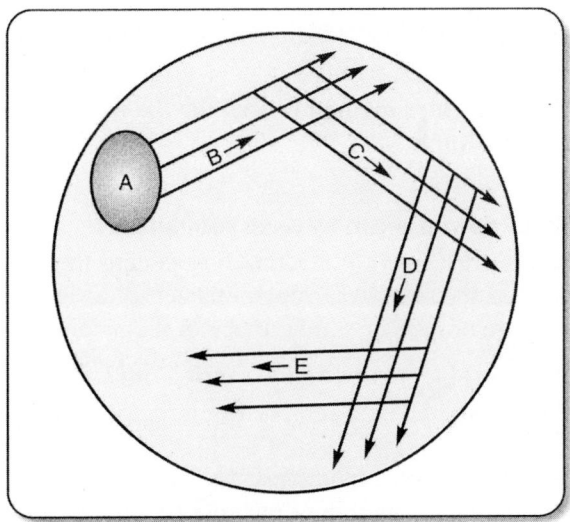

Fig. 12.1. Streak culture.

Lawn culture

Lawn cultures are prepared by flooding the surface of the plate with a liquid culture or suspension of bacteria and pipetting off the excess inoculum or by applying a swab soaked in the bacterial culture or suspension (Fig. 12.2). After incubation, lawn culture provides a uniform surface growth. It is useful for antibiotic susceptibility testing by disc diffusion method and bacteriophage typing.

Stroke culture

Stroke culture is made in tubes containing agar slope or slant. Slopes are seeded by lightly smearing the surface of agar with loop in zig-zag pattern taking care not to cut the agar (Fig. 12.3). It is used for obtaining pure growth for slide agglutination and other diagnostic tests.

Stab culture

Stab cultures in solid media (nutrient, gelatin or glucose agar) are inoculated by plunging the charged wire into the centre

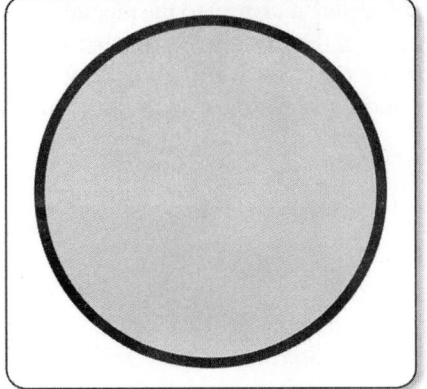

Fig. 12.2. Lawn culture.

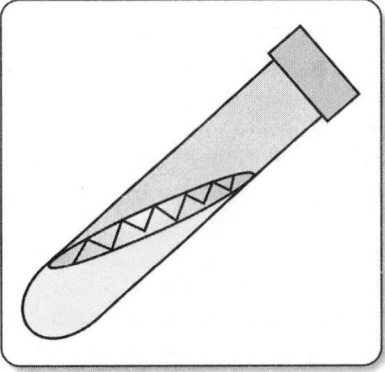

Fig. 12.3. Stroke culture.

of the medium and withdrawing it in the same line to avoid splitting the medium (Fig. 12.4). These are employed mainly for demonstration of gelatin liquefaction and for the maintenance of stock cultures.

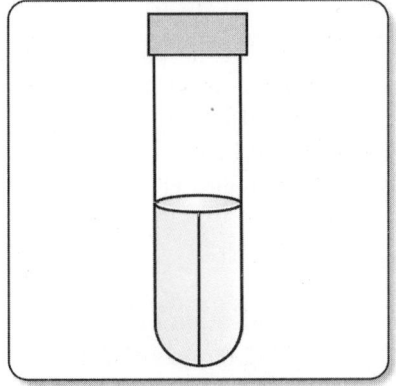

Fig. 12.4. Stab culture.

Shake culture

It is made by melting nutrient agar in a test tube, cooling it to 45°C and inoculating it while molten from a liquid medium with a drop from a capillary pipette. Withdraw the pipette, replace the cap or plug and discard the pipette into disinfectant. Mix the contents of the tube by rotation between the palms of the hands before the agar solidifies and incubate it at 37°C for 24 hours and look for the growth of the organisms.

Pour-plate culture

This method is used for counting the number of living bacteria or groups of bacteria in a liquid culture or suspension. Prepare serial 10-fold dilutions of the bacterial suspension over a range (6–9 tubes) ensuring that one dilution will contain between 50 and 500 viable bacteria/ml (number which can be accurately counted). Starting with the greatest dilution, pipette 1 ml of each dilution into each of three 9 cm petri dishes. Then pour into each dish about 10 ml of clear nutrient agar, melted and cooled to 45–50°C. Mix well by rapidly moving the plate for about 10 seconds. Allow the agar to set and incubate at 37°C for 48 hours. After incubation, colonies will be seen well distributed throughout the depth of the medium and can be enumerated using colony counter. Count the colonies in three plates containing 50–500 colonies/plate. Multiply the average number/plate by the dilution factor to obtain the viable count/ml in the original suspension.

Liquid culture

If the tubes have got cotton plugs, the mouth of the tubes should be heated in flame before and after handling of tube to prevent contamination from the rims of tubes getting into the medium. Incline the tube containing the liquid medium to 45° and deposit the inoculum on its lower end with the use of a straight wire. Return the tube to a vertical position. Now, the inoculum shall be below the surface of the liquid. Liquid cultures may be inoculated by adding the inoculum with pipettes or syringes. Large inocula can be employed in liquid culture and hence this method is adopted for blood culture and for sterility tests, where the concentration of bacteria in inocula are expected to be small. Liquid cultures are also preferred when large yields are desired.

Uses

The purpose of liquid culture is to grow the organism and isolate it in pure form which helps in further identification of organism, antibiotic sensitivity, phage typing, serotyping, etc.

Discussion

1. **What are the specification of nichrome loop?**

   Loop for routine work is made of nichrome, No. 24 SWG. The loop should be flat, circular and completely close with 2–4 mm internal diameter. It is mounted on a handle.

2. **For which test, platinum loop should be used and why?**

   When oxidizing property of a bacterium is to be tested, e.g., oxidase test, platinum loop must be used, as nichrome has oxidizing property.

3. **What are the uses of straight wire?**
   - For stab culture.
   - Picking-up of single colony.
   - Inoculation of liquid media.

4. **Which method is preferred for obtaining isolated colonies?**

   Streak culture.

5. **Why a culture plate should be dried before inoculation?**

   On wet plate, separate colonies do not appear. A sort of spreading or swarming appearance of growth occurs which is difficult to study.

6. **Describe the order in which solid media should be inoculated.**

   Inoculate media without inhibitors, followed by indicator and then selective media.

7. **Which culture method is used for the maintenance of stock cultures?**

   Stab culture.

8. **What do you mean by term subculture?**

   Using a sterile wire or loop, a representative colony is touched and seeded onto appropriate medium by touching the wire or loop onto the surface of the medium.

9. **How aerobic incubation is carried out?**

   For most of the bacteria of medical importance, incubation is carried out at 37°C in an incubator under normal atmospheric pressure. For prolonged incubation, as required for growth of tubercle bacilli, screw-capped bottles should be used instead of test tubes or plates.

10. **Name organisms in which incubation is done in an atmosphere with added carbon dioxide (CO_2).**

    Brucella abortus, pneumococci, gonococci and capnophilic streptococci. They are known as capnophilic organisms.

11. **What is the concentration of CO_2 required for the incubation of capnophilic organisms?**

    5–10%.

12. **How do you provide this 5–10% CO_2?**
    - **Candle jar:** Generate CO_2 inside the jar by lighting a candle in it just before putting on the lid.
    - **CO_2 jars:** The required amount of air is withdrawn with a vacuum pump and replaced with CO_2 from a cylinder.
    - **CO_2 incubators (capnoeic incubator):** They provide a predetermined and regulated amount of CO_2 in a suitably humid atmosphere.
    - **CO_2 generating kits** are also available.

13. **What precaution should be observed for incubating liquid media in CO_2 environment?**

Screw caps on containers of liquid media must not be tight and should preferably be replaced by a closure that allows entry of CO_2.

14. **What are the characters to be studied while examining the growth on solid media?**

Size, shape, surface, elevation, edges, opacity, consistency, emulsifiability in water or saline, pigment production and haemolysis.

15. **Which culture method is used for antibiotic sensitivity testing by disc diffusion method?**

Lawn culture.

Identification of Bacteria (Biochemical Reactions)

Introduction

Most important duty of a medical microbiologist is isolation and accurate identification of disease causing organism from the morbid material and its antibiotic susceptibility. Clinical material is inoculated onto a solid medium in such a way so as to ensure isolated discrete colonies. Enriched, enrichment, selective and differential media, depending upon the organism suspected, are employed. Selective growth conditions, i.e., presence or absence of oxygen and presence of CO_2, etc. are also employed keeping in view the organisms suspected. The culture plates are incubated at optimum temperature.

Identification of the isolate is carried out by following tests:

- Examination of stained and unstained smears of the morbid material.
- Isolation in pure culture on appropriate culture media.
- Study of macroscopic (colonial characters) and microscopic morphology of the isolate.
- Biochemical reactions.
- Serotyping, biotyping, bacteriocin typing, phage typing, etc.
- Animal pathogenicity.
- Nucleic acid probes and polymerase chain reaction (PCR).
- Antimicrobial susceptibility testing.

Requirements

- Bacterial cultures
- Inoculating loop/wire
- Peptone water
- Glucose phosphate broth
- Kovac's reagent
- Methyl red reagent
- Potassium hydroxide and α-naphthol in absolute alcohol
- Simmon's medium or Koser's medium
- Nitrate broth
- Sulphanilic acid
- α-Naphthylamine
- Christensen's medium
- Lead acetate filter paper strip
- 10% H_2O_2
- 1% oxidase reagent (tetramethyl-p-phenylene-diamine dihydrochloride)
- Zinc powder
- Phenylalanine agar
- 10% Ferric chloride
- Potassium cyanide
- Lysine, ornithine and arginine amino acids
- Moeller decarboxylase base
- Sugar media
- Hugh and Leifson medium
- Spirit lamp
- Incubator

Biochemical Reactions

A large number of biochemical tests can be employed for the identification of different bacteria. These include:

1. Indole test

Certain bacteria possessing enzyme tryptophanase, degrade amino acid tryptophan to indole, pyruvic acid and ammonia.

Method

- Inoculate peptone water with the test organism and incubate at 37°C for 48–96 hours.
- Add 0.5 ml of Kovac's reagent and shake gently.
- A red colour in the alcohol layer indicates a positive reaction. Indole is extracted upward by amyl or isoamyl alcohol and forms red-coloured ring by forming a red-coloured complex with paradimethylaminobenzaldehyde. Negative test shows yellow-coloured ring (colour of Kovac's reagent) (Colour Plate III, Fig. 10A).

2. Methyl red (MR) test

This test detects the production of sufficient acid by fermentation of glucose so that pH of the medium falls and it is maintained below 4.5.

Method

- Inoculate the test organism in glucose phosphate broth (5 ml) and incubate at 37°C for 2–5 days.
- Add 5 drops of 0.04% methyl red.
- Mix and read the result immediately. If test is negative after 2 days, repeat it after 5 days.
  - *Positive test:* Bright red colour (Colour Plate III, Fig. 10B)
  - *Negative test:* Yellow colour.

3. Voges-Proskauer (VP) test

Many bacteria ferment carbohydrates with the production of acetyl methyl carbinol (acetoin). In the presence of potassium hydroxide (KOH) and atmospheric oxygen, acetoin is converted to diacetyl, and α-naphthol serves as a catalyst to form a red complex (Colour Plate III, Fig. 10C).

Method

- Inoculate test organism in glucose phosphate broth and incubate at 37°C for 48 hours.
- Add 1 ml KOH and 3 ml of 5% solution of α-naphthol in absolute alcohol.
- Shake the tube for aeration.
  - *Positive test:* Pink colour (2–5 minutes) which becomes crimson in 30 minutes.
  - *Negative test:* Yellow colour.

4. Citrate utilization

This test is used to study the ability of an organism to utilize citrate as a sole source of carbon for the growth. Liquid (Koser's) and solid (Simmon's) media containing citrate as a sole source of carbon can be used. Solid medium contains bromothymol blue as indicator. Citrate utilization results in alkaline pH that turns the indicator from green to blue (Colour Plate III, Fig. 10D).

Method

- Inoculate the test organism with the help of straight wire into either of these media.
- Incubate at 37°C for 24 hours.
  - *Positive test:*
    * Liquid medium: Turbidity
    * Solid medium: Appearance of growth and blue colour.
  - *Negative test:*
    * Liquid medium: No turbidity
    * Solid medium: No growth and original green colour.

5. Nitrate reduction test

This test detects the production of enzyme nitrate reductase which reduces nitrate to nitrite. Nitrite combines with the test reagent to form diazo red dye (Colour Plate III, Fig. 10E).

Method

- Inoculate test organism in 5 ml of nitrate broth.
- Incubate at 37°C for 96 hours.
- Add 0.1 ml test reagent (equal volume of 0.8% sulphanilic acid and 0.5% α-naphthylamine in 5 N acetic acid mixed just before use).
  - *Positive test:* Red colour
  - *Negative test:* Yellow colour.

6. Urease test

This test detects the ability of an organism to produce urease enzyme. This enzyme converts urea into ammonia and CO_2. Ammonia makes the medium alkaline and phenol red indicator changes to purple pink colour (Colour Plate III, Fig. 10F).

Method

- Inoculate test organism on the entire slope of Christensen's medium (contains urea, phenol red and agar).
- Incubate at 37°C and examine after 4 hours, and after overnight incubation.
  - *Positive test:* Purple-pink colour.
  - *Negative test:* Original colour of the medium.

7. Hydrogen sulphide production

This test detects the ability of a few organisms to produce hydrogen sulphide from sulphur-containing amino acids.

Method

- Suspend lead acetate filter paper strip between cotton plug and the tube.
- Incubate at 37°C for 24 hours.
  - *Positive test:* Blackening of filter paper strip (Colour Plate III, Fig. 10G).
  - *Negative test:* Original colour of paper strip.

8. Catalase test

This test detects the presence of enzyme catalase which catalyzes the release of oxygen from hydrogen peroxide (H_2O_2).

Method

- Take a drop of 10% H_2O_2 on clean glass slide.
- Pick-up a colony to be tested from nutrient agar plate with the help of glass rod.
- Dip the glass rod in the drop of H_2O_2.
  - *Positive test:* Production of gas bubbles (Colour Plate III, Fig. 10H).
  - *Negative test:* No gas bubbles.

9. Oxidase test

This test depends on the presence, in bacteria, of certain

oxidases that catalyze the oxidation of reduced tetramethyl-*p*-phenylene-diamine dihydrochloride (oxidase reagent) by molecular O_2.

Method

- Put a drop of freshly prepared 1% solution of reagent on a piece of filter paper.
- Now rub a few colonies of test organism on it with the help of a glass rod.
  - *Positive test:* Purple colour (Colour Plate III, Fig. 10I).
  - *Negative test:* No purple colour.

Alternatively, pour oxidase reagent over the colonies of test organism on the culture plate. The colonies of oxidase-positive organism rapidly develop a deep purple colour.

10. Motility test

This test detects motile organism.

Method

- Inoculate test organism by stab inoculation in a test medium (agar concentration 0.4% or less to allow free spread of organisms) by a single stab.
- Incubate at 37°C for 24 hours.
  - *Positive test:* Movement away from stab line or a hazy appearance throughout the medium indicates motile organism (Colour Plate III, Fig. 10J).
  - *Negative test:* Bacterial growth accentuated along stab line; surrounding medium remains clear.

11. Potassium cyanide test

This test detects the ability of an organism to grow in the presence of potassium cyanide.

Method

- Inoculate test organism in peptone buffered water containing 1 in 13,000 concentration of potassium cyanide.
- Incubate at 37°C for 24–48 hours.
  - *Positive test:* Development of turbidity in the medium indicates the ability of the organism to grow in presence of potassium cyanide (Colour Plate III, Fig. 10K).
  - *Negative test:* No turbidity.

12. Sugar fermentation test

This test detects the ability of an organism to ferment various sugars. This test also detects the production of gas.

Method

- Inoculate test organism in different sugar media (glucose, lactose, mannitol, sucrose, etc.) containing Andrade's indicator.
- Incubate at 37°C for 24 hours.
  - *Positive test:* Red or pink colour (production of acid changes the colour of the medium). Gas, if produced

collects in Durham's tube (a small tube which is kept inverted in the tube containing sugar medium) (Colour Plate III, Fig. 10L).
  - *Negative test:* Original yellow colour.

13. Phenylalanine deaminase test

This test detects the ability of an organism to produce enzyme phenylalanine deaminase that deaminates phenylalanine to phenylpyruvic acid.

Method

- Inoculate test organism in agar slant of medium containing DL-phenylalanine.
- Incubate at 37°C for 18–24 hours.
- Add 4–5 drops of 10% solution of ferric chloride reagent.
  - *Positive test:* Green colour (phenylpyruvic acid reacts with ferric chloride to give green colour) (Colour Plate III, Fig. 10M).
  - *Negative test:* No green colour.

14. Decarboxylase test

This test determines whether the bacterial species possess enzymes capable of decarboxylating specific amino acids in the test medium. The three amino acids commonly used to test for Enterobacteriaceae are lysine, ornithine, and arginine. Specific amine products and CO_2 are products of decarboxylation.

Method

- Inoculate the test organism in Moeller decarboxylase base with amino acid. The former contains glucose, peptone, pH indicator, bromocresol purple and cresol red. The pH is adjusted to 6.0.
- A control tube, consisting of only decarboxylase base without amino acid, must also be set up in parallel.
- Incubate all tubes anaerobically by overlaying with mineral oil at 37°C.
- During the initial stages of incubation, all tubes turn yellow, owing to the fermentation of small amount of glucose in the medium. If amino acid is decarboxylated, alkaline amines are formed and the medium reverts to its original purple colour.
  - *Positive test:* Original purple colour owing to formation of amines from decarboxylation reaction (Colour Plate III, Fig. 10N).
  - *Control tube:* Yellow colour indicates that the organism is viable and pH is sufficiently reduced to activate decarboxylase enzymes.

15. Oxidative-fermentative test (OF test)

This test determines whether a Gram-negative non-glucose fermenting rod is oxidative, fermentative or non-saccharolytic.

Method

- Take two tubes of oxidation-fermentation medium of Hugh and Leifson.
- Inoculate each tube with the test organism using a straight wire, stabbing the medium halfway to the bottom of the tube.
- Cover the inoculated medium in one tube with a 1 cm layer of sterile mineral oil. Leave the other tube uncovered.
- Incubate both tubes at 35–37°C and examine daily for several days.

Result

Result of OF test is given in Table 13.1. (*see also* Colour Plate III, Fig. 10O)

Table 13.1. Result of OF test		
Uncovered tube	**Covered tube**	**Metabolism**
Yellow (acid)	Green	Oxidative
Yellow (acid)	Yellow (acid)	Fermentative
Green	Green	Non-saccharolytic

Discussion

1. **Enumerate oxidase-positive organisms.**
   - *Neisseria*
   - *Pseudomonas*
   - *Aeromonas*
   - *Vibrio*
   - *Alcaligenes*
   - *Campylobacter*

2. **What precautions should be taken for doing oxidase test?**
   - Solution of oxidase reagent must be fresh.
   - Platinum loop or glass rod should be used, as traces of iron catalyze the reaction and give false positive result.
   - Growth should not be picked-up from medium containing catalase, e.g., blood agar.
   - Colour development should be seen within 5–10 seconds.

3. **What is the concentration of oxidase reagent?**
   1%

4. **Which metal can reduce nitrate to nitrite?**
   Zinc

5. **What precautions should be taken for doing citrate test?**
   - Citrate medium should not be inoculated with liquid medium containing growth. On the other hand, a part of a colony is picked-up with a straight wire and inoculated.
   - Keep the inoculum light, since dead organisms can serve as source of carbon, producing a false positive reaction.

6. **Which indicators are used in Simmon's citrate medium and Christensen's medium?**
   Bromothymol blue in Simmon's citrate medium and phenol red in Christensen's medium.

7. **Why red-coloured ring is formed at the top in the indole positive test?**
   Indole formed in the medium is extracted upward by amyl or isoamyl alcohol and reacts with paradimethylamino-benzaldehyde to form red-coloured ring.

8. **If MR test is negative after 2 days, then after how many days test should be repeated?**
   Five days.

9. **Enumerate organisms showing positive phenylalanine deaminase test.**
   - *Proteus* spp.
   - *Morganella* spp.
   - *Providencia* spp.

10. **What are the ingredients of Kovac's reagent?**
    - Paradimethylaminobenzaldehyde (10 g)
    - Amyl or isoamyl alcohol (150 ml)
    - Concentrated hydrochloric acid (50 ml)

11. **Name the organism which shows pseudocatalase test.**
    Enterococcus spp.

Antimicrobial Susceptibility Testing

Introduction

Antimicrobial susceptibility tests are very essential step for the proper treatment of infectious diseases. These are performed on bacteria isolated from clinical specimens. These are not performed on bacteria that are isolated from the anatomic sites of which they are normal inhabitants and on those that are predictably sensitive to the antimicrobial agents commonly used to treat infections caused by these bacteria. Group A β-haemolytic *Streptococcus*, for example, is not routinely tested because it is universally sensitive to penicillin, the drug of choice in treating infections caused by this bacterium. These tests are of two types:

1. **Diffusion methods:**
   - Kirby-Bauer disc diffusion method
   - Stokes disc diffusion method
2. **Dilution methods:**
   - Broth dilution method
   - Agar dilution method

Requirements

- Mueller-Hinton agar/broth
- Antibiotic discs
- Bacterial culture
- Straight wire/loop
- Turbidity standard (0.5 McFarland opacity standard)
- Incubator
- Control strains (ATCC/ NCTC)
- Swab sticks

Kirby-Bauer Disc Diffusion Method

- Sterile Mueller-Hinton agar is poured into plates.
- When the agar has solidified, dry the plates for 10–30 minutes at 37°C by placing them in an upright position in the incubator with the lids tilted.

- To prepare the inoculum from the primary culture plate, touch the tops of 5–10 similar appearing colonies with a straight wire or loop.
- Inoculate them in a suitable broth medium. Incubate at 35–37°C for 4–6 hours when the growth is considered to be in logarithmic phase.
- The density of the organisms is adjusted to approximately 10^8 colony-forming units (cfu)/ml by comparing its turbidity with that of 0.5 McFarland opacity standard (0.5 McFarland opacity standard contains 9.95 ml of 1% sulphuric acid and 0.05 ml of 1% barium chloride). Proper adjustment of the turbidity of the inoculum is essential to ensure that the resulting lawn of growth is confluent or almost confluent.
- Within 15 minutes after adjusting the turbidity of the inoculum suspension to that of the standard, dip a sterile non-toxic cotton swab into the inoculum suspension and remove excess inoculum by pressing and rotating the swab firmly against the side of the tube above the level of the liquid.
- Inoculate the dried surface of Mueller-Hinton agar plate that has been brought to room temperature by streaking the swab in three directions over the entire agar surface.
- Replace the lid of the dish. Allow 3–5 minutes but no longer than 15 minutes for surface of agar to dry before applying the antibiotic discs.
- Place the appropriate antibiotic discs on the surface of agar, using either sterile forceps or multidisc dispenser. After placement, press the disc on the surface of the medium to provide uniform contact. The disc must be evenly distributed on the agar so that they are not closer than 24 mm centre-to-centre. On a plate of 100 mm diameter, seven discs may be placed one in the centre and six in the periphery (Fig. 14.1). The plates are then incubated at 35–37°C for 16–18 hours.

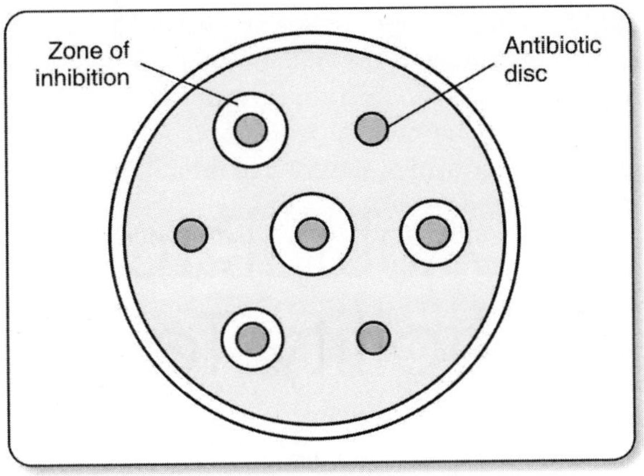

Fig. 14.1. Kirby-Bauer disc diffusion method.

Table 14.1. Interpretation chart of zone size in Kirby-Bauer disc diffusion method

Antimicrobial agent	Diameter of zone of inhibition (mm)		
	Resistant	Moderately susceptible	Susceptible
Benzyl penicillin	≤28	—	≥29
Ampicillin			
• Enterobacteriaceae	≤13	14–16	≥17
• Enterococci	≤16	—	≥17
• *Haemophilus* and *Moraxella* spp.	≤19	—	≥20
Cephalothin	≤14	15–17	≥18
Cefuroxime	≤14	15–17	≥18
Ceftazidime	≤14	15–17	≥18
Cefotaxime	≤14	15–22	≥23
Methicillin	≤9	10–13	≥14
Carbenicillin			
• *E. coli* and *Proteus* spp.	≤17	18–22	≥23
• *P. aeruginosa*	≤13	14–17	≥18
Gentamicin	≤12	—	≥13
Amikacin	≤14	15–16	≥17
Tobramycin	≤12	13–14	≥15
Erythromycin	≤13	14–17	≥18
Clindamycin	≤14	15–20	≥21
Tetracycline	≤14	15–18	≥19
Fusidic acid	≤14	15–18	≥19
Chloramphenicol	≤12	13–17	≥18
Colistin	≤8	9–10	≥11
Nalidixic acid	≤13	14–18	≥19
Nitrofurantoin	≤14	15–16	≥17
Trimethoprim	≤10	11–15	≥16
Trimethoprim/ sulphamethoxazole	≤10	11–15	≥16
Ciprofloxacin	≤15	16–20	≥21
Piperacillin			
• Enterobacteriaceae	≤17	18–20	≥21
• *Pseudomonas*	≤14	15–17	≥18

- By using a caliper or transparent plastic ruler, the zones of complete growth inhibition around each of the discs are carefully measured. The diameter of the disc is included in this measurement. The zone size that is observed in a disc diffusion test has no meaning by itself. The interpretation of zone size is based on the interpretation chart (Table 14.1). Reference strains of *Staphylococcus aureus*, *Escherichia coli*, *Pseudomonas aeruginosa*, etc. (Table 14.2) should be tested each time a new batch of discs or agar is used.

Result

The Kirby-Bauer method recognizes three categories of susceptibility:

- *Susceptible:* An organism is called "susceptible" to a drug when the infection caused by it is likely to respond to treatment with this drug, at the recommended dosage.
- *Intermediate susceptible:* It is applicable to strains that are "moderately susceptible" to an antibiotic that can be used for treatment at a higher dosage because of its low toxicity or because the antibiotic is concentrated at the focus of infection. The term also applies to those strains that are susceptible to a more toxic antibiotic that cannot be used at a higher dosage.
- *Resistant:* The organism does not respond to a given drug, irrespective of the dosage and the location of the infection.

Table 14.2. Control strains for Kirby-Bauer and Stokes disc diffusion methods

Test bacteria	Control strain	
	Kirby-Bauer	Stokes
Coliform organisms	*E. coli* ATCC 25922	*E. coli* NCTC 10418
Pseudomonas	*P. aeruginosa* ATCC 27853	*P. aeruginosa* NCTC 10662
Haemophilus spp.	*Haemophilus influenzae* ATCC 49247	*H. Influenzae* NCTC 11931
Gonococci	*Neisseria gonorrhoeae* ATCC 49226	*N. gonorrhoeae* (sensitive strain)
Enterococci	*Enterococcus faecalis* ATCC 29212	*E. faecalis* NCTC 12697
Other organisms that can grow aerobically	*S. aureus* ATCC 25923	*S. aureus* NCTC 6571

Stokes Disc Diffusion Method

- The Mueller-Hinton agar plate is divided into three parts. The test organism is inoculated on central one-third and control on upper and lower thirds of the plate, however, in modified stokes disc diffusion method, the test organism is inoculated in the upper and lower thirds and control on central one-third.
- An uninoculated gap 2–3 mm wide should separate the test and control areas on which antibiotic discs are applied (Fig. 14.2).
- A maximum of six antibiotic discs can be placed on a single 100 mm diameter plate. The plates are then incubated at 35–37°C for 16–18 hours.
- Measure the zone size, i.e. the distance in mm from the edge of the disc to the zone edge, if that is obvious, if it is not, measure to the point of 80% or more inhibition of growth. However, if the test zones are obviously larger than the control or give no zone of inhibition at all, it is not necessary to perform any measurement.

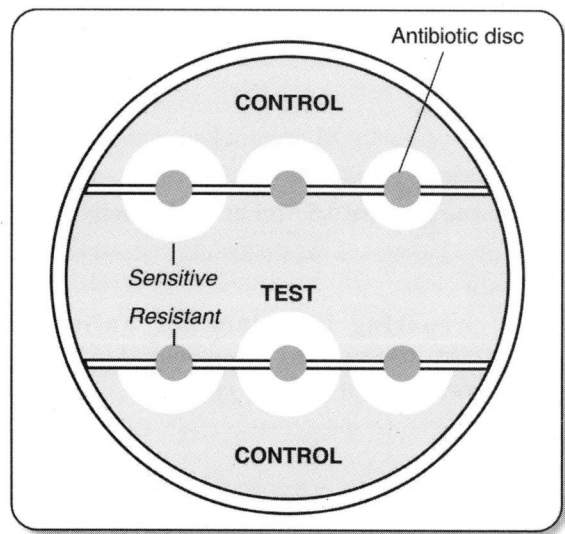

Fig. 14.2. Stokes disc diffusion method.

Result

Zone size is interpreted as follows:

- *Sensitive:* The zone size is equal to, larger than or not more than 3 mm smaller than the control.
- *Intermediate:* The zone size of the test strain is at least 2 mm, but also at least 3 mm smaller than that of the control strain.
- *Resistant:* The zone size of the test strain is smaller than 2 mm.

   For interpretation of the results of Kirby-Bauer and Stokes disc diffusion methods, following points should be borne in mind:

- When β-lactamase-producing staphylococci are tested against penicillin, zones of inhibition are produced with a heaped-up, clearly defined edge; these are readily recognizable when compared with sensitive control, and regardless of the size of the zone of inhibition, they should be reported as resistant.
- Motile organisms such as *Proteus mirabilis* and *P. vulgaris* may swarm when growing on agar surface resulting in a thin veil that may penetrate into the zone of inhibition around antibiotic discs. The zone of swarming should be ignored and outer margin, which is usually clearly outlined, should be measured.
- Methicillin-resistant staphylococci will often appear fully sensitive when tested in an ordinary way. This difficulty can be overcome by incubating the culture at 30°C or by using 5% salt agar and incubating at 37°C.
- With sulphonamides and co-trimoxazole, slight growth occurs within the inhibition zone; such growth should be ignored.
- Polymyxins diffuse poorly in agar, so that zones are small. In this case, by Stokes method, report as:
  - *Sensitive:* Zone size is equal to, wider than, or not more than 3 mm smaller than the control.
  - *Resistant:* The zone size is more than 3 mm smaller than the control.

Determination of Minimum Inhibitory and Minimum Bactericidal Concentrations

The minimum inhibitory concentration (MIC) is the least amount of antimicrobial agent that inhibits visible growth of an organism after overnight incubation. The minimum bactericidal concentration (MBC) is the least amount of antimicrobial agent that prevents growth after subculture of the organism in antimicrobial-free medium. The uses of determination of MIC are:

1. When equivocal results are obtained with disc diffusion tests.
2. In patients with serious infections, e.g., infective endocarditis.

   MIC of an antimicrobial agent may be determined in liquid (Mueller-Hinton broth) or solid medium (Mueller-Hinton agar). Antimicrobial agent is incorporated into the culture medium in the concentrations of 0.25, 0.5, 1, 2, 4, 8, 16, 32, 64, 128 µg/ml, etc. The inoculum is prepared as in case of disc diffusion methods by comparing with 0.5 McFarland opacity standard. For broth dilution, the final inoculum should be 10^5 cfu/ml and for agar dilution method, 1–2 µl of the inoculum is applied on the agar surface. It delivers approximately 10^4 cfu/spot. An organism of known sensitivity should also be titrated. Incubate at 35–37°C for 16–18 hours and read the results. For determination of MIC of methicillin, incubate at 30°C.

MIC is the lowest concentration of antimicrobial agent at which there is no visible growth. For determination of MBC, subculture from each tube showing no growth over a quarter of a nutrient medium free from antimicrobial agent. Incubate and examine them for growth. The tube containing lowest concentration of the antimicrobial agent that fails to yield growth, on subculture, is the MBC of the antimicrobial agent for the test strain.

Discussion

1. **What are the advantages of antimicrobial susceptibility testing?**

   It is used to guide the clinician in selecting the best antimicrobial agent and to accumulate epidemiological information on the resistance of microorganisms of public health importance.

2. **Which medium is preferred for antimicrobial sensitivity testing?**

   Mueller-Hinton agar.

3. **Why Mueller-Hinton agar is preferred for antibiotic sensitivity testing?**

   This medium has minimal inhibitory effect on sulphonamides and trimethoprim due to low concentration of thymidine. Some organisms can use thymidine to bypass the mechanism of action of trimethoprim and grow, even though they are innately sensitive to antibiotics.

4. **Which substance should be added to Mueller-Hinton agar for tests with sulphonamides and trimethoprim, and why?**

   Five per cent lysed horse blood should be added to Mueller-Hinton agar base for tests with sulphonamides and trimethoprim because its content of thymidine phosphorylase neutralizes the inhibitory effect of thymidine in the medium, on the action of these drugs.

5. **What should be the pH of Mueller-Hinton agar medium?**

   The pH of this medium should be between 7.2 and 7.4.

6. **What are the disadvantages of more acidic and more alkaline pH?**

   A more acidic pH decreases the activity of aminoglycosides and macrolide antibiotics, and more alkaline pH favours the action of tetracyclines, novobiocin and fusidic acid.

7. **How much medium should be poured in 100 mm petri dish?**

   Medium should be poured to the depth of 4 mm (25 ml).

8. **What is the size of antibiotic disc?**

   Six mm.

9. **At what temperature these antibiotic disc should be stored?**

   Bulk stock should be stored at $-20°C$ and working ones at $<8°C$.

10. **How many antibiotic discs can be accommodated on a single 100 mm diameter plate?**

    Six and seven in Stokes disc diffusion method and Kirby-Bauer disc diffusion method, respectively.

11. **What do you mean by first-line drugs?**

    These include those antibiotics that are locally available and commonly prescribed and for which routine testing should be carried out for every strain.

12. **In which conditions, second-line/alternative drugs are preferred?**

    • When the causative organism is resistant to the first-line drugs.
    • Allergy to a drug, or its unavailability.

13. **What do you mean by 0.5 McFarland opacity standard?**

    The 0.5 McFarland opacity standard provides a turbidity comparable to that of a bacterial suspension containing 1.5×10^8 colony-forming unit/ml.

14. **How do you prepare 0.5 McFarland opacity standard?**

    The 0.5 McFarland opacity standard contains 9.95 ml of 1% sulphuric acid and 0.05 ml of 1% barium chloride.

15. **While preparing inoculum for antimicrobial susceptibility testing, why it is essential to touch 5–10 colonies rather than a single colony?**

    Five to ten colonies rather than a single colony are selected to minimize the possibility of testing a colony that might have been derived from a suspected mutant.

16. **What are the advantages of Stokes disc diffusion method for antimicrobial susceptibility testing?**

    Reading of test strain is always taken in comparison to that of standard control. All blank discs (without antibiotics) can also be detected.

17. **Name various diffusion methods of antimicrobial sensitivity testing.**

    • Kirby-Bauer method
    • Stokes method

18. **Which diffusion method is recommended by WHO?**

    Kirby-Bauer disc diffusion method.

19. **Enumerate sources of control strains.**

    • American Type Culture Collection (ATCC)
    • National Collection of Type Culture (NCTC)

General Bacteriology

1

Section 2

Serology/Immunology

- Venereal disease research laboratory (VDRL) test
- Widal test
- C-reactive protein (CRP) test
- Rheumatoid factor (RF) test
- Antistreptolysin O (ASO) test
- Complement fixation test
- Weil-Felix test
- Paul-Bunnell test
- Cold agglutination test
- Brucella agglutination test
- Enzyme immunoassay (EIA)

Venereal Disease Research Laboratory (VDRL) Test

Introduction

VDRL test is a nontreponemal test most widely employed for the diagnosis of syphilis. It is a simple and rapid test which requires only a small quantity of serum.

Principle

This is non-specific flocculation test. This test is performed as a slide test in which inactivated patient serum is mixed with a freshly prepared suspension of cardiolipin-lecithin-cholesterol antigen on a glass slide. The mixture is rotated, usually mechanically, for 4 minutes after which the flocculation (aggregation of antigen–antibody complexes in suspension) can be detected under a low power objective of a microscope. Reagin (antibodies that appear in syphilis) in the serum reacts with the VDRL antigen and forms floccules.

Requirements

* Serum
* Water bath (56°C)
* VDRL rotator (180 rpm)
* VDRL glass slides (7.5 × 5 cm) with 12 paraffin rings of approximately 15 mm diameter
* Screw cap bottle of 30 ml capacity with flat inner bottom surface
* Tuberculin syringe
* 18 gauge needle
* Pipettes 1.0, 5.0 ml
* VDRL kit: It contains (a) stock VDRL antigen in ampoules, and (b) buffered saline. It is necessary to prepare carefully a working VDRL antigen fresh before the test. Working VDRL antigen is stable at 0–4°C only for 12 hours.

Method

Preparation of antigen

* Bring the buffered saline and antigen to room temperature.

* Pipette 0.4 ml of buffered saline into a 30 ml round bottomed screw cap bottle.
* Add 0.5 ml of VDRL antigen with the help of a tuberculin syringe, drop by drop rapidly in 6 seconds while gently rotating the bottle in a circle of 5 cm diameter.
* Continue rotation of bottle for 10 more seconds.
* Add 4.1 ml of buffered saline more.
* Replace the top of the bottle and shake it for 10 seconds.
* Allow it to stand for 15–30 minutes. The working antigen suspension may be used during whole working day.

Preparation of serum

Heat the serum in a water bath at 56°C for 30 minutes to inactivate the complement and use within 4 hours. Reinactivate the serum for 10 minutes, if it cannot be processed within 4 hours.

Qualitative Test

Carried on glass slides (7.5 × 5 cm), each with 12 paraffin rings.

* Pipette 50 µl of inactivated patient serum into the paraffin ring on the glass slide.
* Pipette 50 µl each of positive and negative control sera into two other paraffin rings.
* Add one drop of working antigen suspension to each of these paraffin rings from a syringe delivering 60 drops in 1 ml.
* Mix with wooden sticks and rotate slide for 4 minutes with hand on a flat surface in a circular manner in a diameter of about 5 cm or on a mechanical VDRL rotator set at about 180 rpm.
* Read the test results immediately under a low power objective of a microscope (Fig. 15.1). The antigen particles are seen as small fusiform needles which remain more or less evenly dispersed in case of non-reactive serum. Grouping of these particles into small or large clumps denotes the degree of reactivity and is interpreted as follows:

Serology/Immunology

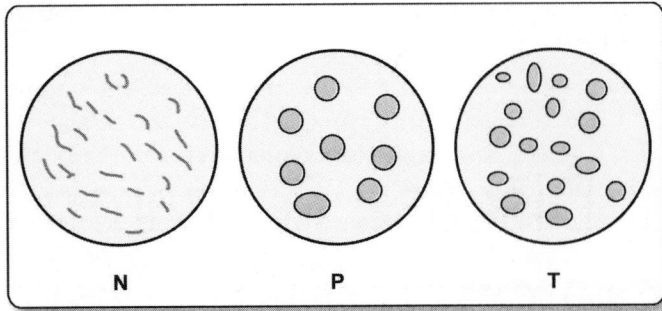

Fig. 15.1. VDRL slide test. N – negative control, P – positive control, T – test serum.

Medium and large clumps	Reactive (R)
Small clumps	Weakly reactive (WR)
No clumps	Non-reactive (NR)

Any specimen giving a weak positive or positive reaction should then be tested quantitatively. It is performed with serial dilutions of patient serum. The highest dilution that can be classified as reactive is reported as the titre.

Quantitative VDRL Test

- Place 6 test tubes in a rack.
- Add 200 μl of physiological saline in each tube.
- Add 200 μl of the patient's serum in first tube and mix well. The dilution will be 1:2.
- Transfer 200 μl from the first up to sixth tube successively. The dilutions will now be 1:2, 1:4, 1:8, 1:16, 1:32, 1:64, respectively.
- Add 50 μl of each dilution to the respective paraffin rings including controls as in qualitative test.
- Add 1 drop of VDRL antigen, i.e., 1/60 ml to each ring from a syringe.
- Rotate the slides on VDRL rotator adjusted at 180 rpm for 4 minutes.

Reporting

Read the test immediately with 10× objective of light microscope. Report the titre as highest dilution of the serum that shows a reactive result. A titre of 1:16 and above for reaginic antibody is interpreted in favour of syphilis.

Interpretation

Since the VDRL antigen is non-specific in nature, the test is often reactive in several other clinical conditions characterized by production of reaginic antibody. These include lepromatous leprosy, malaria, relapsing fever, hepatitis, systemic lupus erythematosus, infectious mononucleosis and tropical eosinophilia and are collectively termed as **biological false positive reactions**. The diagnosis is confirmed by specific treponemal test and quantitative VDRL test.

Advantages

1. VDRL test is used as a screening test and is positive in approximately 70% of primary and 99% of secondary syphilis.
2. It becomes positive in 10–14 days after the appearance of primary chancre.
3. Positive result in VDRL test usually indicates active infection, therefore, it can be used to monitor the efficacy of antibacterial therapy.
4. The VDRL test can be done on CSF, therefore, it is useful in the diagnosis of neurosyphilis.

Disadvantages

1. Antigen has to be prepared fresh.
2. Heat inactivation of sera is necessary to destroy a heat-labile inhibitory factor of IgM class.
3. Microscope is required to read the results.
4. Positive VDRL test should be confirmed by testing with a *Treponema pallidum* specific test.

Rapid Plasma Reagin (RPR) Card Test

RPR card test is a macroscopic non-treponemal flocculation test used for the detection and quantitation of antilipoidal antibodies (reagin).

Principle

VDRL antigen is adsorbed on finely divided carbon particles and suspended in choline which blocks inhibitory factors in the serum thus eliminating the need to heat the serum before testing. The antigen is stabilized with EDTA, allowing it to be used for up to 6 months when stored at 4–10°C. This test is performed by mixing one drop of patient serum or plasma (50 μl), with a drop of this modified antigen (20 μl) on a disposable plastic card (12.5 × 7 cm in size with 10 clearly defined test areas) using a disposable stick. The card is then rocked gently to and fro for 8 minutes and observed under strong source of light. In a positive test, the flocculation of carbon particles (black aggregates) is visible with naked eye. Black aggregates may be deposited at the periphery of the liquid. In a negative case, there is a complete absence of black aggregates with a uniform greyish background.

Any specimen giving a positive reaction should then be tested quantitatively using doubling dilutions of serum.

Advantages

1. Quick and easy to perform.
2. Serum sample does not need to be heat-inactivated.
3. Cards can be read macroscopically.

Disadvantage

It cannot be used to test cerebrospinal fluid.

Discussion

1. **Enumerate various nontreponemal tests or standard tests for syphilis (STS)?**
   - Venereal Disease Research Laboratory (VDRL) test
   - Rapid plasma reagin (RPR) card test
   - Kahn test
   - Wasserman test

2. **Which method is used in VDRL test?**
   Slide flocculation.

3. **Which antigen is used in all nontreponemal tests?**
   The antigen used in nontreponemal tests is an alcoholic extract of beef heart tissue (cardiolipin) to which lecithin and cholesterol are added.

4. **What is the principle of Kahn test and Wasserman test?**
   Tube flocculation test and complement fixation test, respectively.

5. **Why these two tests are not done nowadays?**
   Because of the availability of simple and rapid tests, e.g., VDRL and RPR card tests.

6. **When does 'reagin' antibody develop in syphilitic patients?**
   Ten to 14 days after the appearance of primary chancre.

7. **What is the main difference between VDRL test and Kahn test?**
   In VDRL test, serum is used in various dilutions and antigen is added in a constant volume. In Kahn test, serum is used in constant volume and antigen is used in various dilutions. In addition, VDRL and Kahn tests are slide flocculation and tube flocculation tests, respectively.

8. **Why serum sample is heat inactivated in VDRL test?**
   Heat inactivation of sera is necessary to destroy a heat-labile inhibitory factor of IgM class which may be present in both normal and syphilitic serum.

9. **What is the major advantage of VDRL over RPR test?**
   VDRL test can be used to test cerebrospinal fluid while RPR cannot be used.

10. **What do you mean by biological false positive (BFP) reaction?**
    Detection of antibodies against cardiolipin in the absence of *T. pallidum* infection is known as biological false positive reaction.

11. **How do you differentiate BFP from true positive?**
    In BFP cases, specific treponemal tests are negative and there is no history of present or past treponemal infection.

12. **How do you classify BFP reaction?**

BFP may be divided into acute or transient and chronic BFP reactions:

- *Acute or transient BFP reaction:* It develops shortly after an acute febrile infectious disease and disappears within a few weeks or months after the illness has subsided.
- *Chronic BFP reactions:* It persists longer than six months. These may occur in a wide variety of infectious and non-infectious conditions associated with tissue damage.

13. **Enumerate non-infectious conditions which give BFP reaction?**
    Pregnancy, advanced cancer, multiple myeloma, connective tissue disease and multiple blood transfusions.

14. **When do you get false negative VDRL test?**
    When the patient serum contains high titre of antibody (due to prozone phenomenon).

15. **What is the positivity rate of VDRL test in primary and secondary syphilis?**
    This test is positive in approximately 70% of primary and 99% of secondary syphilis. The titre of antibody may rise to 8 or 16 during primary syphilis and 16–128 during secondary syphilis.

16. **Which class of antibody present in patient serum causes suspension of cardiolipin antigen to flocculate?**
    IgM or IgG

17. **Why heat inactivation of serum is not required in RPR card test?**
    In RPR card test, VDRL antigen is adsorbed on finely divided carbon particles and suspended in choline chloride which blocks inhibitory factors in the serum thus eliminating the need for heat inactivation of the serum before testing.

18. **What do you mean by toluidine red unheated serum test (TRUST)?**
    TRUST is a modification of RPR test. This test has additional advantage in hot climates as the antigen is more stable than RPR antigen on storage at room temperature of 26–31°C. The sensitivity and specificity of this test are similar to that of VDRL and RPR test.

19. **What precautions should be taken while testing CSF by VDRL test?**
    - CSF is not heat inactivated.
    - VDRL antigen is sensitized with 10% saline.

20. **What is the significance of VDRL test in diagnosing a case of neurosyphilis?**

The VDRL test alone is not a reliable indicator of CNS involvement since it is non-reactive in 30–60% of patients with active neurosyphilis.

21. Which test can exclude neurosyphilis?

A negative *Treponema pallidum* haemagglutination (TPHA) test in CSF can exclude neurosyphilis.

22. Does positive TPHA test in CSF indicate active disease?

A positive TPHA test in CSF does not necessarily indicate active disease, since reactivity may be caused by transudation of immunoglobulins from the serum into the CSF.

Widal Test

Introduction

It is a tube agglutination test employed for the serological diagnosis of enteric fever, in which antibodies against *Salmonella* serotype Typhi, *S.* serotypes Paratyphi A and B infections are detected in patient serum. Since two types of agglutinins are generated in the serum which react with 'O' and 'H' antigenic components of the microorganisms, a total of four antigen suspension namely TO, TH, AH and BH are employed in the test.

Principle

Tube agglutination test.

Requirements

- Widal rack
- Dreyer's tubes for 'H' agglutinins (conical bottom)
- Felix tubes for 'O' agglutinins (round bottom)
- Patient serum
- Antigen suspensions (commercially available or locally prepared)
- Physiological saline (0.85% sodium chloride)
- Pipettes
- Water bath at 37°C

Procedure

1. Arrange four rows each containing 7 clean and dry Widal tubes in a Widal rack.
2. Mix 0.1 ml of the patient serum with 1.4 ml of the physiological saline to obtain a 1 in 15 dilution (master dilution).
3. Add 0.4 ml of saline from second to seventh tube with the help of a pipette.
4. Add 0.4 ml of freshly prepared 1 in 15 dilution of serum into the first two tubes of each row.
5. After mixing, transfer 0.4 ml from second tube onwards up to sixth tube and from sixth tube discard 0.4 ml.

6. Add 0.4 ml of respective antigen namely TO, TH, AH and BH in each row from first to seventh tube. The final dilution would be 1:30, 1:60, 1:120, 1:240, 1:480 and 1:960 in the first six tubes respectively, while the last tube would serve as negative control (Fig. 16.1).
7. Incubate the tubes at 37°C in a water bath for 4 hours and read after overnight refrigeration at 4°C.

Results

H agglutination leads to the formation of loose and cotton-woolly clumps, while 'O' agglutination appears as a disc-like granular deposit at the bottom of the tube. Control tube (Felix) shows a compact deposit. The highest dilution of the serum showing agglutination indicates the titre of the antibody.

Interpretation

1. Agglutinins usually appear by seventh to tenth day of illness in enteric fever, so that a negative result at an early stage is inconclusive. The titre then increases steadily till the third or fourth week, after which it declines gradually.
2. Demonstration of rising titre, e.g., four-fold or greater, between tests made in the first and third weeks is highly significant. However, if the first sample is taken late in the disease, a rise may not be demonstrable. Instead a fall in titre may be seen in some cases.
3. Though, it is generally stated that titres of 1:100 or more for O agglutinins and 1:200 or more for H agglutinins are significant, the results in a single test by no means prove the presence of enteric fever nor negative results its absence.
4. Serum from individuals immunized with TAB vaccine may show high titres of antibodies to *S.* serotype Typhi, *S.* serotype Paratyphi A and *S.* serotype Paratyphi B. However, if a marked rise of titre to one serotype is observed, the results may be regarded as diagnostically significant. H agglutinins tend to persist for many months

Serology/Immunology

2

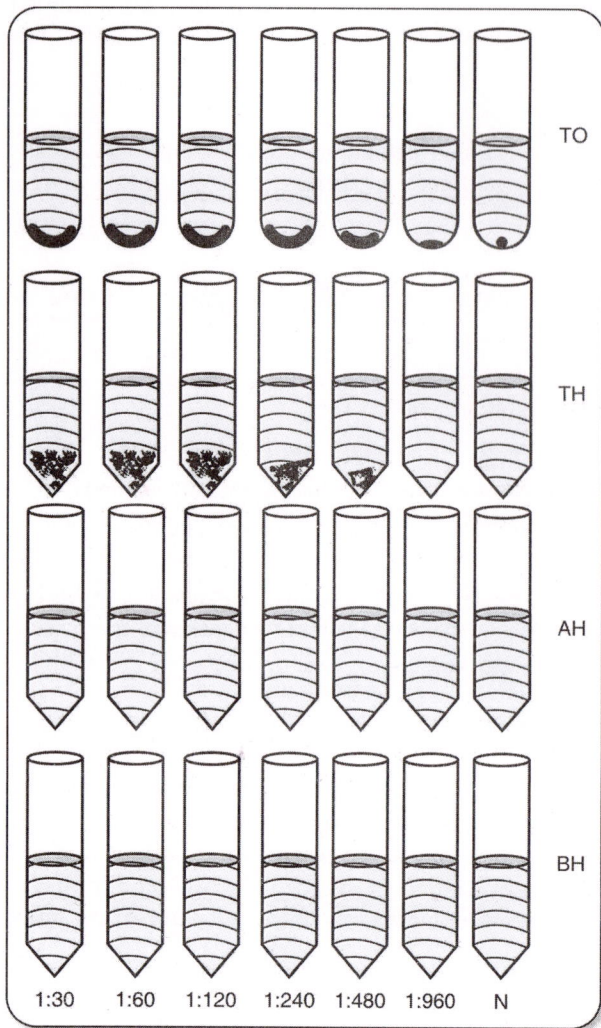

TO

TH

AH

BH

1:30   1:60   1:120   1:240   1:480   1:960   N

Fig. 16.1. Widal test. N – negative control.

after vaccination but O agglutinins tend to disappear sooner, i.e., within 6 months. Therefore, rise in O agglutinins indicate recent infection.

5. For determining the serotype of infecting organism, H agglutinin is more reliable than O agglutinin because the different serotypes have some O antigens in common. Moreover, O antigens are also widely distributed among other enterobacteria.

6. Persons who had past enteric infection or who have been vaccinated may develop **anamnestic** response during an unrelated fever like malaria, influenza, etc. The anamnestic response shows only a transient rise, while in enteric fever, the rise is sustained.

7. Test suspensions of bacteria may contain non-specific antigens such as fimbrial antigens which may produce false positive results.

8. In many healthy individuals, the Widal reaction may be positive in the carrier state. This can be recognized by positive reaction with 'Vi' agglutinin in a titre of ≥1:10.

Discussion

1. **What is the principle of Widal test?**
   Tube agglutination.

2. **What are the uses of Widal test?**
   - This is an important diagnostic test for quantitative estimation of antibodies in enteric fever.
   - Causative salmonellae can be diagnosed, i.e., *S.* serotype Typhi, *S.* serotype Paratyphi A, *S.* serotype Paratyphi B and *S.* serotype Paratyphi C.
   - Declining titre with antibiotics indicates patient is responding to treatment.
   - Progression of disease can be diagnosed with antibody titre.

3. **Why *S.* serotype Paratyphi O antigens of *S.* serotype Paratyphi A and *S.* serotype Paratyphi B are not employed in Widal test?**
   Because they cross react with *Salmonella* serotype Typhi O antigen due to sharing by them of factor 12.

4. **Enumerate antigens of salmonellae.**
   - Flagellar (H) antigens
   - Somatic (O) antigens
   - Fimbrial (F) antigens
   - Surface (Vi) antigens

5. **Which of the somatic and flagellar antigens is more antigenic?**
   Flagellar antigen is more antigenic.

6. **Which of the somatic and flagellar antigens is heat-labile?**
   'H' (flagellar) antigen is heat-labile.

7. **Which strain of *S.* serotype Typhi is used for preparation of O antigen?**
   For the preparation of O antigen *S.* serotype Typhi 901 strain is used.

8. **When do agglutinins appear during the course of enteric fever?**
   Agglutinins usually appear by seventh to tenth day of enteric fever.

9. **In which condition, all tubes show agglutination?**
   In TAB vaccinated person.

10. **Which agglutinins indicate recent infection?**
    Rise in O agglutinins.

11. **Which agglutinins disappear first in the blood after infection?**
    'O' agglutinins appear first after infection. They tend to disappear within 6 months, while 'H' agglutinins tend to persist for nearly 2 years.

12. **How do you differentiate anamnestic reaction from true enteric fever?**

   In both conditions, agglutinins against 'O' and 'H' antigens are raised in the blood. However, the rise is transient in anamnestic reaction whereas in enteric fever, it is sustained.

13. **In which conditions, Widal test is negative in case of enteric fever?**

   • Patient on antibiotic treatment.
   • When Widal test is done in first week.

14. **What are the other serological methods for the detection of antibodies in patient serum in enteric fever?**

   • Indirect haemagglutination test.
   • Counterimmunoelectrophoresis.
   • ELISA
   • Solid-phase RIA

15. **Which agglutinin has been claimed to indicate the carrier state?**

   Vi agglutinin ≥1:10.

16. **How would you diagnose a carrier of *Salmonella*?**

   • Demonstration of Vi agglutinin (≥1:10)
   • Faecal culture
   • Bile culture
   • Urine culture

17. **How much titre of antibodies is diagnostic in Widal test?**

   Rising titres in paired sera is diagnostic. In a single test, ≥1:100 titre of 'O' and ≥1:200 titre of 'H' is diagnostic.

18. **In which conditions, result of Widal test is doubtful?**

   • Past exposure to infection.
   • Previous immunization with TAB vaccine.
   • Early antibiotic treatment.

19. **Which cancer may be seen in chronic typhoid carriers?**

   Hepatobiliary cancer

20. **Which *Salmonella* serotype is more associated with chronic carriers?**

   Salmonella serotype Typhi

21. **Where do the salmonellae reside in a carrier?**

   Salmonellae reside in gallbladder, biliary tract and rarely in intestine and urinary tract.

22. **Why do you collect repeated samples of faeces or bile to diagnose a chronic carrier of *Salmonella*?**

   Because there is intermittent shedding of the organisms.

23. **What is main advantage of detection of carriers?**

   This helps in screening food handlers and cooks. So, detection of carriers is important for epidemiological and public health purposes.

24. **What is the treatment of choice for chronic carriers?**

   • Antibiotics (ampicillin, amoxycillin and co-trimoxazole)
   • Cholecystectomy

C-Reactive Protein (CRP) Test

Introduction

CRP is an abnormal protein (β-globulin). It appears in acute phase sera of cases of pneumonia but disappears during convalescence. It also appears in some other pathological conditions. It is known as C-reactive protein because it precipitates with C antigen of pneumococci. It is not an antibody. Its production is stimulated by bacterial infection, inflammation, malignancy and tissue destruction. It disappears when inflammation subsides. It is used as an index of response to treatment in rheumatic fever and certain other conditions.

Principle

Passive agglutination using latex particles coated with anti-CRP antibody.

Requirements

- Latex CRP kit
  - Latex CRP reagent
  - Positive and negative serum controls
  - Dark slide or test plate
  - Disposable applicator sticks
- Normal saline
- Patient serum
- Pipettes

Procedure

1. Bring serum sample and reagents to room temperature.
2. Dilute patient serum 1:5 with normal saline.
3. Add one drop each of diluted patient serum, and positive and negative control sera in the respective zones of the test plate.
4. Then add one drop each of latex CRP reagent (antigen) to each of these sera.
5. Mix well with disposable applicator sticks and observe for agglutination within 2 minutes (Fig. 17.1).

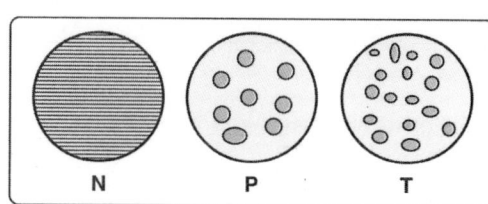

Fig. 17.1. C-reactive protein test. N – negative control, P – positive control, T – test serum.

Interpretation

Marked agglutination generally indicates presence of CRP concentration >5 µg/ml in serum. In negative serum control, no agglutination is observed.

Uses

1. CRP is used as an index of response to treatment in rheumatic fever and certain other conditions.
2. The detection of CRP is more sensitive and more reliable indicator for inflammatory processes than the ESR.
3. It detects the activity of inflammatory process in acute disease.

Discussion

1. **What is the principle of C-reactive protein test?**
   Passive agglutination.

2. **Why is it known as C-reactive protein?**
   It is known as C-reactive protein because it precipitates with C antigen of pneumococci.

3. **What is the nature of this protein?**
   β-globulin.

4. **What is the upper limit of C-reactive protein in healthy person?**
   5 µg/ml.

5. **What is the diameter of latex particle?**

0.8–1 µm in diameter.

6. **Name tests which are based on the principle of latex agglutination.**

C-reactive protein (CRP), antistreptolysin O (ASO), rheumatoid factor (RF), human chorionic gonadotrophin (HCG); and latex particles coated with antibodies to meningococci, *Haemophilus influenzae* type b and pneumococci can be used to detect corresponding antigens in cases of pyogenic meningitis.

7. **Which other carrier molecules can be used besides latex?**

Bentonite, gelatin and RBCs.

8. **What is the diagnostic importance of CRP test?**

It detects the activity of inflammatory processes in the body. Its level decreases with appropriate treatment.

Rheumatoid Factor (RF) Test

Introduction

In rheumatoid arthritis, rheumatoid factor (an antigamma-globulin autoantibody) appears in the serum of the patient. It acts as an antibody to human immunoglobulin G (IgG). Latex polystyrene beads coated with denatured human IgG when mixed with patient serum leads to agglutination of latex polystyrene beads.

Principle

Passive agglutination. RF in patient serum reacts with IgG-coated latex particles resulting in agglutination.

Requirements

- Normal saline
- Patient serum
- Commercially available RA kit with positive and negative controls.
- Latex RF reagent consists of an aqueous suspension of polystyrene particles coated with human IgG. When 1:5 diluted serum is tested, the positive result indicates the limit of detection about 20 IU/ml.
- Test plate or dark slide.
- Stirring rods

Procedure

1. Bring the reagents and serum samples to room temperature.
2. Dilute patient serum 1:5 with normal saline.
3. Add one drop each of diluted patient serum, and negative and positive controls on the respective zones of a test plate.
4. Add one drop of latex rheumatoid reagent to each of these drops.
5. Mix well with stirring rods.
6. Look for agglutination within 2 minutes.

Interpretation

Marked agglutination indicates the presence of rheumatoid factor ($\geq$20 IU/ml). For quantitative test, prepare further dilutions of serum (1:10, 1:20, 1:30, 1:40) which indicate RF concentration 40, 80, 120, 260 (IU/ml), respectively.

Uses

1. Presence of rheumatoid factor is of significant diagnostic value.
2. High titres indicate more severe disease and a generalized pathological process.
3. Seropositive cases have less favourable prognosis than seronegative.

Discussion

1. **Rheumatoid factor belongs to which class of immuno-globulins?**
   It is IgM. It acts as an antibody to human IgG.

2. **What is the principle of RF test?**
   Passive agglutination.

3. **Name the disease for which RF is used as a diagnostic test.**
   Rheumatoid arthritis.

4. **Name the other conditions where RF test is positive.**
   Systemic lupus erythematosus, hepatitis, dermato-myositis, cirrhosis liver, syphilis, etc.

5. **Does negative RF test rule out rheumatoid arthritis?**
   No. Negative result is observed in one-third of the patients of rheumatoid arthritis.

6. **What is the nature of latex rheumatoid factor antigen?**
   It is an aqueous suspension of polystyrene particles coated with human IgG.

7. **Which test was used earlier for detection of RF?**

Rose-Waaler test. This is an agglutination test in which sheep erythrocytes coated with a subagglutinating dose of antierythrocyte antibody (amboceptor) are used as the antigen.

8. **Define rheumatoid arthritis?**

This is a symmetric polyarthritis with muscle wasting and subcutaneous nodules, commonly associated with serositis, myocarditis, vasculitis and other disseminated lesions.

Antistreptolysin O (ASO) Test

Introduction

This test is important in the investigation of post-streptococcal disease. Most complications develop at a stage when it is not possible to isolate streptococci (group A) in culture. In 80–85% of the patients with rheumatic fever, there is a rise in ASO antibody, which is highest soon after the onset of the disease. Infection with group 'C' and group 'G' streptococci can also produce a rise in ASO titre.

Principle

The qualitative slide test reagent contains an aqueous suspension of polystyrene latex particles which are sensitized with streptolysin O. The particles agglutinate in the presence of ASO present in patient serum.

Requirements

- Latex ASO reagent kit
- Positive and negative serum controls
- Normal saline
- Test plate or dark slide
- Patient serum

Procedure

1. Bring reagents and serum samples to room temperature.
2. Dilute patient serum 1:5 with normal saline.
3. Place one drop each of diluted patient serum, and positive and negative control sera on the respective zones of a test plate.
4. Add one drop of latex ASO reagent to each of these drops.
5. Mix well with stirring rods and look for the agglutination within 2 minutes.

Interpretation

Marked agglutination indicates the presence of ASO. The results are reported in Todd units/ml or international units (IU). ASO titres higher than 200 Todd units/ml are indicative of prior streptococcal infection. For quantitative test, prepare further dilutions of serum (1:10,1:20,1:30,1:40,) which indicates ASO concentration 400, 800, 1200, 1600 Todd units/ml, respectively.

Uses

1. Simple to perform.
2. Rising titre indicates active and progressive streptococcal infection.
3. Declining titre indicates recovery of the patient.

Discussion

1. **In which conditions, ASO titres are elevated?**
   - Rheumatic fever
   - Glomerulonephritis
   - Scarlet fever

2. **What is streptolysin O?**
   Streptolysin O is a heat-labile protein with a molecular weight of 50,000 to 75,000 daltons. It binds to the cholesterol-containing erythrocyte membrane and produces large holes in it, leading to complete lysis. It is strongly antigenic. It induces brisk antibody response, usually within 10–14 days. In addition to group A streptococci, this haemolysin is also produced by streptococci of groups C and G.

3. **Which factors inhibit the activity of streptolysin O?**
   - Cholesterol in the serum
   - Bacterial contamination of serum
   - Chemical treatment of serum

   Therefore, all these factors make serum unfit for ASO test.

4. **Which titre of ASO test is significant?**

An ASO titre in excess of 200 Todd units is considered significant and suggests either recent or recurrent infection with streptococci.

5. **Why this lysin is called streptolysin 'O'?**

Because it is oxygen-labile.

6. **Why plasma should not be used for ASO test?**

Fibrinogen in the plasma can lead to nonspecific agglutination of the latex particles.

7. **What are the supporting evidences for acute rheumatic fever?**

- Recent scarlet fever.
- Increased titre of ASO, CRP and ESR.
- Positive throat culture for group 'A' streptococci.

8. **What is the disadvantage of latex antistreptolysin O test?**

Latex antistreptolysin O titre also rises in streptococcal group 'C' and 'G' infection.

9. **Why ASO titre is not raised in skin infection.**

The ASO response following skin infection is poor, presumably because of inactivation of antigen by cholesterol present in the skin.

10. **What is the principle of ASO test by tube method?**

This is a neutralization test for the detection of ASO. In this test, a constant amount of streptolysin O antigen reagent (reduced form) is added to the series of dilutions of the serum. Following period of incubation, group 'O' washed red cells (human or rabbit) are added. The tubes are then examined for lysis of red cells. Haemolysis occurs in those tubes in which there is insufficient antibody to neutralize the antigen. The highest dilution of serum which indicates no haemolysis is the ASO titre.

11. **Which other test may be performed for the diagnosis of rheumatic fever?**

Anti-deoxyribonuclease B assay may be performed since >15% of patients with acute rheumatic fever do not have an increased ASO titre.

12. **Anti-deoxyribonuclease B increased titre is significant in which condition?**

Anti-deoxyribonuclease B is useful in the retrospective diagnosis particularly of skin infection, where ASO titre may be low.

13. **What is the significant titre of anti-deoxyribonuclease B?**

Titres higher than 300 or 350 Todd units are taken as significant.

Complement Fixation Test

Introduction

The term complement (C) is applied to a system of components present in the serum of man and animals. It consists of nine different proteins denoted C_1–C_9, some of which are heat-labile and are destroyed by heating at 56°C for 30 minutes. Serum deprived of C activity is said to be inactivated. Complement takes part in many of the immunological reactions and gets fixed during the combination of antigen (Ag) and antibody without any visible effect. This property of antigen and antibody complex to fix the complement is used in complement fixation test (CFT) for the identification of specific antibodies and antigens. The haemolytic system containing sheep erythrocytes and its corresponding antibody (amboceptor) is used as an indicator which shows the utilization or availability of the complement.

Principle

Complement lyses antibody coated red cells. If the complement is fixed, then there will be no lysis of erythrocytes, thus denoting a positive test. If the complement is available, then there will be haemolysis which is a property of complement, thus denoting a negative test.

Requirements

- Patient serum (inactivated by heating in water bath at 56°C for 30 minutes)
- Physiological saline
- Complement (pooled guinea pig serum)
- Sheep RBCs
- Amboceptor (antisheep red cell antibody)
- Centrifuge machine
- Antigen (soluble or particulate)
- Microtitre plates and micropipettes

Procedure

The procedure is carried out in two stages:

1. In stage 1, test serum (for the detection of antibody) and the antigen are mixed in the presence of carefully measured amount of complement and then incubated at 37°C for 1 hour. If the test serum contains antibody, then antigen–antibody complexes are formed and complement gets fixed on it.

2. In stage 2, indicator system, antibody-coated sheep red cells, is added to determine whether the complement has been fixed in stage 1 reaction or not. If the complement is taken up during stage 1 reaction, then it will not be available to lyse the red cells, whilst a negative test, with unused complement, is shown by lysis of the red cells (Fig. 20.1).

Interpretation

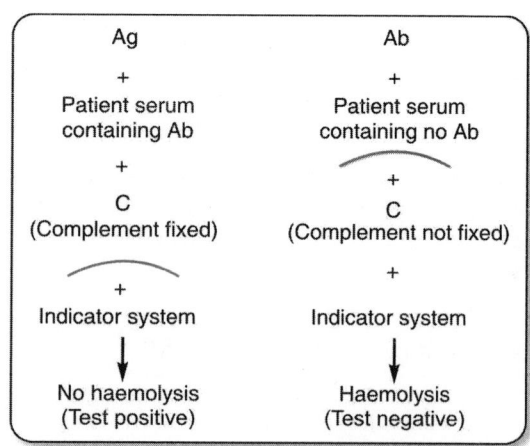

Fig. 20.1. Complement fixation test.

Uses

1. This is a very sensitive test and can detect as little as 0.04 µg of antibody and 0.1 µg of antigen.
2. Wasserman reaction and Reiter protein complement fixation test (RPCFT) for serodiagnosis of syphilis are based on this test.

3. CFT is useful for the identification of bacterial, viral, fungal, chlamydial and parasitic antigen.

Discussion

1. **Why do you heat serum at 56°C for 30 minutes for CFT?**

   To inactivate complement present in the serum. It also inactivates certain non-specific factors which are likely to interfere with antigen–antibody reaction.

2. **What is the source of complement used in CFT?**

   It is pooled serum obtained from 4 to 5 guinea pigs. It should be fresh or specially preserved, as the complement activity is heat-labile (may be stored at –30°C in small fractions).

3. **What is the principle of Wassermann reaction?**

   Complement fixation test.

4. **Which test is more specific (Wassermann or VDRL)?**

   Wassermann.

5. **What do you mean by amboceptor?**

   Rabbit antibody to sheep red cells prepared by inoculating sheep erythrocytes into rabbit under standard immunization protocol, is known as amboceptor.

6. **Define minimum haemolytic dose (MHD) of complement.**

   MHD or one unit of complement is the highest dilution of guinea pig serum that lyses one unit volume of washed sheep RBCs in the presence of excess of haemolysin (amboceptor) within a fixed time (usually 30–60 minutes) at 37°C.

7. **Define MHD of haemolysin.**

   One MHD of haemolysin may be defined as highest dilution of the serum that lyses one unit volume of washed sheep RBCs in the presence of excess complement within a fixed time (usually 30–60 minutes) at 37°C.

8. **Name pathways of complement activation.**

   Classical pathway and alternative pathway.

9. **Which class/es of immunoglobulins is/are involved in classical pathway?**

   IgM and IgG (IgG 3, 1, 2).

10. **Which subclass of IgG cannot fix complement?**

    IgG 4.

11. **Which class of immunoglobulin can activate alternative pathway of complement activation?**

    IgA.

12. **Name the factors which can activate alternative pathway of complement activation.**

    - Bacterial endotoxin
    - Rabbit RBCs
    - Snake venom proteins
    - Nephritic factor
    - Yeast cell wall

13. **What is the percentage of complement in the serum?**

    Complement constitutes about 5% of normal serum proteins.

14. **Can you increase the complement level in the body by immunization?**

    No.

15. **Who coined the term "complement"?**

    Ehrlich.

16. **Where is the complement binding site located in the immunoglobulin?**

    Complement binding site is located on the Fc piece of the immunoglobulin molecule (C_H2 domain on IgG and C_H4 on IgM).

17. **Can complement from one species react with antibodies from other species?**

    Yes, it can react.

18. **In which state, complement is normally present in serum?**

    Complement, in serum, is normally present in inactive state. Its activity is induced by antigen–antibody interaction.

19. **What happens if there is complement deficiency in the serum?**

    There are recurrent bacterial and fungal infections. Collagen diseases also occur in complement deficiency.

Weil-Felix Test

Introduction

Weil-Felix test is a heterophile agglutination test. It is useful in the serodiagnosis of rickettsial infections, e.g., epidemic typhus, endemic typhus, spotted fevers and scrub typhus.

Principle

The test is based upon the sharing of an alkali stable carbohydrate antigen between some rickettsiae and certain non-motile strains of *Proteus*, *P. vulgaris* OX19 and OX2, and *P. mirabilis* OXK. The antibodies against the pathogen appear around the 5th day of onset of disease. These can be detected by slide or tube agglutination test.

Requirements

- Physiological saline (0.85% sodium chloride)
- Patient serum
- Antigenic suspension of *Proteus* (OX19, OX2 and OXK)
- Pipettes
- Test tubes
- Test tube rack
- Water bath

Procedure

1. Arrange 3 rows each containing 7 clean and dry tubes in a rack (total 21 tubes).
2. Mix 0.1 ml of the patient serum with 0.9 ml of saline to obtain a 1 in 10 dilution (master dilution).
3. Add 0.4 ml of physiological saline from second to seventh tube with the help of pipette.
4. Add 0.4 ml of freshly prepared 1:10 dilution of serum into first 2 tubes of each row.
5. After mixing well, go on transferring 0.4 ml from second tube onwards up to sixth tube and from sixth discard 0.4 ml accordingly.

6. Add 0.4 ml of the respective *Proteus* antigen namely OX19, OX2 and OXK in each row from first to seventh tube. The final dilution would read as 1: 20, 1: 40, 1:80, 1:160, 1:320 and 1: 640 from the first to sixth tubes respectively, while the last tube serves as a negative control (Fig. 21.1).

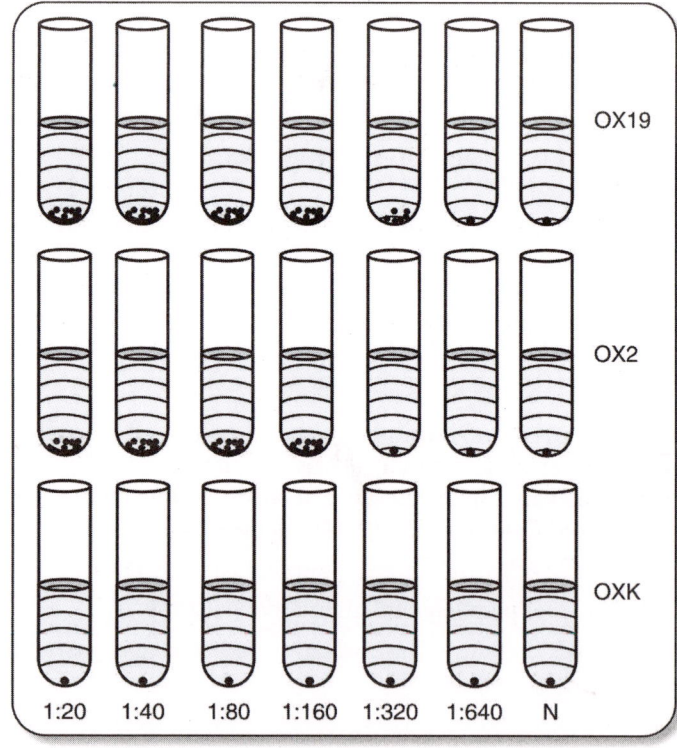

Fig. 21.1. Weil-Felix test. N – negative control.

7. Incubate the tube at 50°C in an incubator for nearly 4 hours. Then keep at 37°C overnight.
8. Read the test results next day and observe for granular clumps (agglutination)

Interpretation

A single titre of ≥160 is considered clinically significant. An increasing value of titre in the subsequent samples indicates recent infection.

Uses

Diagnosis of rickettsial infection. Sera from patients with epidemic and endemic typhus strongly agglutinate OX19 and weakly agglutinate OX2. In Brill-Zinsser disease, the test is negative or weakly reactive. In spotted fevers, both OX19 and OX2 are agglutinated. OXK agglutinins are present only in scrub typhus (Table 21.1)

Table 21.1. Weil-Felix reaction in rickettsial disease

Disease	Agglutination with		
	OX19	OX2	OXK
Epidemic typhus	++++	+	–
Endemic typhus	++++	+	–
Brill-Zinsser disease	+/–	–	–
Spotted fevers	++++ to +	+ to ++++	–
Scrub typhus	–	–	+++

Discussion

1. **What is the principle of Weil-Felix test?**
   Heterophile tube agglutination test.

2. **What is the source of antigens in this test?**
   These are somatic (O) antigens of certain non-motile strains of *Proteus*, *P. vulgaris* OX19 and OX2, and *P. mirabilis* OXK.

3. **What is the nature of the antigen shared by rickettsiae and *Proteus*?**
   Alkali-stable carbohydrate antigen.

4. **In which rickettsial infections, this test is of no use?**
   Rickettsial pox, Q fever and trench fever.

5. **In which conditions, Weil-Felix reaction is false positive?**
   Typhoid fever, liver diseases and infections by *Proteus*.

6. **Which is the most frequently used serological method using rickettsial antigen?**
   Complement fixation test (using group-specific soluble antigen or type-specific washed rickettsial antigen).

7. **What do you mean by heterophile antigens?**
   Same or closely-related antigens occurring in different biological species, classes and kingdoms are known as heterophile antigens.

8. **Which test is used to differentiate epidemic typhus and endemic typhus?**
   Complement fixation test.

9. **Name various serological tests utilizing rickettsial antigens.**
   - Complement fixation test
   - Immunofluorescence
   - Enzyme immunoassay
   - Latex agglutination test

10. **What is the significant titre in Weil-Felix test?**
    A single titre of ≥1:160 is considered clinically significant. However, titre may rise up to 1:1000 or 1:5000 during second week and decline rapidly during convalescence.

11. **Name serological tests based on the principle of heterophile antigens.**
    - Weil-Felix reaction
    - Paul-Bunnell test
    - Cold agglutination test
    - Agglutination of *Streptococcus* MG.

Paul-Bunnell Test

Introduction

This is one of the most widely used haemagglutination test for the diagnosis of infectious mononucleosis. Infectious mononucleosis or glandular fever is an acute febrile illness characterized by fever, malaise, headache, generalized lymphadenopathy, sore throat, a mononuclear blood picture and heterophile antibody in blood. This disease is caused by Epstein-Barr virus (EBV).

Principle

This is a heterophile tube agglutination test. The heterophile antibody develops in the blood which agglutinates sheep erythrocyte.

Requirements

- Patient serum (inactivated at 56°C for 30 minutes in a water bath)
- Physiological saline
- Sheep blood
- Test tubes (3″ × ½″)
- Pipettes
- Test tube rack
- Centrifuge machine
- Water bath

Preparation of Sheep Erythrocytes (Antigen)

1. Collect 10–20 ml sheep blood in a citrated flask with all aseptic precautions by puncturing the external jugular vein with a wide bore needle.
2. Wash the sheep RBCs three to four times in physiological saline by centrifuging at 2000 rpm, for 5 to 10 minutes.
3. Discard the supernatant.
4. Take 1 ml of RBCs from the button and add to 99 ml of physiological saline to obtain 1% suspension of RBCs.

Procedure

1. Arrange 11 tubes in a rack.
2. Add 0.4 ml of physiological saline from second to eleventh tube.
3. Prepare 1 in 16 dilution of the patient serum by taking 0.1 ml of serum in 1.5 ml of saline (master dilution).
4. Add 0.4 ml from master dilution to the first 2 tubes. The first tube will have 1:16 dilution while the dilution in second tube is 1:32.
5. After mixing well, go on transferring 0.4 ml from second tube onwards up to the tenth tube and from tenth tube discard 0.4 ml accordingly.
6. Add 0.4 ml of 1% sheep RBCs suspension from first tube to eleventh tube.
7. The final dilutions will be 1:16, 1:32, 1:64, 1:128, 1:256, 1:512, 1:1024, 1:2048, 1:4096, 1:8192 from first tube to tenth tube while the last tube will serve as a negative control.
8. Shake the tubes thoroughly and incubate at 37°C for 4 hours.
9. Keep the tubes in a refrigerator at 4°C overnight.
10. Read the test next day after incubation at 37°C for 2 hours. This avoids fallacious results from "cold agglutination" which is reversible at 37°C and, is not associated with infectious mononucleosis.
11. Note which tubes show agglutination of RBCs and state the titre of reaction in terms of the final dilution of the serum.

Interpretation

A positive reaction is denoted by carpet formation and negative reaction is indicated by formation of button having regular well-defined margin. Normal serum may show agglutination in lower dilutions. Suggestive titre is 1:128, while a titre of 1:256 is diagnostic of infectious mononucleosis.

Use

Diagnosis of infectious mononucleosis caused by EBV.

Discussion

1. **What is the principle of Paul-Bunnell test?**
   Heterophile tube agglutination test.

2. **What is the significant titre of Paul-Bunnell test?**
   A suggestive titre is 1:128 and a significant titre is 1:256.

3. **In which other conditions, heterophile agglutinins may be present in the blood?**
   - In persons who have recently received an injection of a therapeutic serum (from the horse), an apparently similar heterophile antibody (Forssman's antibody) may be present in considerable amount in the blood, since horse serum contains the appropriate heterophile antigen and stimulates production of an antibody for sheep red cells.
   - Normal serum may agglutinate in low dilutions.

4. **What is Paul-Bunnell differential absorption test?**
   The type of antibody present in infectious mononucleosis differs in certain respects from the Forssman antibody, and also from that found in normal serum. This difference can be determined by Paul-Bunnell differential absorption test (Table 22.1).

5. **Why do you keep the tubes at 37°C for 2 hours after overnight refrigeration at 4°C.**

Table 22.1. Paul-Bunnell differential absorption test

Antibody	Treated with emulsion of guinea pig kidney	Treated with ox red cells
Normal serum	Absorbed	Not absorbed
After serum therapy	Absorbed	Absorbed
Infectious mononucleosis	Not absorbed	Absorbed

To avoid the fallacious results on account of cold agglutination.

6. **What is the percentage of sheep red cells used in Paul-Bunnell test?**
   1% suspension.

7. **What is the nature of these heterophile antibodies in infectious mononucleosis?**
   IgM.

8. **When do heterophile antibodies appear in the blood of patient suffering from infectious mononucleosis?**
   These appear early during the acute phase of illness, reaching peak levels 2 weeks after the onset. The titre decreases rapidly after fourth week and is not detectable after 3 months.

9. **Name other serological tests used for the diagnosis of infectious mononucleosis?**
   More reliable indicator of EBV infection is the demonstration of IgM antibody to the EBV viral capsid antigen by ELISA or indirect immunofluorescence tests.

Cold Agglutination Test

Introduction

This test detects antibody to human O group erythrocytes. Since these antibodies react best at 4°C, the test is referred to as cold agglutination test. The test is frequently positive in patients suffering from primary atypical pneumonia caused by *Mycoplasma pneumoniae*.

Principle

Tube agglutination test.

Requirements

- Patient serum
- 2% suspension of human O group erythrocytes [0.2 ml packed red cells + 9.8 ml normal saline]
- Normal saline
- Test tubes
- Test tube rack
- Centrifuge machine
- Refrigerator
- Pipettes

Procedure

1. Arrange 9 tubes in a rack.
2. Add 0.2 ml saline from second to ninth tube.
3. Prepare 1 in 4 dilution of the patient's serum by taking 0.1 ml of serum in 0.3 ml saline (master dilution).
4. Add 0.2 ml each from master dilution to the first 2 tubes. The first tube will have 1:4 dilution while the dilution in second tube is 1:8.
5. After mixing well, go on transferring 0.2 ml from second tube onwards up to eighth tube and from eighth tube discard 0.2 ml accordingly.
6. Add 0.2 ml of 2% red cell suspension in each tube already containing saline and serum.
7. The final dilutions will be 1:4, 1:8, 1:16, 1:32, 1:64, 1:128,

1:256, 1:512, from first tube to eighth tube while the last tube will serve as a negative control.
8. Shake the tubes and refrigerate at 4°C overnight.
9. Next day read immediately before tubes warm up.

Interpretation

The highest final dilution of serum giving agglutination is taken as the titre (the agglutination should disappear on warming). A titre of ≥1:64 is suggestive but demonstration of rise in titre in paired serum sample is more reliable.

Uses

Cold agglutination test is useful for the diagnosis of atypical pneumonia. However, cold agglutinins are occasionally induced in other diseases such as infectious mononucleosis, rubella, adenovirus infection, psittacosis, tropical eosinophilia, trypanosomiasis, cirrhosis of liver, paroxysmal haemoglobinuria and haemolytic anaemia.

Discussion

1. **Do all patients of primary atypical pneumonia develop cold agglutinins?**

   No, demonstrable cold agglutinin titres develop in 50% of the patients only.

2. **Does agglutination occur at 37°C?**

   Agglutination occurs at low temperature, i.e., 4°C. At 37°C, the clumping is dissociated.

3. **Which blood group RBCs are taken for cold agglutination test?**

   Human O group RBCs.

4. **What is the diagnostic titre?**

   A four-fold rise in cold agglutinin titre or a single titre of ≥1:64 is suggestive of *M. pneumoniae* infection.

5. **What precaution should be taken while dealing with the blood sample of the patient submitted for cold agglutination test?**

The patient blood sample should not be refrigerated before separation of the serum, as the agglutinins are readily absorbed by the homologous erythrocytes at low temperature.

6. **When do cold agglutinins appear during the course of primary atypical pneumonia?**

Cold agglutinins appear about one week after infection with a peak at 4–5 weeks. Thereafter, titre declines rapidly and the test becomes negative after about 5 months.

7. **Name other serological tests used for the diagnosis of atypical pneumonia?**

- Detection of antigen in respiratory exudate by:
  - direct immunofluorescence,
  - counterimmunoelectrophoresis,
  - immunoblotting with monoclonal antibodies, and
  - enzyme immunoassay.
- Detection of antibody by:
  - agglutination of *Streptococcus* MG,
  - complement fixation test, and
  - enzyme immunoassay.

8. **What is the advantage of cold agglutinin test over other specific tests?**

Cold agglutinin titre may increase before a specific antibody response can be seen.

Brucella Agglutination Test

Introduction

Brucellosis is a zoonosis, primarily affecting animals and transmitted to humans by contact with infected animals or through their products. Three species namely *Brucella abortus*, *B. suis* and *B. melitensis* are pathogenic to man. They are responsible for Malta fever or undulant fever.

Principle

Standard tube agglutination test (SAT).

Requirements

- Patient serum
- Pipettes
- Test tubes
- Test tube rack
- Standard antigen suspension of *B. abortus*
- Phenol saline
- Incubator

Procedure

1. Arrange 9 tubes in a rack.
2. Add 0.5 ml of phenol saline in tubes second to ninth.
3. In tube No. 1 add 0.1 ml of patient serum and 0.9 ml of phenol saline.
4. Mix and transfer 0.5 ml from tube first to second and then tube second to third till the eighth tube.
5. Finally discard 0.5 ml from eighth tube.
6. Add 0.5 ml of *Brucella* antigen to each tube.
7. Dilutions are 1:10, 1:20, 1:40, 1:80, 1:160, 1:320, 1:640, and 1:1280. Last ninth tube acts as a control.
8. Mix well and incubate at 37°C for 24 hours or 50°C for 18 hours.
9. Next day record agglutination.

Interpretation

The test is read by observing the clearing and sedimentation and is graded as follows:

(a) Complete agglutination and sedimentation or 100% clearing.
(b) About 75% clearing or nearly complete agglutination.
(c) About 50% clearing and marked sedimentation.
(d) About 25% clearing and distinct sedimentation.

A titre of ≥1:160 is considered significant. Most patients with acute brucellosis develop titres of ≥1:640 by 3–4 weeks of illness. In normal individuals, agglutinin titres vary with geographical location and exposure to the organisms but it is usually <1:100.

Uses

Diagnosis of brucellosis.

Discussion

1. **What is the source of antigen for standard tube agglutination test?**

   Brucella abortus somatic antigen.

2. **Which class of antibody is mainly identified by standard tube agglutination test?**

   IgM.

3. **What do you mean by prozone phenomenon?**

   In first few tubes, agglutination may be negative but in later tubes agglutination is seen. This may be due to antibody excess or due to the presence of blocking or non-agglutinating antibodies.

4. **Which test is used to identify blocking antibodies?**

   Anti-human globulin (Coombs') test.

5. **Blocking antibodies belong to which class/es of immunoglobulins?**

IgG and IgA.

6. **When do the antibodies appear following *Brucella* infection?**

Antibodies appear within 7–10 days of onset of disease. IgM antibodies appear first. They are rapidly followed and superseded by IgG and to a lesser extent by IgM antibodies.

7. **Name various serological tests for the detection of *Brucella* antibodies.**

- Standard tube agglutination test (SAT)
- 2-mercaptoethanol (2 ME) agglutination test
- Complement fixation tests
- Anti-human globulin (Coombs') test
- ELISA
- RIA (radioimmunoassay)

8. **Which of the above is the most widely used test?**

Standard tube agglutination test.

9. **What is the significant titre of standard tube agglutination test?**

A single titre ≥1:160 by SAT is presumptive evidence of recent *Brucella* infection.

10. **How do you express agglutinin titres in international units (IU)?**

The reciprocal of serum dilution is doubled, e.g., if the end point dilution is 1:160, then the corresponding IU would read as 320 IU/ml.

11. **What is the disadvantage of standard tube agglutination test?**

This test cannot detect chronic cases.

12. **Which tests are better to differentiate between acute and chronic brucellosis?**

ELISA and RIA are very sensitive tests and can distinguish IgM, IgG and IgA *Brucella* antibodies. Therefore, these tests are helpful to distinguish acute and chronic brucellosis.

13. **What is the other advantage of ELISA test?**

For screening a large number of serum samples.

Enzyme Immunoassay (EIA)

Introduction

The term enzyme immunoassay (EIA) includes all assays based on the measurement of enzyme labelled antigen, hapten or antibody. EIAs are of two basic types—homogeneous and heterogeneous. In homogeneous EIA, there is no need to separate the bound and free fractions so that the test can be completed in one step, with all reagents added simultaneously. Heterogeneous EIA requires the separation of the free and bound fractions either by centrifugation or by absorption on solid surface and washing. It is, therefore, a multistep procedure, with reagents added sequentially. The major type of heterogeneous EIA is enzyme-linked immunosorbent assay (ELISA).

ELISA

ELISA is a highly sensitive and specific test used for the detection of a variety of antigens and antibodies of microbial and human origin. ELISA test is classified into 3 types depending upon the source of antigen used in the test proper. They are:

1. First generation ELISA,
2. Second generation ELISA, and
3. Third generation ELISA.

Principle

Antigen or antibody is adsorbed on the solid phase which may be polystyrene or polyvinyl microtitre plates. Test serum with antigen or antibody is added and incubated at 37°C for 2 hours for formation of antigen–antibody complex and unbound components are finally removed by washing. The amount of bound fraction is subsequently measured by addition of enzyme-linked anti-human globulin or specific antibody and an appropriate substrate to produce colour and products detected by the ELISA reader.

Requirements

- Patient serum
- Diagnostic kit
  - Microtitre plate
  - Enzyme conjugate (peroxidase labelled purified antigen)
  - Buffered substrate (contains H_2O_2)
  - Chromogen solution (tetramethylbenzidine in dimethyl-sulfoxide)
  - Stopping solution (sulphuric acid)
  - Washing solution
  - Sample diluent
  - Negative control
  - Positive control
  - Cut-off-serum
  - Conjugate diluent
  - Diluents for reagents and specimen.
- Microplate ELISA reader

Procedure

1. Add appropriate volume of diluent in each well.
2. Add appropriate volume of test serum and equal volume of positive and negative controls into the respective wells of microtitre plate.
3. Cover the plate with adhesive film and incubate at 37°C for specified time.
4. Aspirate the contents and wash the wells 4 times by using working wash solution. Now add appropriate volume of the conjugate. Mix well and incubate at 37°C for specified time.
5. Aspirate the contents and wash the wells five times by using wash solution.
6. Add appropriate volume of buffered substrate and chromogen solutions. Incubate at 37°C for specified time.
7. Add stop solution and read absorbance biochromatically at 450 nm and 660 nm by using a microplate reader.

Uses

ELISA kits have been developed for the detection of:

- HIV-1 and HIV-2 antigens and antibody.
- *Entamoeba histolytica* antigens in stools.
- *Toxoplasma* antigens in patient serum.
- *Haemophilus influenzae* antigens in spinal fluid.
- β-haemolytic streptococcal antigen in spinal fluid.
- Hepatitis A virus in stools.
- Respiratory syncytial virus in pharyngeal secretions.
- Adenovirus antigens in nasopharyngeal specimens.
- Labile enterotoxin of *Escherichia coli* in stools.
- Hepatitis-B surface antigen and its antibody.
- Cytomegalovirus antigen.
- Rubella IgG and IgM.
- Thyroid hormones T_3, T_4 and TSH.

Discussion

1. **What do you mean by first, second and third generation ELISA?**

   - *First generation ELISA:* Here the antigen is prepared by propagating viruses in mammalian cell line. It is coated on microwell plates after disrupting and inactivating the viral concentrate.
   - *Second generation ELISA:* Here the antigen is prepared either by bacterial recombinant DNA technology or proteins which corresponds to viral component.
   - *Third generation ELISA:* Here the synthetic peptides are used as antigen source and they generally correspond to viral antigenic epitopes.

2. **What do you mean by immunosorbent in term ELISA?**

   An absorbing material specific for one of the components of the reaction, the antigen or antibody.

3. **Enumerate immunosorbents.**

Particulate	• Cellulose
	• Agarose
Solid phase (tubes or microwell)	• Polystyrene
	• Polyvinyl
	• Polycarbonate
Membranes or disc	• Polyacrylamide
	• Paper
	• Plastic

4. **Name different types of ELISA.**

   - Indirect ELISA
   - Competitive ELISA
   - Sandwich ELISA (direct and indirect)

   The diagrammatic representation of these is given in Fig. 25.1.

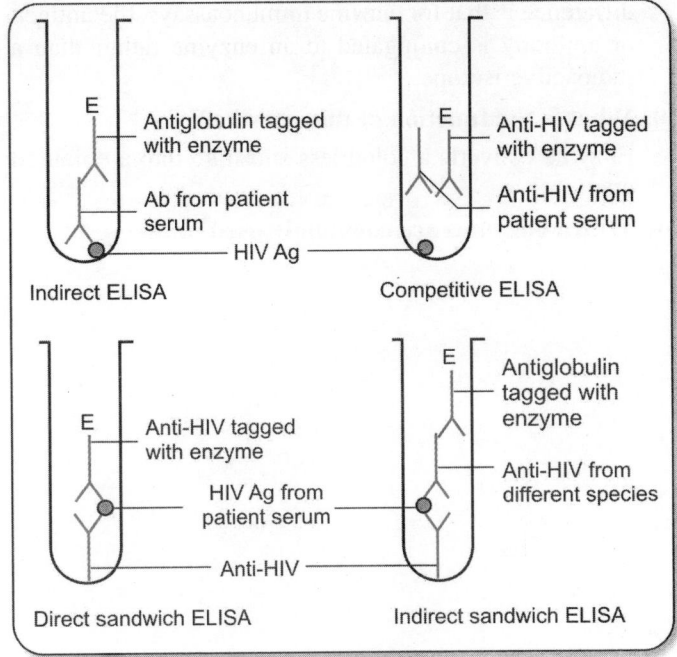

Fig. 25.1. Different types of ELISA.

5. **What do you mean by indirect ELISA?**

   This is used for the detection of antibody and, therefore, the solid phase is conjugated with antigen.

6. **Describe briefly competitive ELISA.**

   This method can be used for the detection of antigen or antibody. For the detection of antibodies, solid phase is coated with antigen. Test sample and enzyme labelled specific antibody conjugate are added at the same time for specific period. During incubation, there is competition between antibodies of patient serum and specific antibody conjugate for sharing of antigen. Intense colour suggests the binding of specific antibody conjugate and hence a non-reactive reaction, while lack of colour indicates binding of patient serum antibodies and hence a reactive reaction.

7. **What is the advantage of competitive over indirect ELISA?**

   - It takes less time.
   - No predilution of test serum is required.

8. **How many types of sandwich ELISA are known to you?**

   Two types:

   - Single antibody or direct sandwich ELISA.
   - Double antibody or indirect sandwich ELISA.

9. **What is the difference between EIA and radio-immunoassay (RIA)?**

   These tests are based on the same principle. The key

difference is that for enzyme immunoassays, the antigen or antibody is conjugated to an enzyme rather than a radioactive isotope.

10. What is the function of this enzyme?

Enzyme converts a colourless substrate into a coloured one.

11. Which enzymes are commonly used in this test?

- Horseradish peroxidase.
- Alkaline phosphatase.

12. What are the advantages of ELISA test?

- Highly sensitive.
- Safe and economical.
- Simple instrument required.
- Many tests can be performed at the same time.

Section
3

Parasitology

- Collection and preservation of stool specimen
- Examination of stool
- Identification of faecal eggs
- Identification of faecal trophozoites, cysts and oocysts
- Culture techniques
- Examination of blood

Collection and Preservation of Stool Specimen

Introduction

Stool or faeces sample is the most common specimen used for the diagnosis of intestinal parasitic infections. Depending on the nature of the parasite, the microscopic observations include the identification of cysts, ova, trophozoites, larvae or portions of the adult structure. The ability to detect and identify human parasite is directly linked to the quality of the clinical specimen.

Collection of Specimen

1. Specimen should be collected in a wide-mouthed clean container without contamination with urine, water or disinfectants.
2. The collection of three faecal specimens usually suffice to make the diagnosis of intestinal parasitic diseases, two obtained on successive days during normal bowel movement and a third after magnesium sulphate purge. A total of six specimens, collected on successive days, may be required, if intestinal amoebiasis or giardiasis is suspected.
3. The specimen should be free of oil and other non-faecal substances such as barium or bismuth. Patients who have received a barium enema may not excrete organisms in their stool for at least 1 week following barium enema, therefore, stool examination must be delayed for at least 1 week following the enema.
4. Cathartics with an oil base should be avoided because oils retard the motility of trophozoites and distort the morphology of the parasite.
5. The specimen should be properly labelled with patient's name, age, sex and date of collection.
6. Liquid stool specimens should be examined within 30 minutes after collection or semiformed stool within 60 minutes to detect motile trophozoites, particularly in suspected infections with *Entamoeba histolytica* and *Giardia lamblia*. Formed stools, in which trophozoites are not expected, may be examined up to 24 hours after passage.

7. Specimen should not be kept at the warm temperature, and drying of the specimen should be prevented.

Preservation of Specimen

Preservation of stool helps in maintaining morphology of protozoan parasites and preventing further development of some helminth eggs and larvae. Since the preservatives kill parasites, therefore, characteristic motility of trophozoites cannot be seen. Following are the commonly used preservatives.

Formalin solution

Faecal sample can be preserved in 10% formalin saline (100 ml formaldehyde in 900 ml 0.85% sodium chloride). Three parts of formalin preservative solution is thoroughly mixed with one part of stool specimen. It adequately preserves protozoan cysts, and helminth eggs and larvae. One disadvantage of formalin-fixed stool specimens is the unsuitability for the preparation of permanent stained smears.

Polyvinyl alcohol (PVA)

It preserves intestinal protozoa especially trophozoite stage. It is prepared by mixing 62.5 ml of 95% ethyl alcohol, 125 ml of saturated aqueous solution of mercuric chloride, 10 ml of glacial acetic acid, and 3 ml of glycerine in a 500 ml beaker. Then 10 g of PVA powder is added, without stirring. The beaker is then covered and allowed to soak overnight. It is then heated slowly to 75°C. When this temperature is reached, the mixture is removed from heat and it is stirred until a homogenous, slightly milky solution is obtained. For the preservation of stool, three parts of PVA is mixed with one part of the specimen.

Merthiolate-iodine-formalin (MIF) solution

MIF solution is prepared in two separate stock solutions to be mixed immediately before use. Solution I is prepared by

Parasitology

3

mixing 250 ml of distilled water, 200 ml of thiomersal, 25 ml of formaldehyde, and 5 ml of glycerol. Solution II is Lugol's iodine (5% iodine in 10% potassium iodide solution in distilled water). Before use, 2.35 ml (94 parts) of solution I is mixed with 0.15 ml (6 parts) of solution II. A small amount of the faecal specimen is added to this solution and mixed by stirring and shaking. It stains and fixes all microscopic parasite cysts, eggs, and larvae in the stool without any need for further staining by wet mounts. These are well preserved for 1 year or more.

Schaudinn's solution

It is prepared by mixing 45 g of mercuric chloride, 310 ml of 95% ethyl alcohol, 50 ml of glacial acetic acid, 15 ml of glycerol and 625 ml of distilled water. In a 20 ml screw-capped vial, 1 ml of stool sample is mixed and stirred in 14 ml of Schaudinn's solution. The vial is then closed and shaken vigorously for 20–30 seconds. It fixes and preserves the specimen for 1 year or more.

Sodium acetate acetic acid-formalin (SAF) fixative

It is prepared by mixing 1.5 g of sodium acetate, 2 ml of glacial acetic acid, 4 ml of formaldehyde (37–40% solution) and 92 ml of distilled water. This is a fixative from which a permanent stained smear of stool can be easily prepared and has the advantage of not containing mercuric chloride. The smear of the stool, preserved with SAF fixative tends to give better result when stained with iron-haematoxylin, than with that of trichrome stain.

Discussion

1. **Which type of container is used for collecting faecal samples?**

   Samples should be collected in a wide-mouthed clean container.

2. **Why contamination with urine and water should be avoided while collecting faecal sample?**

   Because urine can destroy motile trophozoites and water may contain free-living organisms, which may be mistaken for human parasites.

3. **Enumerate some medications which interfere in the detection of parasites.**

   - Bismuth
   - Mineral oil
   - Kaolin
   - Barium sulphate
   - Certain antibiotics – tetracyclines, sulphonamides
   - Anti-diarrhoeal agents.

4. **What precautions should be followed before collection of the faeces?**

   - The person should not have received medications which interfere in the detection of parasites.
   - Any radiological studies involving barium sulphate should not be performed at least 1 week before the collection of stool specimens.
   - The specimen should not be contaminated with urine or water.

5. **How many faecal specimens are sufficient to make the diagnosis of intestinal parasitic diseases?**

   Three faecal specimens usually suffice to make the diagnosis of intestinal parasitic diseases. However, if intestinal amoebiasis or giardiasis is suspected, then a total of six specimens, collected on successive days, may be required.

6. **When should you examine the faecal specimens after collection?**

   The liquid stool specimens should be examined immediately within 30 minutes of passage and the semiformed and soft specimens within 60 minutes of passage.

7. **How do you confirm whether the parasites have been eliminated after treatment or not?**

   In order to confirm the elimination of parasites after treatment, the faecal specimens should be examined 3–4 weeks after therapy in cases of protozoan infections, and 1–2 weeks after therapy in case of helminth infections. Absence of the parasite in the faecal specimen indicates that the parasite has been eliminated.

8. **How many faecal specimens are collected after treatment?**

   Three specimens (same as for the diagnosis).

9. **In case of delay in processing, at what temperature you should keep the faecal specimen?**

   In the refrigerator at 4°C.

10. **What are the disadvantages of freezing or incubating the faecal specimens?**

    Freezing the specimen will lead to loss of motility of the trophozoites and they will disintegrate with time. Incubation of faecal sample will lead to growth of bacterial flora. Keeping the samples at room temperature for long period should also be avoided.

11. **What are the advantages of preservation of faecal specimens?**

    Preservation of stool helps in:

    - Maintaining morphology of protozoan parasites.
    - Preventing further development of some helminth eggs and larvae.

12. **Enumerate the commonly used preservatives.**

    - Formalin solution
    - Polyvinyl alcohol (PVA)

Parasitology

3

- Merthiolate-iodine-formalin solution (MIF)
- Schaudinn's solution
- Sodium acetate acetic acid-formalin fixative (SAF).

13. Why do we need preservatives?

We need preservatives in the following conditions:

- In case of lag time between collection and examination.
- To preserve specimens for teaching purposes.
- Transportation of specimens to referral laboratory for confirmation.

14. Which is the most common chemical used for preservation of faecal specimen?

Formalin.

15. What are the disadvantages of preservation?

Preservatives kill the parasite, therefore, characteristic motility of the trophozoites cannot be seen.

16. What are the advantages of formalin as preservative?

- It preserves protozoan cysts, and helminth eggs and larvae.
- It is easy to prepare and is economical.

17. What is the major disadvantage of formalin?

Formalin preserved specimens are unsuitable for the preparation of permanent stained smears.

18. What are the major advantages of MIF as preservative?

- It is very useful for field surveys.
- Long shelf life and contains no mercury compound.

19. What is the disadvantage of MIF?

Morphology of organisms on permanent stained smear is not good.

20. What are the advantages of SAF?

- Concentration and permanent staining can be done on SAF preserved specimens.
- Easy to prepare
- Long shelf life
- Contains no mercury compounds.

21. What are the disadvantages of SAF?

- Staining quality with trichrome is not good.
- Albumin-coated slides are recommended to prepare the smear due to poor adhesive property of 'SAF' preserved specimen.

22. What are the advantages of polyvinyl alcohol (PVA)?

- PVA can preserve cysts, ova, larvae and even trophozoites of parasites.
- Concentration and staining can be done on PVA preserved specimens.
- Long shelf life.
- PVA can be used to preserve even liquid stools.

23. What are the disadvantages of PVA?

- It is difficult to prepare in the laboratory.
- It may turn white and gelatinous when it begins to dehydrate or when refrigerated.
- It contains mercury compounds.
- *Trichuris trichiura* eggs and *Giardia lamblia* cysts are not concentrated as easily as in formalin-based fixatives. *Cytoisospora* (*Isospora*) *belli* oocysts may not be visible in PVA preserved material.
- Morphology of *Strongyloides stercoralis* is not well preserved.

24. What are the advantages of Schaudinn's fixative?

- Concentration and staining (permanent) can be done from fixed material.
- It can be used with fresh stool samples or samples from intestinal mucosa.

25. What are the disadvantages of Schaudinn's fixative?

- It contains mercuric chloride, so there is a disposal problem.
- It has poor adhesive qualities with liquid or mucoid specimens.

26. Enumerate preservatives which contain mercury compounds.

- PVA
- Schaudinn's fixative.

Examination of Stool

Examination of stool consists of macroscopic and microscopic examination.

MACROSCOPIC EXAMINATION

Consistency

It may indicate types of organisms present. Trophozoites are usually found in soft or liquid specimens and cysts are found in semisolid or solid specimens.

Consistency	Reasons
1. Well formed	Normal
2. Hard	Constipation
3. Watery	Bacterial infection, purgative
4. Rice water stools	Cholera
5. Pale, bulky and frothy	Steatorrhoea
6. Flattened and ribbon-like	Obstruction in the lumen of bowel
7. Semisolid	Mild diarrhoea, after taking laxative, digestive upset

Adult Worms

Following adult worms may be present in the stool:

- Roundworm
- Pinworm
- Hookworm
- Tapeworm

Colour

Normal colour of the stool is light to dark brown (due to the presence of bile pigments).

Abnormal colour	Reasons
1. Black	Bleeding in the upper gastro-intestinal tract (GIT), iron intake
2. Bright red	Bleeding at the lower GIT level
3. Blood and mucus	Dysentery
4. Clay coloured	Obstruction to the flow of bile to intestine
5. White or light tan	After barium meal

MICROSCOPIC EXAMINATION

Intestinal protozoa, and eggs and larvae of helminths can be detected and identified by microscopic examination of the stool using:

1. Direct smear
2. Smear after concentration
3. Permanent stained smear.

Direct Smear

Saline wet mount

Saline wet mount is made by mixing a small quantity (about 2 mg) of faeces in a drop of saline placed on a clean glass slide. Remove any gross fibres or particles and cover with a coverslip. Avoid air bubble by drawing one edge of coverslip slightly into the suspension and lowering it almost to the slide before letting it fall. The mount should be just thick enough that newspaper print can be read through the slide. The smear is then examined under microscope. Begin at one corner of the smear and systematically examine successive adjacent swaths with the low power of the microscope (Fig. 27.1). When a parasite-like object comes into view, it should be more closely examined and identified under high power. Saline wet mount is used for the detection of trophozoites and cysts of protozoa, and eggs and larvae of helminths. It is particularly useful for detection of live motile trophozoites of _Entamoeba histolytica_, _Giardia lamblia_ and _Balantidium coli_.

Iodine wet mount

Stool is emulsified in a drop of five times diluted solution of Lugol's iodine on a clean glass slide, covered with a clean coverslip and examined under microscope as above. Both saline and iodine wet mounts may be prepared on the same slide (Fig. 27.1). For the preparation of Lugol's iodine, 10 g of potassium iodide is dissolved in 100 ml distilled water and 5 g of iodine crystals are then added slowly. The solution is filtered and kept in a stoppered bottle of amber colour. It should be prepared every two weeks.

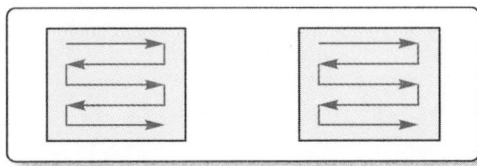

Fig. 27.1. Examination of a faecal smear (saline and iodine mount).

Iodine wet mount is used for the study of the nuclear character of cysts and trophozoites for the identification of the species. However, iodine immobilizes trophozoites. Iodine stained cysts of _E. histolytica_ show pale refractile nuclei, yellowish cytoplasm and brown glycogen mass. The chromidial bars do not stain with iodine. Helminth eggs and larvae are readily identified without stain, but the iodine stain can be used advantageously in the examination of larvae as it immobilizes and kills them and stain some parts differentially.

Buffered methylene blue wet mount

In the wet mount preparation of the stool, Nair's buffered methylene blue is used for demonstration of nuclei in the trophozoites of protozoa. Prepare a smear as for wet mount using buffered methylene blue instead of saline. Wait for 5–10 minutes before examination. Buffered methylene blue stained trophozoites show pale blue cytoplasm and dark blue nuclei. Cysts are not stained.

Smear after Concentration

The concentration of stool allows the detection of small number of parasites present in stool specimens. This procedure allows the increased recovery of eggs and larvae of helminths, and cysts of protozoa. Trophozoites of the protozoa are destroyed during the concentration procedure. Two commonly used methods are:

- Floatation techniques
- Sedimentation techniques

Both these methods are designed to separate intestinal protozoa and helminth eggs from excess of faecal debris by their differences in the specific gravity.

Floatation techniques

Floatation involves suspending the specimen in a medium of greater density than that of the helminth eggs and protozoan cysts. The eggs and cysts float to the top and are collected by placing a glass slide on the surface of the meniscus at the top of the tube. Following floatation techniques can be used:

- **Saturated salt floatation technique:** About 1 g of faeces is placed in a flat-bottomed vial (50 mm tall and 20 mm wide) and a few drops of saturated salt solution (specific gravity 1.20) are added. It is then stirred with a glass rod to make an even emulsion. More salt solution is added, so that the container is nearly full, stirring the solution throughout. Any coarse matter, which floats up, is removed. At this stage, the container is placed on a level surface. The final filling of container is carried out by means of a dropper, until a convex meniscus is formed. A glass slide 7.5 × 5 cm is carefully laid on the top of the container so that the centre is in contact with the fluid (Fig. 27.2). The preparation is allowed to stand for 20–30 minutes, after which the glass slide is quickly lifted, turned over smoothly so as to avoid spilling of the liquid, and examined under the microscope. A coverslip may not be placed over the fluid.

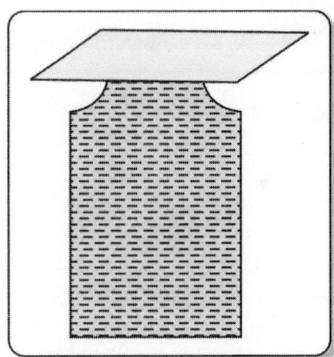

Fig. 27.2. Saturated salt floatation technique.

It has been observed that all the helminth eggs float in the saturated salt solution except unfertilized eggs of _Ascaris lumbricoides_, eggs of _Taenia solium_, _T. saginata_, and all intestinal flukes. _Strongyloides stercoralis_ larvae also do not float in salt solution.

- **Zinc sulphate centrifugal floatation technique:** About 1 g of faeces is thoroughly mixed in 10 ml of lukewarm distilled water. The coarse particles are removed by straining through gauze. The filtrate is poured into a 15 ml conical centrifuge tube and centrifuged at 2,500 revolutions per minute (rpm) for one minute. The supernatant fluid is poured off and distilled water is added to the sediment. It is shaken well, centrifuged and process is repeated 2 or 3 times till the supernatant fluid is clear. The clear supernatant is poured off and 3–4 ml of 33% zinc sulphate (specific gravity 1.18) is added to the sediment and more zinc sulphate solution is added to fill the tube up to the top and centrifuged again at 2,500 rpm for one minute. With a platinum wire loop, sample is taken from the surface (Fig. 27.3), onto a clean glass slide, a coverslip is put on and examined under microscope. For protozoal cysts, one drop of iodine solution is added before the coverslip is put on.

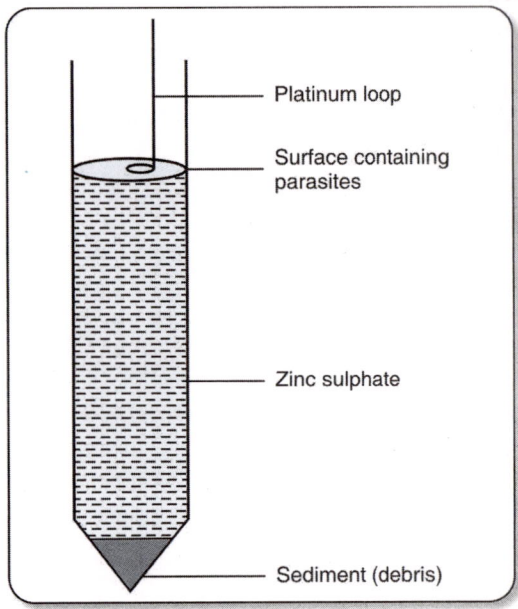

Fig. 27.3. Various layers observed after zinc sulphate floatation technique.

Zinc sulphate centrifugal floatation technique effectively concentrates cysts of protozoa, eggs of nematodes, and small tapeworms. This method is not suitable for unfertilized eggs of *A. lumbricoides* and eggs of most trematodes and large tapeworms.

Sedimentation technique

Concentration of intestinal parasites by sedimentation techniques, using either gravity or centrifugation, leads to a good recovery of cysts of protozoa, and eggs of helminths. Cysts and eggs of parasites settle and are concentrated at the bottom because they have greater density than the suspending medium.

Following are the commonly used sedimentation techniques:

- **Simple sedimentation:** A sufficient amount of faeces is thoroughly mixed with 10 to 20 times its volume of tap water and allowed to settle in a cone-shaped flask for an hour or two. This process is repeated several times till the supernatant fluid is clear. The clear supernatant fluid is discarded and the sediment at the bottom is examined for the eggs. This method is not suitable for protozoal cysts.
- **Formalin-ether sedimentation:** Half teaspoonful of faeces is thoroughly mixed in 10 ml of water and strained through

two layers of gauze in a funnel. The filtrate is centrifuged at 2,000 rpm for 2 minutes. The supernatant is discarded and the sediment is resuspended in 10 ml of physiological saline. It is again centrifuged and the supernatant is discarded. The sediment is resuspended in 7 ml of formalin saline and allowed to stand for 10 minutes or longer for fixation. To this is added 3 ml of ether. The tube is stoppered and shaken vigorously to mix. Then the stopper is removed and the tube is centrifuged at 2,000 rpm for 2 minutes.

The tube is allowed to rest in a stand. Four layers become visible, top layer consists of ether and dissolved fat, second is a plug of faecal debris, third is a clear layer of formalin saline and the fourth is sediment containing parasites (Fig. 27.4). The plug of faecal debris is detached from the side of the tube with the aid of a glass rod and the liquid is poured off. With a pipette, the sediment is removed and the saline and iodine mounts are made and examined under microscope.

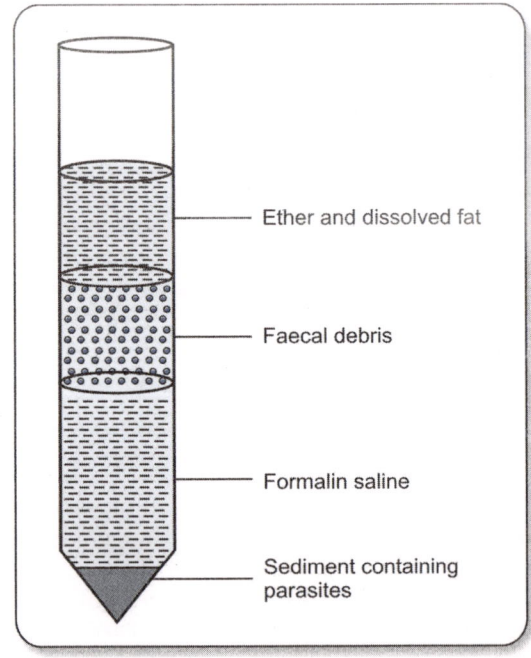

Fig. 27.4. Various layers seen in tube after formalin-ether sedimentation.

Ether dissolves faecal fats and formalin fixes the parasites and removes faecal odour. Risk of laboratory acquired infection from faecal organism is minimized because organisms are killed by formalin saline.

Permanent Stained Smear

Permanent stained smears are essential for cytological details for accurate diagnosis. These can be prepared with both fresh and polyvinyl alcohol preserved stool specimens. Iron-haematoxylin, trichrome and modified acid-fast stain are commonly used methods.

Iron-haematoxylin stain

A thin smear of faeces is made on a clean glass slide. It is fixed by keeping it in Schaudinn's solution for 15 minutes or longer. The smear is then immersed successively in 70% alcohol, 70% alcohol to which enough iodine has been added to give it the colour of urine, 70% alcohol, and 50% alcohol, 2–5 minutes in each.

It is washed in running tap water for 2–10 minutes and immersed in 2% aqueous ferric ammonium sulphate solution for 5–15 minutes followed by washing in running water for 3–5 minutes. It is then stained with 0.5% aqueous haematoxylin for 5–15 minutes and washed in running water for 2–5 minutes. Then it is differentiated in saturated aqueous solution of picric acid for 10–15 minutes and dehydrated by immersion for 2–5 minutes each in 50%, 70%, 80% and 95% alcohol, and 5 minutes each in two changes of absolute alcohol. Stained smear is then cleared in two changes of xylol for 3–5 minutes each, mounted in Canada balsam and covered with coverslip.

Morphology of parasites after staining with iron-haematoxylin stain:

- *Background:* Grey
- *Protozoa:* Light blue
- *Nuclei:* Bluish black

Trichrome stain

The trichrome stain contains chromotrope 2R, 0.6 g; light green SF, 9.3 g; and phosphotungstic acid, 0.7 g. These dry components are mixed with 1.0 ml of glacial acetic acid and allowed to stand for 30 minutes, then diluted with 100 ml of distilled water. Faecal smear is prepared and fixed as in case of iron-haematoxylin staining. It is washed in 70% alcohol and in 70% alcohol containing enough iodine, to give it a yellow colour, for 1–5 minutes each. Then it is stained with trichrome solution for 10 minutes and differentiated in acid alcohol (99 parts 90% alcohol: 1 part glacial acetic acid) for 2–3 seconds. It is rinsed in absolute alcohol several times and dehydrated in two changes of absolute alcohol for 2–5 minutes each. Stained smear is then cleared in two changes of xylol for 2–5 minutes each, mounted in Canada balsam and covered with coverslip.

Morphology of parasites after staining with trichrome stain:

- *Background:* Green
- *Protozoa:*
  - *Cytoplasm:* Bluish green to purple
  - *Nucleus, chromatoid bodies:* Red to purplish red

Modified acid-fast stain

Modified acid-fast stain is used for detection and identification of oocysts of *Cryptosporidium parvum*, *Cystoisospora (Isospora) belli* and *Cyclospora cayetanensis*. The staining solution contains:

1. *Carbol fuchsin:* 4 g basic fuchsin is dissolved in 20 ml 95% ethanol. To this mixture, 100 ml distilled water is added slowly while shaking. Phenol is melted in a water bath at 56°C and 8 ml of this is added to above solution.
2. *Decolourizer:* It is 5% sulphuric acid.
3. *Counterstain:* It is 0.3% methylene blue in distilled water.

A thin smear of faeces is made on a clean glass slide. It is fixed by heat at 70°C for 10 minutes. It is kept on the staining rack and flooded with carbol fuchsin. The slide is heated till carbol fuchsin starts steaming. More carbol fuchsin is added to prevent slide from drying. The slide is allowed to stain for 9 minutes and washed with tap water. It is then decolourized with 5% aqueous sulphuric acid for 30 seconds, followed by washing with tap water and counterstaining it with methylene blue for 1 minute. Finally, it is washed with tap water, dried, mounted in Canada balsam and covered with coverslip.

The acid-fast oocysts of *C. parvum*, *C. belli* and *Cyclospora cayetanensis* stain red with carbol fuchsin and non-acid-fast background stains blue.

QUANTIFICATION OF WORM BURDEN

For quantitative estimation of worm burden, two methods are commonly used:

- Direct smear egg count
- Stoll's method

Direct Smear Egg Count

Two mg of faeces is mixed in a small drop of saline on a slide and a coverslip is applied avoiding formation of air bubbles. The entire preparation is examined under low power of the microscope and the number of eggs (in 2 mg faeces) is counted and then the number of eggs per g of faeces is calculated.

Stoll's Method

This is commonly used method for determining the number of helminth eggs in faeces. Four g of faeces is thoroughly mixed with 56 ml of N/10 NaOH in a flask to make a uniform suspension. This is facilitated by adding a few glass beads and closing the mouth with a rubber stopper and then shaking vigorously. 0.15 ml of the emulsion is removed with measuring pipette and is placed on a glass slide, a coverslip is put over it and all the eggs in the preparation are counted under low power of the microscope. The number of eggs per g of faeces is calculated by multiplying the count with 200. The total eggs production per day can then be calculated by multiplying the number of eggs/g with a 24-hour faecal sample. Considering the consistency of faecal specimen, a correction factor (CF) is employed to convert the estimate to formed stool.

Stool sample	Correction factor
Mushy-formed stool	×1.5
Mushy stool	×2

Mushy diarrhoeic	×3
Frankly diarrhoeic	×4
Watery stool	×5

ANAL SCRAPINGS AND SWABS

Amoebiasis cutis of the perianal area may be diagnosed by demonstrating motile trophozoites of *E. histolytica* in material scraped from ulcers and examined in a saline suspension on a slide under a coverslip.

Enterobius vermicularis infection is usually diagnosed by demonstrating the presence of eggs on the perianal skin. This can be done by following methods:

• Scotch cellulose adhesive tape method
• NIH swab

Scotch Cellulose Adhesive Tape Method

Hold clear (not frosted) scotch cellulose adhesive tape approximately 10 cm long between thumbs and forefingers with sticky surface facing outward. Before the patient has arisen from the bed in the morning (preferably when the child is still asleep), press the sticky side of the tape against the skin across the anal opening with even, thorough pressure. Gently, place the sticky side of the tape down against the surface of a clear glass slide for examination. A drop of toluene may be placed between the tape and slide. The toluene clears essentially everything except eggs and hair. Eggs of other helminths may also be seen in this preparation.

NIH Swab

NIH swab consists of a glass rod at one end of which a piece of transparent cellophane (with sticky surface out) is wrapped and held in place with a rubber band (Fig. 27.5). The other

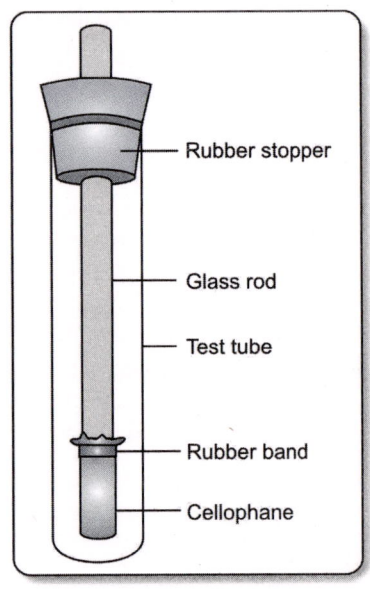

— Rubber stopper

— Glass rod

— Test tube

— Rubber band

— Cellophane

Fig. 27.5. NIH swab.

end of the glass rod is fixed in a rubber stopper and kept in a test tube. The cellophane part is used for swabbing by rolling over the perianal area. Then the cellophane is detached, spread over glass slide and examined microscopically. This procedure should be repeated on three successive days. Eggs may also be recovered from under the fingernails and the washings from garments.

ENTERO TEST

Entero test is used to obtain duodenal contents without intubation. In this test, the patient is asked to swallow a gelatin capsule which contains a nylon string at one end (Fig. 27.6). The free end of the string is fixed at the mouth. In the stomach, the capsule is dissolved and the string remains in the duodenum and jejunum. After overnight, the string is removed, the bile-stained mucus is collected on the glass slide and examined microscopically for motile trophozoites of *Giardia lamblia* and larvae of *Strongyloides stercoralis*.

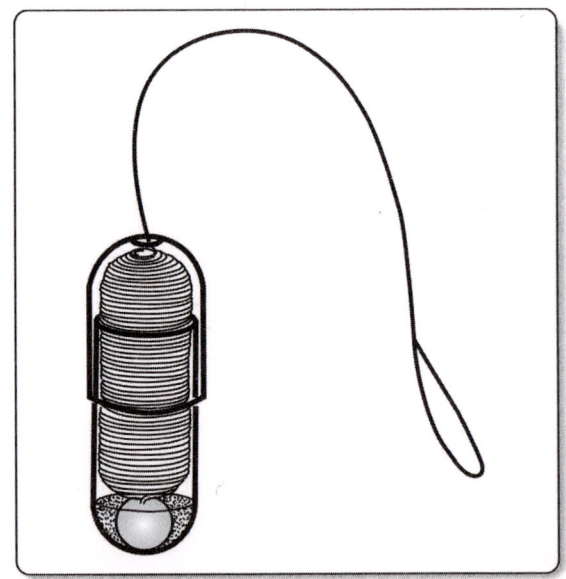

Fig. 27.6. Entero test capsule for sampling duodenal contents.

Discussion

1. **How do you assess best smear for faecal examination?**
   Direct smear for faecal examination should be so thin that newsprint can be read through the smear.

2. **Enumerate various parasites which can be observed in saline wet mount.**
   • Trophozoites and cysts of *E. histolytica, Giardia lamblia* and *Balantidium coli.*
   • Eggs and larvae of helminths.

3. **Which iodine solution should be used for iodine staining?**
   Weak iodine solution should be used. Gram's iodine is

unsuitable. Five-times diluted Lugol's iodine solutions should be used.

4. **Why weak iodine solution should be used for iodine staining?**

Because too strong solution of iodine can obscure the details of the parasite.

5. **What is the appearance of *Entamoeba histolytica* cysts on iodine staining?**

- *Body of parasite:* Yellow to light brown, and the nucleus is clearly seen with a central karyosome
- *Cytoplasm:* Smooth and hyaline
- *Glycogen mass:* Brown
- *Chromatoid bars:* Not stained

6. **Enumerate artifacts observed in faecal specimens which may mimic parasitic ova and cysts.**

- Yeast cells
- Plant cells
- Pollen grains
- Plant fibres

7. **What is the advantage of concentration methods for examination of faecal specimens?**

Concentration methods help to increase the sensitivity of ova and cysts detection in faeces.

8. **Enumerate methods of stool concentration.**

- Floatation techniques
- Sedimentation techniques

9. **Enumerate commonly used floatation techniques.**

- Saturated salt floatation
- Zinc sulphate centrifugal floatation

10. **What are the characteristic features of vial used for saturated salt floatation technique?**

Vial should be flat-bottomed and it should be 50 mm tall and 20 mm wide.

11. **Enumerate eggs and larvae which do not float in saturated salt solution.**

- Unfertilized eggs of *Ascaris lumbricoides*.
- Eggs of *Taenia solium*, *T. saginata* and all intestinal flukes.
- *Strongyloides stercoralis* larvae.

12. **What is the concentration and specific gravity of zinc sulphate in floatation technique?**

The concentration is 33% and specific gravity is 1.18 for fresh samples and 1.20 for formalin preserved sample.

13. **What are the advantages of zinc sulphate floatation technique?**

- It effectively concentrates cysts of protozoa, and eggs of nematodes, and small tapeworms.
- Easy to prepare and cheap.
- Simple technique.

14. **What are the disadvantages of zinc sulphate floatation?**

- Unfertilized eggs of *A. lumbricoides*, and eggs of most trematodes and large tapeworms do not float.
- Protozoal cysts and thin-walled ova are subject to collapse and distortion when left for more than a few minutes in contact with the zinc sulphate.

15. **Name commonly used sedimentation technique.**

Formalin-ether sedimentation.

16. **What is the role of formalin and ether in formalin-ether sedimentation technique?**

Formalin fixes the parasites and removes faecal odour. Ether dissolves faecal fat.

17. **What are the advantages of formalin-ether sedimentation technique?**

- It concentrates all types of protozoal cysts, ova and larvae.
- Easy to perform.
- Risk of laboratory-acquired infection from faecal organism is minimized because organisms are killed by formalin.

18. **Enumerate disadvantages of formalin-ether sedimentation.**

- Ether is highly inflammable.
- Morphology of trophozoites gets distorted.

19. **Why there is a need of permanent staining of faecal specimens?**

- It provides a permanent record.
- It is a good method for detection and correct identification of parasites.
- Small protozoans can be identified which are usually missed in a wet smear.
- Stained slides can be used for teaching purpose.
- Slides can be sent to reference laboratory for confirmation.

20. **Enumerate commonly used methods of permanent staining of faecal specimens.**

- Iron-haematoxylin stain
- Trichrome stain
- Modified acid-fast stain

21. **What is the morphology of parasites after staining with iron-haematoxylin stain?**

Cytoplasm of the parasite is light grey and nuclei are bluish black while background is grey in colour.

22. **What are the disadvantages of iron-haematoxylin and trichrome permanent stain?**

- They are not recommended for staining helminth eggs or larvae as they stain too dark or distorted.
- Oocysts of *Cytoisospora belli*, *C. parvum* and *Cyclospora cayetanensis* are not detected by these methods.

23. What is the major advantage of permanent stained smear?

It stains the intestinal protozoa (both trophozoite and cysts).

24. Which stain is better for SAF preserved faecal specimen?

Iron-haematoxylin stain

25. Enumerate parasites which are stained by modified acid-fast stain?

- *Cryptosporidium* spp.
- *Cyclospora cayetanensis*
- *Cystoisospora belli*

26. What is the concentration of sulphuric acid used in modified acid-fast staining technique?

Five per cent.

27. What is the colour of oocysts in faecal smears stained with modified acid-fast staining technique?

Oocysts stain bright pink against blue background.

28. Name the swab used for the diagnosis of *Enterobius vermicularis* infection.

NIH swab.

29. Name other method used for the diagnosis of *Enterobius* infection.

Scotch cellulose adhesive tape method.

30. What is Charcot-Leyden crystal?

This is a breakdown product of granules of eosinophils.

31. Can you observe trophozoites of protozoa with iodine preparation of stool?

Yes, morphology of trophozoites can be observed but iodine preparation kills them, therefore, their motility can not be seen.

32. Which consistency of stool is best for examination of trophozoites?

Trophozoites are best seen in liquid stool.

33. Name parasite whose trophozoites can be seen in formed stool as well as liquid stool.

Dientamoeba fragilis

34. Enumerate the differences between a macrophage and trophozoite of *E. histolytica*.

Differences between a macrophage and trophozoite of *E. histolytica* are given in Table 27.1.

Table 27.1. Differences between a macrophage and trophozoite of *E. histolytica*

Features	Trophozoite of *E. histolytica*	Macrophage
Average size	20 μm	30–60 μm may be 5–10 μm
Ratio of nuclear material to cytoplasm	1:10–1:12	1:4–1:6
Cytoplasm	May contain red blood cells and some debris, no polymorphonuclear leucocytes	Usually contains ingested debris, red blood cells and polymorphonuclear leucocytes
Nucleus	One nucleus. It is round with central karyosome and peripheral fine chromatin granules	One large nucleus that may be irregular

35. Why both normal saline and iodine preparation are required for examination of stool specimen?

Cysts are observed better in iodine preparation, while normal saline preparation is useful to examine trophozoites, bile-stained and non bile-stained eggs, and to observe motility of trophozoites.

36. Which methods are used for determining the number of helminth eggs in faeces?

- Direct smear egg count
- Stoll's method

Identification of Faecal Eggs

Ascaris lumbricoides (Roundworm)

Fertilized eggs

The fertilized eggs are round or oval in shape and measure 60–75 µm in length and 40–50 µm in breadth. They are bile-stained and brown in colour. They are surrounded by a thick, transparent shell, consisting of a relatively nonpermeable innermost lipoidal vitelline membrane; a thick transparent middle layer and an outermost coarsely mammillated albuminoid layer (Colour Plate IV, Fig. 11). Outer mammillated coat is sometimes lost. Such eggs are called decorticated eggs. Each egg contains a large conspicuous unsegmented ovum with a clear crescentic area at each pole. Fertilized eggs float in saturated solution of common salt.

Unfertilized eggs

In the absence of a male worm, the female produces unfertilized (infertile) eggs. These are narrower and longer and measure 90 µm in length and 55 µm in breadth. They are bile-stained and brown in colour. Each egg contains a small atrophied ovum and a thin shell within an irregular coating of albumin. The innermost lipoidal vitelline membrane of the shell is absent (Colour Plate IV, Fig. 12). The unfertilized eggs are heaviest of all the helminth eggs, therefore, they do not float in saturated solution of common salt.

Enterobius vermicularis (Pinworm/Threadworm)

The eggs are colourless, not bile-stained and flattened on one side (planoconvex). They measure 60 µm in length and 30 µm in width. They are surrounded by a thin, smooth, transparent shell and usually contain fully developed larvae (Colour Plate IV, Fig. 13). They float in saturated solution of common salt.

Ancylostoma duodenale and Necator americanus (Hookworms)

Eggs are oval or elliptical measuring 60 µm in length and 40 µm in width. They are colourless (not bile-stained) and are surrounded by a thin transparent hyaline shell. They possess a segmented ovum with usually four blastomeres (Colour Plate IV, Fig. 14). There is a clear space between the segmented ovum and the egg shell. The eggs float in saturated salt solution.

Trichuris trichiura (Whipworm)

The eggs are barrel-shaped with a mucous plug at each pole. Shell is yellow to brown (bile-stained) and plugs are colourless. They measure 50–54 µm × 22–23 µm in size (Colour Plate IV, Fig. 15). They float in saturated solution of common salt. When freshly passed, they contain unsegmented ova and are not infective to man.

Strongyloides stercoralis

The eggs measure 50–58 µm × 30–34 µm. They are thin shelled, transparent and oval. They contain larvae ready to hatch. As soon as the eggs are laid, the rhabditiform larvae start hatching and bore their way out of the mucous membrane into the lumen from where they are passed in the faeces. As a result, it is the larvae, which are excreted in faeces, and the eggs are not routinely detected. Rhabditiform larvae measure 200–250 µm in length by 16 µm in width. They have short mouth and double-bulb oesophagus.

Diphyllobothrium latum (Fish Tapeworm)

Egg of *Diphyllobothrium latum* is yellowish-brown in colour (bile-stained), oval or elliptical in shape, measures 70 µm in length and 45 µm in breadth and has thin and smooth shell. It contains an immature embryo. There is an inconspicuous operculum at one end (operculated egg) with a small knob at the other end. It does not float in saturated solution of common salt. The egg is not infective to man.

Taenia saginata (Beef Tapeworm) and Taenia solium (Pork Tapeworm)

Eggs of both these species are indistinguishable. They are

spherical, brown in colour (bile-stained) and measure 31–43 μm in diameter. They are surrounded by embryophore which is brown, thick-walled and radially striated. Outside this may be present thin transparent shell which represents the remnant of yolk mass. Inside the embryophore is present hexacanth embryo (oncosphere) with three pairs of hooklets (Colour Plate IV, Fig. 16). It does not float in saturated solution of common salt. The eggs of *T. solium* are infective to pig and also to man, while those of *T. saginata* are infective only to cattle.

Hymenolepis nana (Dwarf Tapeworm)

Egg is spherical or oval, hyaline, 35–40 μm in diameter. It has a smooth, thin and colourless outer shell and an inner membrane (embryophore), containing a hexacanth embryo (oncosphere). The space between two membranes is filled with yolk granules and 4–8 polar filaments emanating from polar thickenings at either end of embryophore. It is non-bile-stained and floats in saturated solution of common salt (Colour Plate IV, Fig. 17).

Dipylidium caninum (Double-pored Dog Tapeworm)

The eggs are spherical measuring 25–40 μm in diameter. They have thin, hyaline, brick-red tinged shell. Gravid proglottids separate singly or in groups from the strobila and are passed out of anus. Disintegration of these proglottids does not commonly occur within the bowel and at times groups of eggs within the embryonic membrane are passed in the faeces.

Echinococcus granulosus (Dog Tapeworm)

The eggs are indistinguishable from those of other *Taenia* species. These measure 32–36 μm in length and 25–32 μm in breadth and contain hexacanth embryos with three pairs of hooklets.

Schistosoma haematobium

Egg is elongated, 110–170 μm long and 40–70 μm wide. It has a thin, smooth shell, a rounded anterior end and a characteristic terminal spine from the tapered posterior end.

Schistosoma mansoni

Egg is elongated, 115–180 μm long and 40–70 μm wide. It has a thin, smooth shell with a prominent lateral spine near the more rounded posterior end. Its anterior end tends to be somewhat pointed and curved.

Schistosoma japonicum

Egg is oval or subspherical, 70–80 μm long and 55–65 μm wide. It has a smooth relatively thick shell. A small lateral knob may be seen. Because it is often located in a depression in the shell, this is often difficult to see.

Fasciola hepatica (Sheep Liver Fluke)

Eggs are large, elliptical to oval, operculate, light yellowish-brown and measure 140 μm × 80 μm. The shell is thin with a smooth surface. Each egg contains an immature larva, the miracidium, which extends to the shell margins without leaving a clear space.

Fasciolopsis buski (Giant Intestinal Fluke)

The eggs are almost identical with those of *F. hepatica*. Each worm lays about 25,000 eggs per day.

Clonorchis sinensis (Chinese Liver Fluke; Oriental Liver Fluke)

The eggs are broadly ovoid, have a moderately thick, light yellowish-brown shell (bile-stained) and are provided with a distinct convex operculum resting on shoulders. A small knob is often seen at the posterior end. They measure 28–35 μm × 12–19 μm (average 29 μm × 16 μm). They contain ciliated embryos (miracidia) when discharged into the bile ducts. They hatch only after ingestion by suitable molluscan hosts. They do not float in saturated solution of common salt.

Paragonimus westermani (Oriental Lung Fluke)

The eggs of *P. westermani* are oval, yellowish-brown, measure 90 μm × 50 μm and have a flattened operculum resting on shoulders. Shell is smooth and thick. They are unembryonated when laid.

Discussion

1. **Enumerate parasites whose eggs do not float in saturated salt solution.**
   - Unfertilized eggs of *A. lumbricoides*
   - *D. latum*
   - *Taenia solium* and *Taenia saginata*
   - Eggs of all intestinal flukes

2. **Enumerate parasites whose eggs are non-bile-stained.**
   - *Ancylostoma duodenale*
   - *Necator americanus*
   - *Enterobius vermicularis*
   - *Hymenolepis nana*

3. **Classify oviparous nematodes.**
   Laying unsegmented eggs
   - *A. lumbricoides*
   - *Trichuris trichiura*

   Laying eggs with segmented ova
   - *Ancylostoma duodenale*
   - *Necator americanus*
   - *Trichostrongylus* spp.

Laying eggs containing larva
- *Enterobius vermicularis*
- *Strongyloides stercoralis*

4. **Name ovoviviparous nematode.**

   Strongyloides stercoralis

5. **Name parasite whose eggs are detected in urine.**

   Schistosoma haematobium

6. **Name parasite whose egg is planoconvex.**

   E. vermicularis

7. **Eggs of which parasite are considered heaviest of all the helminth eggs?**

   Unfertilized eggs of *A. lumbricoides*

8. **What do you mean by decorticated eggs of *A. lumbricoides*?**

   If outermost mammillated albuminoid layer of eggs is lost, then they are called decorticated eggs.

9. **Name parasite whose eggs can be detected in sputum.**

Paragonimus westermani

10. **What is the infective form of *Ascaris lumbricoides*?**

    Embryonated egg.

11. **What is the mode of infection of *Ascaris lumbricoides*?**

    By ingestion of embryonated eggs.

12. **How do you differentiate the egg of *Ancylostoma duodenale* from that of *Necator americanus*?**

    They cannot be differentiated on the basis of egg morphology.

13. **Name the infective form of hookworms.**

    Filariform larva.

14. **What is the mode of infection of *Trichuris trichiura*?**

    It is by ingestion of embryonated eggs.

15. **How do you differentiate the egg of *Taenia solium* from that of *T. saginata*?**

    They cannot be differentiated on the basis of egg morphology.

Identification of Faecal Trophozoites, Cysts and Oocysts

Entamoeba histolytica

Trophozoite

It measures 10–60 μm (average 20–30 μm) in diameter. The cytoplasm of the trophozoite can be divided into a clear outer ectoplasm and an inner finely granular endoplasm in which red blood cells, leucocytes and tissue debris are found within the food vacuoles. Trophozoites are motile. Movement results from long finger-like pseudopodial extensions of ectoplasm into which endoplasm flows. Trophozoite is the only form present in the tissues. It usually appears only in diarrhoeic faeces in active cases and survives only for a few hours. Nucleus is spherical in shape varying in size from 4–6 μm in diameter. In stained preparations, it shows a central dot-like karyosome which is surrounded by a clear halo. The nuclear membrane is delicate and is lined by a single layer of fine chromatin granules. The space between the karyosome and the nuclear membrane is traversed by linin network (achromatic fibrils) having spoke-like radial arrangement (Fig. 29.1).

Cyst

It is spherical, 10–15 μm in diameter. It is surrounded by a thick chitinous wall which makes it highly resistant to the gastric acid, adverse environmental conditions and the chlorine concentration found in potable water. It starts as a uninucleate body, but later the nucleus divides to form two and then four nuclei (Fig. 29.1). Uninucleate and binucleate cysts in addition also possess a glycogen mass, which stains brown with iodine, and 1–4 chromidial or chromatoid bars (Colour Plate IV, Fig. 18). These do not stain with iodine but appear as refractile oblong bars with rounded ends in normal saline preparations. With iron-haematoxylin stain, they stain black in colour.

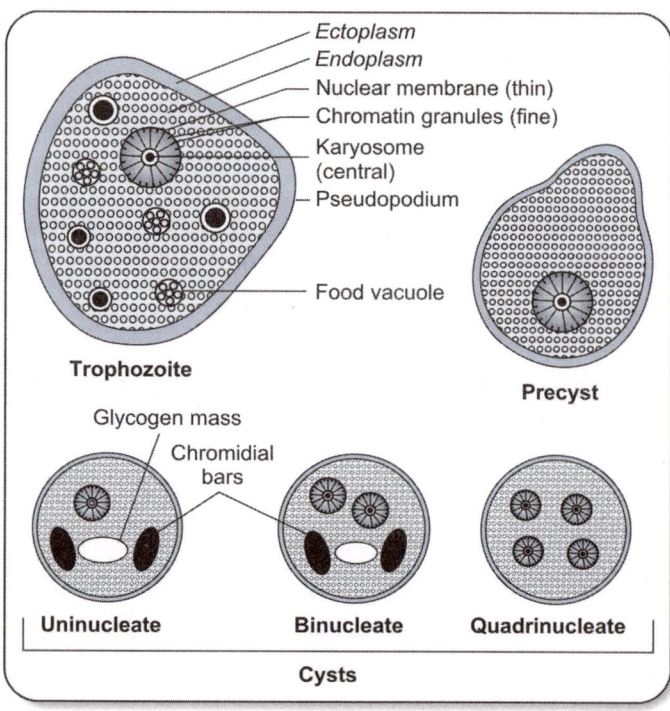

Fig. 29.1. Morphological forms of *Entamoeba histolytica*.

Entamoeba coli

Trophozoite

It measures 20–50 μm in diameter. The cytoplasm is not defined into ectoplasm and endoplasm, and contains bacteria and cellular debris but never red blood cells (Fig. 29.2). Trophozoites are motile. They extend pseudopodia in multiple planes and 'wander' aimlessly in one direction then the other. Nucleus shows eccentric karyosome. The nuclear membrane is thick and is lined by coarse chromatin granules. Nucleus is visible in unstained preparation.

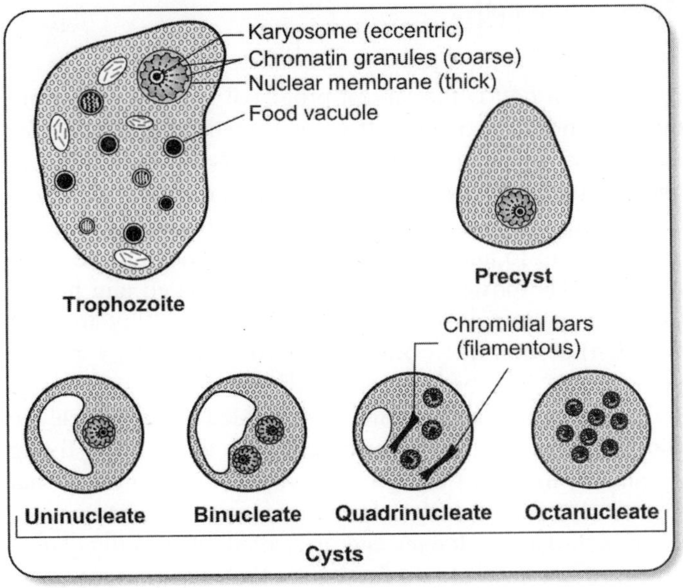

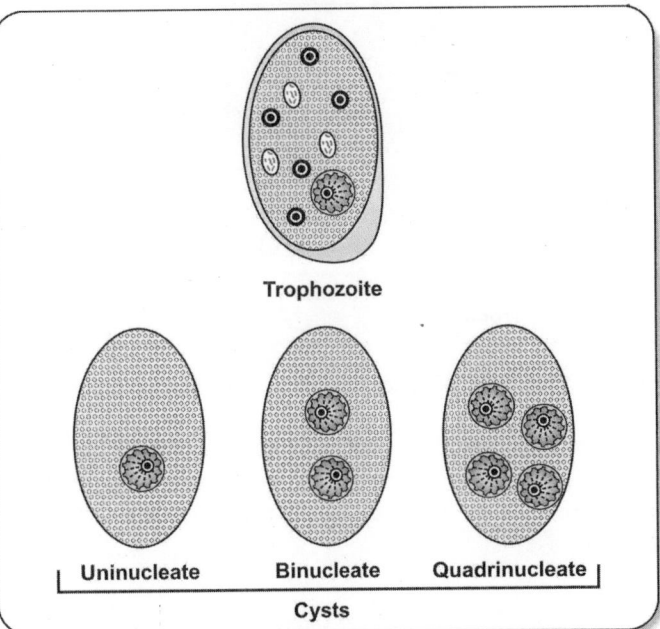

Fig. 29.2. Morphological forms of *Entamoeba coli*.

Fig. 29.3. Morphological forms of *Endolimax nana*.

Cyst

It is spherical and 15–20 μm in diameter (Fig. 29.2 and Colour Plate IV, Fig. 19). It contains 1–8 nuclei and chromidial bars are filamentous. It lives freely in the lumen of large intestine of man and is nonpathogenic.

Entamoeba hartmanni

E. hartmanni is morphologically similar to *E. histolytica*, but both its trophozoites and cysts are smaller and the former never contain ingested red blood cells. Earlier it was regarded as small race of *E. histolytica*. The trophozoites and the cysts of *E. hartmanni* range from 4–12 μm and 5–10 μm in diameter, respectively. It is nonpathogenic amoeba.

Endolimax nana

Trophozoite

It is small, measuring 6–15 μm (average 10 μm) in diameter. The cytoplasm has an inner finely granular endoplasm and a clear outer ectoplasm. It exhibits sluggish motility by means of short, blunt, hyaline pseudopodia. Cytoplasmic inclusions contain bacteria, small vegetable cells, and crystals but never red blood cells. Nucleus is minute spherical with a large irregular karyosome lying eccentrically from which several achromatic strands extend to the nuclear membrane (Fig. 29.3).

Cyst

It is oval measuring 8–10 μm in diameter. The number of nuclei varies from 1–4 but mature cyst is quadrinucleate. Chromidial bars and glycogen vacuole are absent (Fig. 29.3). It is nonpathogenic and produces no symptoms.

Iodamoeba bütschlii

Trophozoite

Trophozoites vary in size from 6–20 μm in diameter and are fairly active in freshly evacuated unformed stools and show sluggish movement in older stools. The clear ectoplasm is not usually well differentiated from denser endoplasm that contains coarse and fine granules and has bacteria and yeast cells in food vacuoles. Occasionally, a discrete glycogen vacuole, which stains golden brown with iodine may be demonstrated in the cytoplasm of the trophozoite (Fig. 29.4). The nucleus is relatively large measuring 2.0–3.5 μm in diameter. The karyosome is a large circular mass, central in position and surrounded by refractile globules. Peripheral chromatin lining is absent.

Cyst

Cyst of *I. bütschlii* is ovoid or irregularly pyriform in shape, uninucleate and measures 8–15 μm in longest diameter. The cytoplasm contains a large glycogen vacuole. Chromidial bars are absent (Fig. 29.4 and Colour Plate IV, Fig. 20).

Giardia lamblia

Trophozoite

It is pear-shaped with rounded anterior and pointed posterior end (Fig. 29.5 and Colour Plate IV, Fig. 21). It measures 10–20 μm in length and 5–15 μm in width. The dorsal surface is convex while on the ventral surface it has a shallow posteriorly notched concavity (sucking disc) that embraces anterior half of the organism. It acts as an organelle of attachment. It is bilaterally symmetrical and has one pair of nuclei, one on

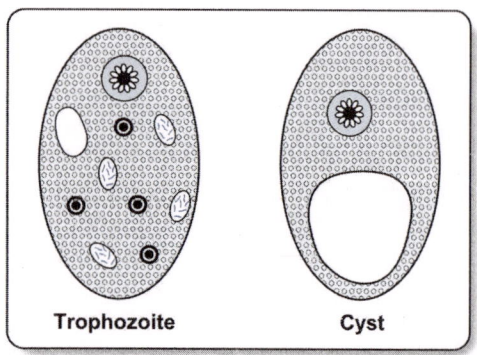

Fig. 29.4. Morphological forms of *Iodamoeba bütschlii*.

each side of the midline, one pair of axostyles, one pair of parabasal bodies present on the axostyles, four pairs of flagella and probably four pairs of blepharoplasts from which the flagella arise.

Cyst

Mature cyst is oval in shape and measures 11–14 μm × 7–10 μm in size. It has two pairs of nuclei which may remain clustered at one end or lie in pairs at opposite ends. The remains of the flagella and margins of the sucking disc may be seen inside the cytoplasm of the cyst (Fig. 29.5 and Colour Plate IV, Fig. 22).

Balantidium coli

Trophozoite

Balantidium coli is the largest protozoal parasite inhabiting the large intestine of man. It is oval in shape and measures 60 μm × 45 μm or more. The anterior end is somewhat pointed and has a groove (*peristome*) leading to a mouth (*cytostome*) terminating in a short funnel-shaped gullet (*cytopharynx*) extending up to anterior one-third of the body. There is no intestine. The posterior end is broadly rounded and has an excretory opening known as *cytopyge* (Fig. 29.6) through which the residual contents of food vacuoles empty periodically. The body is covered with a delicate pellicle showing longitudinal striations. Embedded in the pellicle are short cilia of relatively uniform length that, in the living organism, maintain a constant synchronized motion that vigorously propels the protozoan forward. The cilia that line the mouth part are longer and are called adoral cilia. These are used for propelling food into the cytopharynx. The cytoplasm of trophozoite has two nuclei (macronucleus and micronucleus), two contractile vacuoles and numerous food vacuoles.

Cyst

The cyst of *B. coli* is spherical or oval measuring 40–60 μm in diameter. It is surrounded by a thick and transparent double-

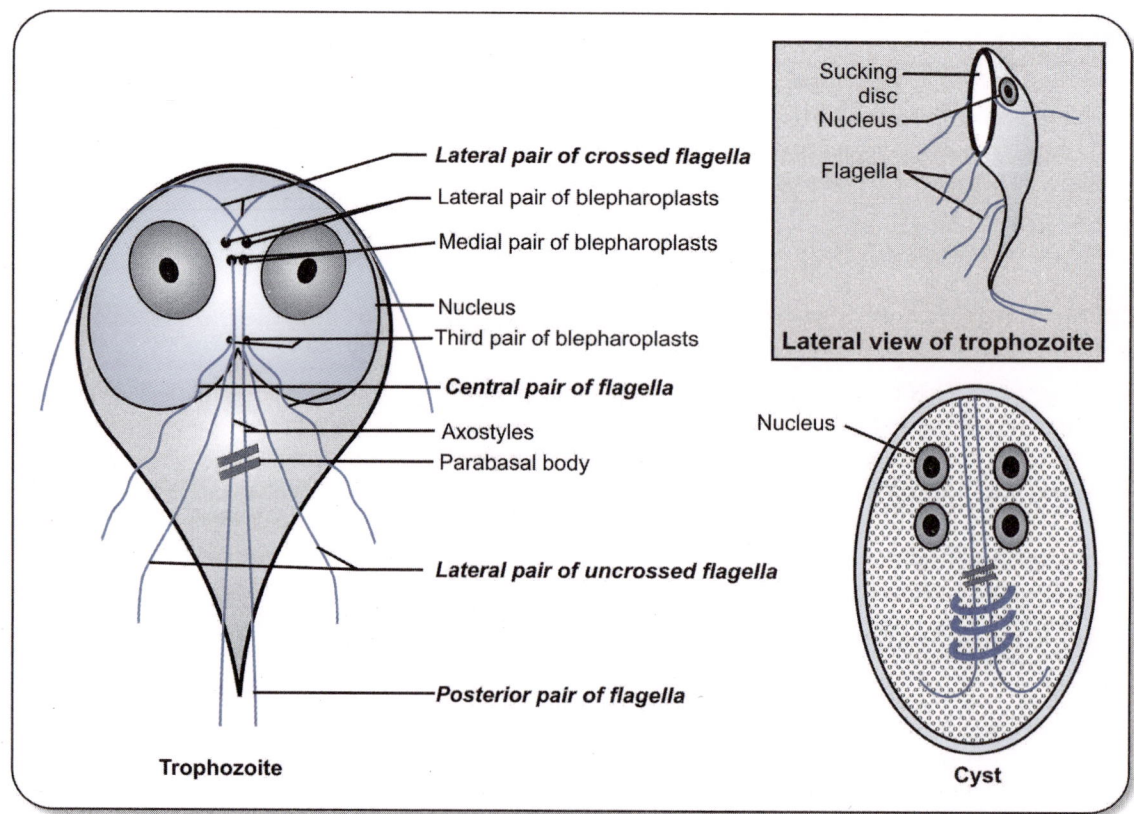

Fig. 29.5. Morphological forms of *Giardia lamblia*.

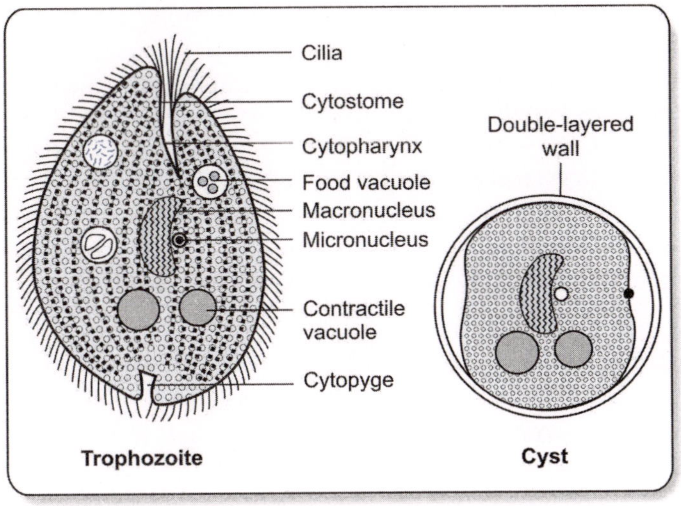

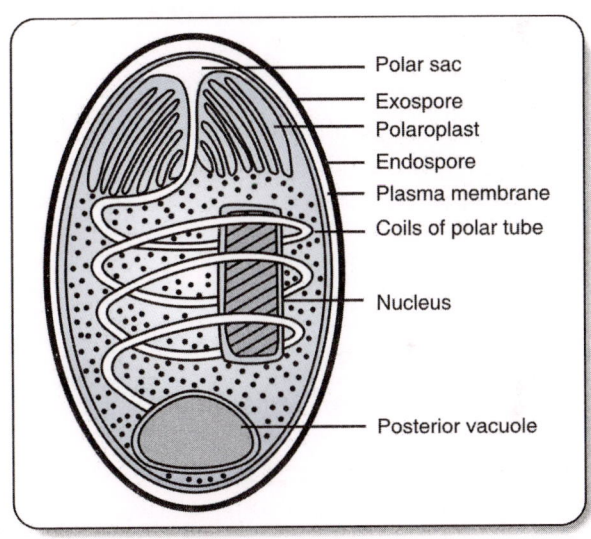

Fig. 29.6. Morphological forms of *Balantidium coli.*

layered wall (Fig. 29.6). Newly formed cyst shows movement, but as the cyst matures the cilia are absorbed and the movement ceases. The macronucleus, micronucleus and vacuoles are present in the cyst also. Unlike encystation in amoebae, in *B. coli* this is not preceded by complete discharge of undigested foods.

Cystoisospora belli

Unsporulated oocysts of *C. belli* are elongate-ovoidal, measuring 20–33 µm × 10–19 µm. Inside each oocyst develop two sporoblasts which later on covert into sporocysts. Each sporocyst is 9–14 × 7–12 µm and contains four crescent-shaped sporozoites. The oocyst is surrounded by a thin, smooth, two-layered cyst wall. Man acquires infection by ingestion of food or water contaminated with faeces containing oocysts.

Cyclospora cayetanensis

Oocysts of *C. cayetanensis* are nonrefractile, spherical to oval, slightly wrinkled bodies (mulberry appearance) measuring 8–10 µm in diameter. They contain two ovoid sporocysts, 4 µm × 6 µm in size. Each sporocyst contains four sporozoites. Unsporulated oocysts are excreted in the faeces. Sporulation occurs outside the body. Man acquires infection by ingestion of food or water contaminated with faeces containing oocysts.

Cryptosporidium parvum

Oocyst is colourless, spherical or oval and measures 4–5 µm in diameter. It contains four crescent-shaped naked or nonencysted sporozoites (sporocysts not present). The anterior end of the sporozoite is pointed and the posterior end which contains a prominent nucleus is rounded. The oocyst wall of *C. parvum* is composed of an electron-lucent middle zone surrounded by two electron-dense layers. Oocyst does not stain with iodine and is acid-fast (Colour Plate IV, Fig. 23).

Microsporidia

Spores

Spores are highly resistant and are the only life cycle stage able to survive outside the host cell and is the infective stage. They are small, ranging from 1.5–2.5 µm × 2.5–4.0 µm. They are oval to cylindrical and possess a thick double-layered spore wall that renders it environmentally resistant. The outer layer, or exospore, is proteinaceous and electron-dense and, the inner layer, or endospore, is chitinous and electron-lucent. The plasma membrane lines the inside of the spore wall. Within the cytoplasm, the spore possesses a coiled polar tube. It has a spring-like tubular extrusion mechanism by which the infective material, 'sporoplasm' is injected into host cell (Fig. 29.7). Inside the host cell, the invading parasite grows into a spherical or oblong schizont, with two to eight or more nuclei which become separate merozoites, followed by a complex series of sexual and asexual divisions leading to more spore production.

Fig. 29.7. Microsporidian spore.

The spores stain poorly with haematoxylin and eosin but can be better visualized with Gram, acid-fast, periodic acid-Schiff, Giemsa, or modified trichrome stains. They are Gram-positive and acid-fast. Identification of species and genera is based upon electron microscopic morphology of the spore, nuclei, and coiled polar filament.

Discussion

1. **Which morphological form of *E. histolytica* is seen in the tissues?**

   Trophozoite

2. **Define the term 'amoeboma'.**

   Amoeboma is pseudotumoural lesion caused by *E. histolytica* whose formation is associated with necrosis, inflammation and oedema of the mucosa and submucosa of the colon.

3. **What is the appearance of pus of liver abscess produced by *E. histolytica*?**

Anchovy sauce.

4. **What is the shape of trophozoite of *Giardia lamblia*?**

Pear shape.

5. **How many pairs of blepharoplasts are present in trophozoite of *Giardia lamblia*?**

Four.

6. **How many sporocysts are seen in sporulated oocyst of *Cystoisospora belli*?**

Two.

7. **How many sporozoites are seen in each sporulated oocyst of *Cyclospora cayetanensis*?**

Four.

8. **What is the colour of oocysts of *Cryptosporidium parvum* in modified acid-fast staining?**

Red.

9. **Enumerate parasites causing diarrhoeal disease in persons with HIV infection.**

- *Cryptosporidium* spp.
- *C. cayetanensis*
- *C. belli*
- Microsporidia
- *E. histolytica*
- *G. lamblia*

10. **Enumerate parasites causing traveller's diarrhoea.**

- *E. histolytica*
- *G. lamblia*
- *C. cayetanensis*
- *C. parvum*

11. **Enumerate infectious protozoans which may be present in the faecal specimen received in the laboratory.**

- *E. histolytica*
- *G. lamblia*
- *Cryptosporidium* spp.

12. **Enumerate parasites causing infection by ingestion of contaminated food and water.**

- *E. histolytica*
- *G. lamblia*
- *C. cayetanensis*
- *Cryptosporidium* spp.
- *Cytoisospora belli*
- *B. coli*

13. **Which sporozoan parasite may cause autoinfection?**

C. parvum.

14. **Enumerate protozoan parasites causing CNS infection.**

- *E. histolytica*
- *Naegleria fowleri*
- *Acanthamoeba* spp.
- *Balamuthia mandrillaris*
- Microsporidia

15. **Enumerate protozoan parasites causing eye infection.**

- *Acanthamoeba* spp.
- *Encephalitozoon* spp.

16. **Enumerate parasites causing dysentery.**

- *E. histolytica*
- *B. coli*
- *Schistosoma japonicum*
- *Trichuris trichiura*

17. **Which protozoan parasite is associated with malabsorption syndrome?**

G. lamblia.

18. **Enumerate protozoan parasite transmitted by sexual contact.**

- *Trichomonas vaginalis*
- *E. histolytica*
- *G. lamblia*

19. **In which stage of *E. histolytica* glycogen mass and chromidial bars are absent?**

Quadrinucleate cyst.

20. **Which is the most common organ involved in extra-intestinal amoebiasis?**

Liver.

Culture Techniques

The culture methods are frequently useful for accurate diagnosis of the organism, as a supplement to other methods or to provide positive diagnosis when routine methods have failed. These are also essential for preparation of antigen for immunodiagnosis of parasitic infections and for *in vitro* screening of drugs. Laboratory culture methods are available for many parasites.

Cultivation of *Entamoeba histolytica*

Polyxenic and monoxenic cultures

In all these cultures, it is necessary to include certain associates such as enteric bacteria or the flagellates (*Trypanosoma cruzi*), as well as starch or rice flour for the amoebae to grow and multiply.

1. Balamuth's aqueous egg yolk infusion medium

This medium is used to detect the presence of amoebae. The specific solutions required are phosphate buffer and whole-liver concentrate solution. The addition of rice flour (prerinsed with distilled water) to Balamuth's medium is reported to support abundant growth of *Balantidium coli*.

2. Boeck and Drbohlav Locke-egg-serum (LES) medium

This diphasic medium consists of an egg slant base with an isotonic overlay. This egg-serum medium containing Locke's solution was the first medium used for successful cultivation of *Entamoeba histolytica* in the presence of bacterial flora.

Axenic culture

In 1961, Diamond first reported the successful cultivation of *E. histolytica* in the absence of bacteria. In 1965, he described a clear liquid medium for initiation, maintenance and mass cultivation of the amoebae. This medium consists of trypticase, ox-liver digest, glucose, cysteine, ascorbic acid, and salts supplemented with horse serum and a vitamin mixture. This medium yields 100–150 million *E. histolytica* from an inoculum of 10 million amoebae. Axenic cultivation of *E. histolytica* is essential for study of its:

- pathogenicity,
- immunological and biochemical properties,
- *in vitro* drug susceptibility testing,
- preparation of axenic amoebic antigen for use in immunodiagnosis of amoebiasis, and
- to maintain quality control strains.

Culture of Pathogenic Free-Living Amoebae and *Naegleria fowleri*

Naegleria fowleri may be cultivated by placing some of the CSF on non-nutrient agar (1.5%) spread with a lawn of washed *Escherichia coli* or *Enterobacter aerogenes* and incubated at 37°C. The amoebae grow on the moist surface and use the bacteria as food, producing plaques as they clear the bacteria. As colonies grow and expand, cysts that survive moderate desiccation are formed; thus, strains can be maintained by transfer of either trophic or cystic forms. In case of *Acanthamoeba*, the method of cultivation is the same as for *N. fowleri*, but incubation is done at 30°C instead of 37°C. *Acanthamoeba* does not have a flagellate stage but its tropho-zoites are identified by small spiky acanthopodia and cysts are readily identified by their double-walled wrinkled appearance. *Balamuthia mandrillaris* can be grown in tissue culture, preferably Vero cells and cytopathic effects can be seen. Besides these, peptone-yeast extract glucose medium and Nelson's medium are liquid media for *Acanthamoeba* spp. and *N. fowleri*, respectively.

Cultivation of Flagellates

Trussell and Johnson's medium

This is a simple medium that gives good growth of *Tricho-monas vaginalis*. It consists of proteose peptone, sodium

Parasitology

3

chloride, sodium thioglycollate and normal human serum. Simplified trypticase serum medium is also suitable for the isolation of *T. vaginalis*. It is also used to maintain bacteria-free cultures of the flagellate. It grows best at 35–37°C under anaerobic conditions and less well aerobically. The optimum pH for growth is 5.5–6. Culture is very sensitive (95%) procedure for diagnosis of trichomoniasis. It is recommended when direct smear is negative.

Cultivation of *Leishmania donovani*

NNN medium

L. donovani can be cultured on NNN medium which was first introduced by Novy and MacNeal (1904) and later modified by Nicolle (1908). It consists of two parts of salt agar and one part of defibrinated rabbit blood. The tubed salt agar medium is melted and then cooled to 48°C. To each tube of medium, one-third of its volume of sterile defibrinated rabbit blood is added and mixed thoroughly by rotating the tubes. The tubes are slanted and allowed to cool preferably on ice, as more water of condensation is obtained. Blood, aspirates, or small biopsy samples from spleen, liver or bone marrow obtained aseptically are inoculated into water of condensation of the medium and incubated at 22–25°C. The amastigote form changes into promastigote form which then multiplies rapidly by longitudinal fission to produce a large number of flagellates, particularly in the water of condensation at the bottom of the tube (Fig. 30.1 and Colour Plate IV, Fig. 24).

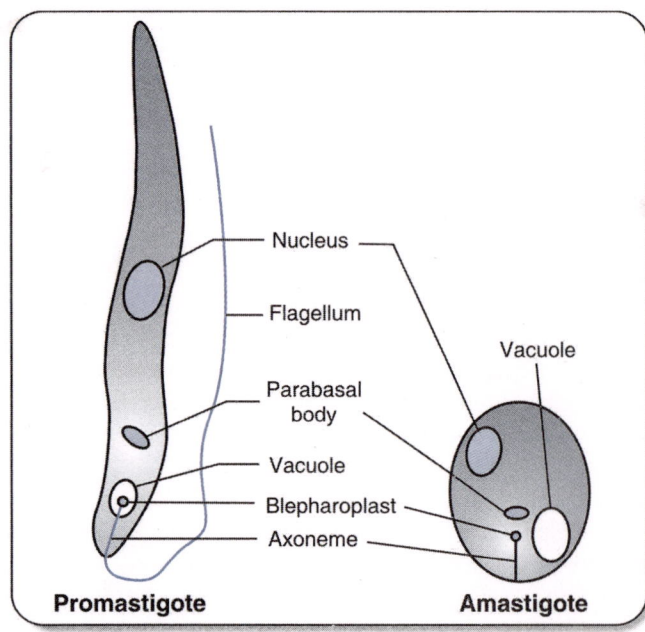

Fig. 30.1. Morphological forms of *Leishmania donovani*.

Hockmeyer's medium

This liquid medium consists of Schneider's commercially prepared insect cell culture medium, supplemented by the addition of 30% heat inactivated foetal calf serum and with 100 IU penicillin and 100 μg streptomycin per ml. The medium is inoculated with the specimen, incubated at 22–25°C, and examined microscopically daily for the presence of promastigotes. The latter can usually be detected after 2–3 days of incubation but the cultures should be held for four weeks.

Cultivation of *Trypanosoma brucei gambiense*

Weinman's medium

T.b. gambiense can be grown in Weinman's medium. This medium consists of 100 ml of citrated human plasma and human haemoglobin (made by mixing 1 part of blood and 3 parts of distilled water), 900 ml of distilled water and 8 g of sodium chloride. The medium is adjusted to pH 7.4–7.5 and dispensed in rubber-stoppered test tubes. It is inoculated and incubated at 26–28°C. The culture becomes positive in 7–10 days. Long slender forms of trypomastigote, similar to midgut forms of tsetse fly, are encountered in culture (Fig. 30.2).

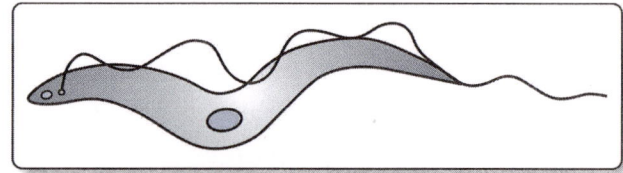

Fig. 30.2. Trypomastigote form of *Trypanosoma brucei gambiense*.

Cultivation of *Trypanosoma cruzi*

It can be easily cultivated in the epimastigote form in NNN medium. Blood and other specimens are inoculated in NNN medium and incubated at 22–24°C and subcultured every 1–2 weeks. Centrifuged material is examined microscopically for trypanosomes (Fig. 30.3).

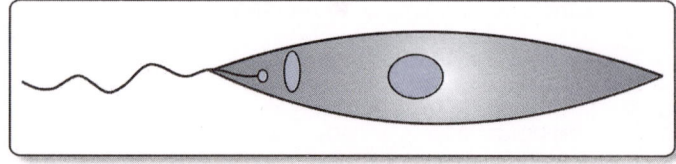

Fig. 30.3. Epimastigote form of *Trypanosoma cruzi*.

Cultivation of *Plasmodium falciparum*

Trager and Jensen successfully cultivated and maintained *P. falciparum in vitro* in human red blood cells. They used medium RPMI 1640 in a continuous flow system in which human erythrocytes were in a shallow stationary layer covered by shallow layer of medium. The medium was made to flow slowly and continuously over the layer of settled red cells, under an atmosphere with 7% carbon dioxide and 1–5% oxygen. This culture system is now widely used for production of antigen.

Culture of Larval Stage of Nematodes

Nematode infections giving rise to larval stages that hatch in soil or tissues may be diagnosed by using certain faecal culture methods. Culture of faeces for larvae is useful to:

- Detect light infections caused by hookworms, *Strongyloides stercoralis* and *Trichostrongylus* spp. infections.
- Specific diagnosis of hookworms and *Trichostrongylus* spp. infections because their eggs are identical and specific identifications are based on larval morphology.
- Allow development of larvae into the filariform stage for further differentiation.

    Different culture techniques are:

- Harada-Mori filter paper strip culture
- Filter paper or slant culture
- Charcoal culture
- Baermann culture.

Harada-Mori filter paper strip culture

This technique requires filter paper to which fresh faecal material is added and a test tube into which the filter paper is inserted (Fig. 30.4A). Moisture is provided by adding water to the tube. The tube is incubated at 25–28°C for 10 days. Distilled water is added to maintain the original level. The tube is checked daily by withdrawing a small amount of fluid from the bottom of the tube. Smear is prepared on a glass slide and examined under 10× objective. The larvae are examined for typical morphological features to reveal presence of hookworms, *Strongyloides stercoralis*, or *Trichostrongylus* spp. larvae.

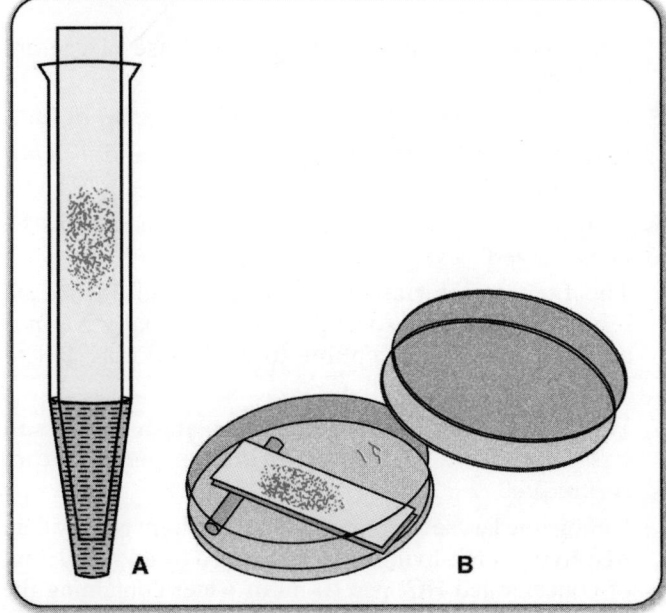

Fig. 30.4. (A) Harada-Mori filter paper strip culture, and (B) Slant culture.

Note:

- Faecal material to be cultured should not be refrigerated, since some parasites, especially *Necator americanus*, are susceptible to cold and may fail to develop after refrigeration.
- Also, caution must be taken in handling the filter paper strip itself, since infective *Strongyloides stercoralis* larvae may migrate upward as well as downward on the paper strip, therefore, hold the filter paper strip with forceps.
- Both pathogenic and free living larvae can grow in the culture, hence these should be differentiated.
- Preserved stool specimens or specimens obtained after barium meal are not suitable. Fresh stool should be taken for the culture.

Filter paper or slant culture

Fresh stool material is placed on the filter paper, which is cut to fit the dimensions of a standard microscope slide. The filter paper is then placed on a slanted glass slide in a petri dish containing water (Fig. 30.4B). This technique allows direct examination of the culture system with a dissecting microscope to look for larvae in the faecal mass or surrounding water. There may be infective larvae in the moisture that accumulates under the petri dish lid, so be careful not to allow the water to touch the skin when the lid is raised.

Charcoal culture

The conditions of this culture provide an environment for larval development that mimics conditions in nature. It provides an efficient way to harvest large numbers of infective-stage larvae. Faecal material suspension prepared in tap water is mixed with granulated hard wood charcoal in a dish (4″ × 3″). Dish is covered and placed in dark for 5–6 days. To harvest the larvae, prepare a round gauze pad (10–12 layers thick) stapled at the edges and cut to fit the dish. Moisten the pad (not dripping wet) and apply it carefully with forceps so that it snugly covers the surface of the charcoal. Expose the dish, with lid off, to a light source. The lamp should be 6–8 inch from the surface of charcoal. After 1 hour, remove the pad with forceps and invert onto the surface of water in a glass filled with water. The gauze pad will remain at the top, and the larvae will make their way through the pad, enter the water, and fall to the bottom of the glass, where they can be harvested with pipette after another 30–60 minutes.

Baermann culture

The Baermann technique, in which a funnel apparatus is used, relies on the principle that active larvae will migrate from a fresh faecal specimen that has been placed on a wire mesh with several layers of gauze which are in contact with tap water (Fig. 30.5). Larvae migrate through the gauze into the water and settle to the bottom of the funnel, where they can be collected and examined.

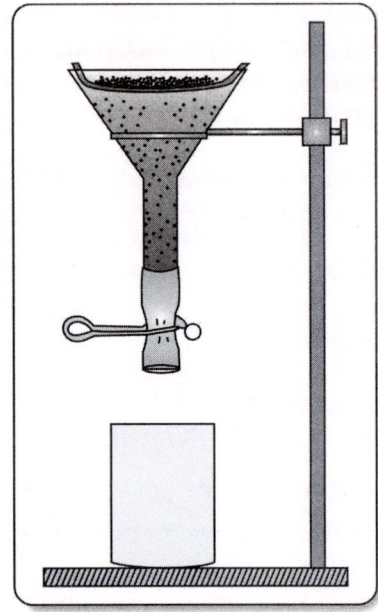

Fig. 30.5. Baermann culture apparatus.

Discussion

1. **What do you mean by polyxenic, monoxenic and axenic culture?**
   - *Polyxenic:* When the parasite grows along with a number of other organisms.
   - *Monoxenic:* When the parasite grows along with one other organism.
   - *Axenic:* No organism is required for growth of parasite.

2. **Enumerate some media of polyxenic/monoxenic cultivation of intestinal protozoa.**
   Balamuth's aqueous yolk infusion medium, Boeck and Drbohlav Locke-egg-serum (LES) medium.

3. **Who first reported the axenic cultivation of *E. histolytica*?**
   Diamond in 1961

4. **What are the advantages of axenic cultivation of *E. histolytica*?**
   Axenic cultivation of *E. histolytica* is essential for study of its:
   – pathogenicity,
   – immunological and biochemical properties,
   – *in vitro* drug susceptibility testing,
   – preparation of axenic amoebic antigen for use in immunodiagnosis of amoebiasis, and
   – to maintain quality control strains.

5. **Which medium is used for culture of pathogenic free-living amoebae and *Naegleria fowleri*?**
   Non-nutrient agar overlaid with a culture of *Escherichia coli* or *Enterobacter aerogenes*.

6. **What is the role of *Escherichia coli* in the culture media for free-living amoebae and *Naegleria fowleri*?**
   Escherichia coli acts as a source of nutrition for the parasites.

7. **Name medium used for cultivation of *Trichomonas vaginalis*.**
   Trussell and Johnson's medium

8. **Which medium is used for cultivation of *Leishmania* spp.?**
   NNN medium (Novy, MacNeal and Nicolle)

9. **Which morphological form of *Leishmania* is seen in culture media?**
   Promastigote

10. **Name any other parasite besides *Leishmania* spp. which can be cultivated in NNN medium.**
    Trypanosoma cruzi

11. **Who did first culture of *P. falciparum* successfully in the laboratory?**
    Trager and Jensen

12. **Which medium is used for cultivation of *P. falciparum*?**
    RPMI 1640.

13. **Enumerate methods used for culture of larval stage of nematode.**
    - Harada-Mori filter paper strip culture
    - Filter paper or slant culture
    - Charcoal culture
    - Baermann culture

14. **Why precautions should be taken while handling larval culture?**
    The precautions should be taken because larvae are infectious.

15. **Enumerate nematodes whose larvae develop in soil.**
    Hookworms, *Strongyloides stercoralis* and *Tricho-strongylus* spp.

16. **Why faecal material to be cultured should not be refrigerated?**
    The faecal material to be cultured should not be refrigerated because some parasites, especially *Necator americanus*, are susceptible to cold and may fail to develop after refrigeration.

17. **How do you differentiate between pathogenic and free-living larvae of nematodes in filter paper culture technique?**
    Pathogenic larvae are more resistant to slight acidity than free-living. Free-living larvae are killed by adding 0.3 ml of concentrated HCl per 10 ml of water containing the larvae, while pathogenic species live for about 24 hours.

18. **How do you observe rapidly moving larvae in cultures?**

It is often difficult to observe details in rapidly moving larvae. Therefore, the larvae can be killed by slight heating or formalin. Iodine can also be used to kill larvae.

19. What is the main advantage of Baermann culture technique over Harada-Mori filter paper culture?

Baermann culture provides a better chance of larval recovery in a light infection as larger amount of stool is used.

20. Why S. stercoralis larvae must be differentiated from hookworm larvae in culture?

These larvae must be differentiated since therapies for the two infections are different.

21. How do you differentiate rhabditiform larvae of S. stercoralis from those of hookworms?

These larvae are differentiated on the basis of length of buccal cavity. The length is extremely short in S. stercoralis larvae while the length of buccal cavity in hookworm larvae is three times long.

22. How do you differentiate filariform larvae of S. stercoralis from those of hookworms?

S. stercoralis filariform larvae have a slit in the tail (notched tail), while hookworm filariform larvae have a pointed tail.

23. How do you differentiate Trichostrongylus spp. eggs from those of hookworm eggs?

Eggs of Trichostrongylus spp. are longer and narrower (measuring 75–91 μm × 39–47 μm), with one end more pointed than the other.

Examination of Blood

The blood provides the most common medium for recovery of various stages of animal parasites, e.g., *Plasmodium* spp., *Babesia* spp., *Leishmania* spp. *Trypanosoma brucei gambiense*, *Trypanosoma brucei rhodesiense*, *Trypanosoma cruzi*, *Wuchereria bancrofti*, *Brugia malayi*, *Brugia timori*, *Loa loa* and *Mansonella ozzardi*. However, in any particular infection, the parasites may not be consistently present. Following methods can be used for the examination of parasites in the blood.

Wet Preparation

A drop of anticoagulated blood can be placed on a clean glass slide, a coverslip put in place and examined microscopically for large, often motile, exoerythrocytic parasites, such as trypanosomes and microfilariae.

Permanent Stained Blood Smear

Permanent stained blood smear is essential for accurate identification of blood parasites. Two types of blood films are used:

- Thin blood film
- Thick blood film
- Combined thick and thin films on the same slide

Thin blood film

Thin blood film is used primarily for the definitive species identification of plasmodia (Colour Plate V, Fig. 25) and other intraerythrocytic parasites. The pulp of a finger or lobe of an ear is wiped with spirit and allowed to dry. Thereafter, it is pricked with surgical cutting needle under aseptic condition. A drop of blood, about the size of pinhead, is taken on a grease-free clean glass slide at about 2 cm from the right end. The drop of blood is touched with the edge of another slide. It is held at an angle of 30° and pushed gently to the left, till the blood is exhausted. As the blood is exhausted, the film begins to form 'tails' which end near about the centre of the slide. The film is allowed to dry. The thin film ideally is one cell thick, with erythrocytes lying flat on the glass surface. If the stain to be used in an aqueous solution, e.g., Giemsa stain, the film must be fixed by covering it with absolute methyl or ethyl alcohol for 2–3 minutes to prevent dehaemoglobinization. For alcohol stains, e.g., Leishman stain, this treatment is not required.

Thick blood film

Thick blood film, many cells thick, contains 6–20 times as much blood per unit area as a thin film. A thick drop of blood is taken on a slide and spread with a needle or with a corner of another slide to form an area of about 12 mm square. It may also be prepared by taking four small drops of blood and joining the corners of the drop with a needle. The blood is continuously stirred for about 30 seconds to prevent formation of fibrin clots. If anticoagulated blood is used, stirring is not necessary because fibrin strands do not form. Potassium EDTA is the anticoagulant of choice. The film is allowed to air-dry in the dust-free areas. The thickness of the film should be such as to allow a newspaper print to be read or the hands of the wrist watch to be seen through the dry preparation.

Once the film is dry, it should be dehaemoglobinized by placing the film in distilled water in a vertical position in a glass cylinder for 5–10 minutes. When the film becomes white, it is taken out and allowed to dry in an upright position. The disruption of the erythrocytes and the loss of their haemoglobin from the slide permits the remaining structures, including blood parasites, to be seen microscopically even when lying deep in the film. Dehaemoglobinization should be done as promptly as possible to assure total dehaemoglobinization. Thick blood films are especially useful in detecting malaria parasites in light infections.

Combined thick and thin films on the same slide
(Fig. 31.1)

This method is of special value in survey work. Two drops of blood are taken; one, 1 cm and another, 2.5 cm from the right end of the slide. The former is made into a thick film and the latter into a thin film.

Fig. 31.1. Combined thick and thin films on the same slide.

Staining Blood Film

Both thin and thick smears can be stained by Leishman and Giemsa stains. In addition, thick smear can be stained by Field stain.

Leishman stain

Leishman stain is prepared by dissolving 0.15 g of Leishman dry powder in 100 ml of absolute methyl alcohol in a bottle. The bottle is shaken until the powder is dissolved and allowed to stand for 48 hours with frequent shaking in between.

The smear is covered with 5–10 drops of stain. After 2 minutes, the stain is diluted by adding twice as many drops of buffered distilled water. The diluted stain is allowed to remain on the slide for 15–20 minutes for staining. The slide is washed with buffered distilled water, dried in air and examined under oil-immersion lens.

Giemsa stain

0.75 g of Giemsa stain powder is placed in a mortar and 25 ml of glycerol is added to it and is grinded with a pestle until a paste is formed. To this is added 75 ml of methanol and stirred to make a solution. It is then poured in a dark-coloured bottle and incubated at 37°C for 24 hours.

The film is fixed by covering it with absolute methyl alcohol for 2–3 minutes. The slide is allowed to dry and immersed in 1:10 dilution of Giemsa stain in buffered distilled water for 30 minutes. It is then washed in buffered distilled water to remove excess stain and allowed to drain by keeping in the upright position and dried in air. The stained film is examined under oil-immersion lens.

For staining thick and thin films on the same slide, the thick film is first dehaemoglobinized and then stained along with the thin film. A line with a grease pencil is drawn between the films. The undiluted Leishman stain is poured over the thin film and after dilution the stain is flooded over the thick film. If the slide is to be stained with Giemsa stain, then the thin part of the film is first fixed with methyl alcohol and

after drying, the whole slide is flooded with dilute Giemsa stain and allowed to remain for half to two hours.

Field stain

This is a quick method of staining of malaria parasites in thick films (without fixation). This requires two solutions:

- Solution A
- Solution B

Solution A

Methylene blue	0.8 g
Azure I (or Azure B)	0.5 g
Disodium hydrogen phosphate (anhydrous)	5.0 g
Potassium hydrogen phosphate (anhydrous)	6.25 g
Distilled water	500 ml

Solution B

Eosin	1.0 g
Disodium hydrogen phosphate (anhydrous)	5.0 g
Potassium hydrogen phosphate (anhydrous)	6.25 g
Distilled water	500 ml

The phosphate salts are first dissolved in water, then the stain is added. Solution of azure I or azure B is facilitated by grinding in a mortar with the phosphate solvent. The solutions are set aside for 24 hours and after filtration are ready for use.

The thick film is placed in solution A for 1–2 seconds. It is removed and immediately rinsed by waving gently in clean water for a few seconds. It is then placed in solution B for 1 second. It is removed and rinsed gently in clean water for 2–3 seconds. It is then allowed to stand upright to drain and dry. Field stain is useful where large number of blood films have to be examined.

JSB (Jaswant Singh, Bhattacharjee) stain

This is a rapid Romanowsky method of staining malaria parasites by water-soluble stain. It consists of two solutions:

- Solution I
- Solution II

Solution I

This is prepared by dissolving methylene blue 0.5 g in 500 ml distilled water in a narrow-mouthed flask. 1% sulphuric acid 3 ml and potassium dichromate 0.5 g are added one after another, with the formation of a heavy deposit of amorphous purple-coloured precipitate of methylene blue chromate. The solution is heated in a water-bath at boiling point for 2–3 hours. At the end of this period, the solution turns blue. This indicates almost complete polychroming. The solution is allowed to cool at room temperature and the precipitate appears as steel-blue needle-like branched crystals. At this stage, 10 ml of 1% potassium hydroxide is added, drop by drop, with the flask being shaken continuously. The liquid is filtered several times till the dye remaining on the filter paper is completely dissolved. The filtrate is blue having a violet iridescence and is a mixture of the azures with only a trace of methylene blue. It is left to mature at room temperature for 48 hours.

Solution II

This is prepared by dissolving 1 g eosin in 500 ml distilled water.

Staining of thin film

Thin film is fixed with methyl alcohol for 3–5 minutes and allowed to dry. It is then immersed in solution I for 30 seconds, washed with acidulated tap water (pH 6.2–6.6), stained with solution II for 1 second, washed again with acidulated tap water for 4 seconds, immersed in solution I again for 30 seconds, washed again with acidulated water for 10 seconds, dried and examined under microscope.

Staining of thick film

The procedure for staining thick film is the same as for thin film except that the first step of fixation with methyl alcohol is omitted.

If an anticoagulated blood specimen is required, use a suitable anticoagulant, e.g., sodium citrate for microfilariae and EDTA for malaria parasites and trypanosomes. Mix blood well but gently with the anticoagulant. Smears should be prepared on anticoagulated blood sample as soon after collection as possible because the long exposure to the anticoagulant may compromise staining. Morphology of mature schizonts and gametocytes in particular may be altered. Sexual stages continue to develop during storage of blood sample in a warm laboratory environment, or following exposure of the blood sample to air. Gametocytes may exflagellate, releasing gametocytes into plasma. Merozoites, particularly those of *P. vivax*, may be released from mature schizonts and reinvade erythrocytes in which they may appear similar to the small accolé forms of *P. falciparum*.

Blood Concentration Methods

Several concentration methods can be used for the detection of haemoparasites. These include:

1. Microhaematocrit centrifugation

Blood is collected in haematocrit tube up to its two-thirds of the volume. The end of the tube is sealed and centrifuged at 1,500 g for 7 minutes. The RBC-plasma interface is then examined under oil-immersion lens for malaria parasites and trypanosomes.

2. Triple centrifugation

9 ml of venous blood is mixed with 1 ml of 6% sodium citrate and centrifuged at 100 g for 10 minutes. The supernatant is collected and centrifuged at 250 g for 10 minutes. The supernatant is centrifuged again at 700 g for 10 minutes and

sediment is examined as a wet film or as stained smear. This method is useful for detection of trypanosomes.

3. Buffy coat concentration

5 ml of citrated or oxalated blood is centrifuged in a tube. Buffy coat present between the plasma and packed red cells is collected and stained for parasites. This method is used for detection of *L. donovani* and trypanosomes in the blood.

4. Knott concentration

2 ml of blood is thoroughly mixed with 10 ml of 2% solution of formalin and allowed to stand for 10 minutes or longer. It is then centrifuged at 200 g for 2 minutes and the sediment is examined microscopically for microfilariae (Colour Plate VI, Fig. 26).

5. Membrane filtration

1 ml of venous blood is drawn into a 10 ml syringe containing 0.1 ml of a 5% solution of sodium citrate. Then in the same syringe, 9 ml of 10% solution of Teepol in physiological saline is drawn and shaken gently for 1 minute. Needle of the syringe is removed and attached to a Swinney filter holder containing a 25 mm membrane filter of 5 μm porosity placed over a supporting filter paper pad of the same size, moistened with saline. With gentle and steady pressure, blood is forced through the filter. Filter is washed three times by passing 10 ml of physiological saline through it. Filter is removed and stained for 5 minutes in hot, but not boiling, Harris' haematoxylin, then it is briefly 'blued' in running tap water. It is dried, covered with mounting medium and coverslip, and examined under microscope. This method is used for detection of microfilariae in the peripheral blood.

6. Gradient centrifugation

4 ml of Ficoll-Hypaque solution is mixed with an equal volume of heparinized blood. This is centrifuged at 150 g for 40 minutes. This shows three layers—white cell layer in the bottom, Ficoll-Hypaque layer in the middle and plasma layer on the top. Middle layer is examined for microfilariae.

Rapid Diagnostic Tests (RDTs)

RDTs are based on the detection of antigens derived from malaria patients in lysed blood, using immunochromatographic methods. Most frequently they employ a dipstick or test strip bearing monoclonal antibodies directed against the target parasite antigens. The tests can be performed in about 15 minutes. Several commercial test kits are currently available.

Antigens targeted by currently available RDTs

- Histidine-rich protein II (HRP-II) is water-soluble protein produced by trophozoites and young (but not mature) gametocytes of *P. falciparum*. Commercial kits currently available detect HRP-II from *P. falciparum* only.

- Parasite lactate dehydrogenase (pLDH) is produced by asexual and sexual stages (gametocytes) of malaria parasites. Test kits currently available detect pLDH from all four *Plasmodium* species that infect humans. They can distinguish *P. falciparum* from the non-*falciparum* species, but cannot distinguish between *P. vivax*, *P. ovale* and *P. malariae*.
- Other antigen(s) that are present in all four species are also targeted in kits that combine detection of the HRP-II antigen of *P. falciparum* together with that of an, as yet unspecified, "pan-malarial" antigen of other species.

General test procedure

- Test strip (most often nitrocellulose) (Fig. 31.2) consists of a sample pad, three detection lines containing capture antibodies specific for *P. falciparum*, all *Plasmodium* spp. and control antibody respectively and an absorbent pad.
- Depending on the kit, 2–50 µl of finger prick blood specimen is collected. Some manufacturers state that anticoagulated blood or plasma can also be used.
- The blood specimen is mixed in a separate test tube or a well, or on a sample pad with a buffer solution that contains a haemolysing compound as well as specific antibody that is labelled with a visually detectable marker such as colloidal gold. If the malaria antigen is present, an antigen–antibody complex is formed.
- The labelled antigen–antibody complex migrates up the test strip by capillary action towards the detection lines containing capture antibodies that have been pre-deposited during manufacture.
- A washing buffer is then added to remove the haemoglobin and permit visualization of any coloured line on the strip.
- If the blood contains malaria antigen (*P. falciparum* or all *Plasmodium* spp.), the labelled antigen–antibody complex will be immobilized at the corresponding predeposited line of capture antibody and will be visually detectable. The complete test run time varies from 5–15 minutes.

Some RDTs detect the four *Plasmodium* spp. that infect humans, depending on the antigens on which they are based. Some RDTs detect *P. falciparum* only, while others detect *P. falciparum* and the other malaria parasites on two separate bands. No commercial RDTs have been reported to differentiate reliably between *P. vivax*, *P. ovale* and *P. malariae*, although research to develop such a test is continuing.

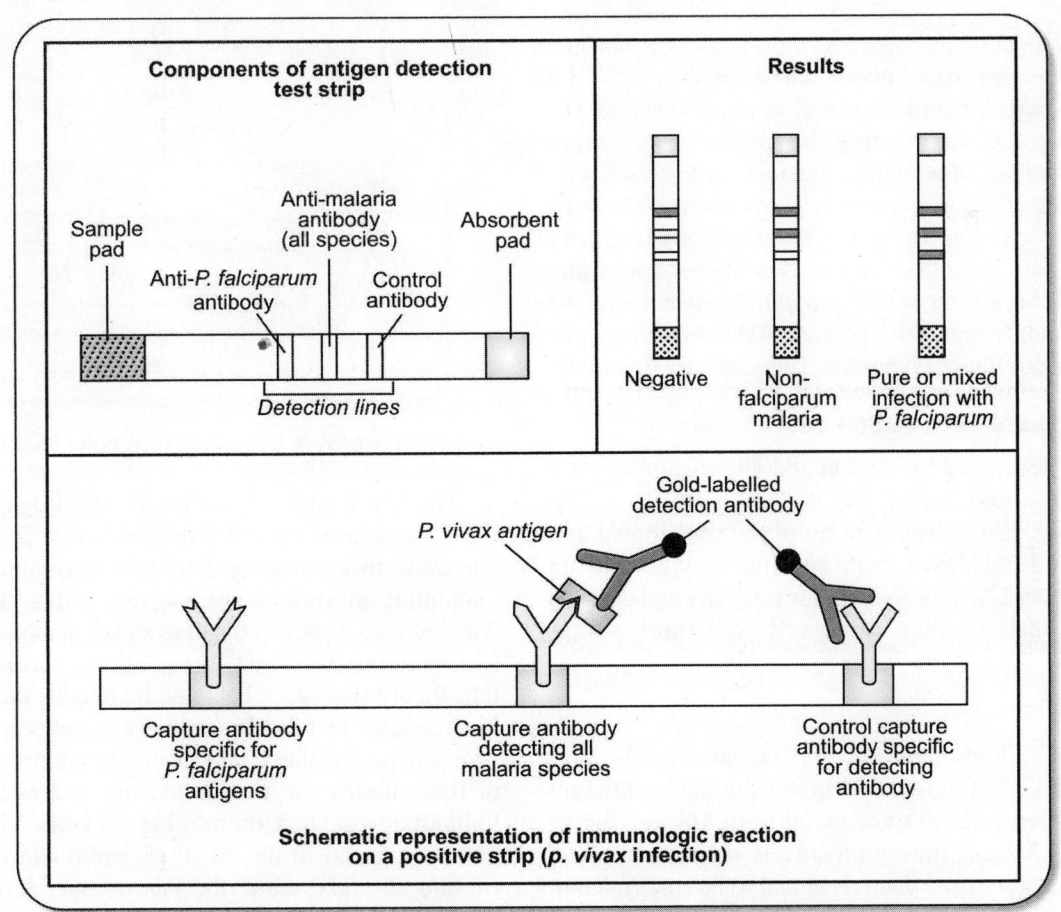

Fig. 31.2. General test procedure of rapid diagnostic test for the diagnosis of malaria.

The sensitivity of the RDTs has been most studied for *P. falciparum*, since the *P. falciparum* kits, targeting mostly *P. falciparum* HRP-II, have been available for a longer time. RDTs for *P. falciparum* generally achieve a sensitivity of >90% at parasite densities above 100 parasites per µl of blood. Below the level of 100 parasites per µl of blood, sensitivity decreases markedly. RDT sensitivity for non-*falciparum* spp. has been less extensively studied. The specificity of RDTs is also >90%. The predictive values, both positive and negative, vary with parasite prevalence and are often found to be acceptable.

Advantages of RDTs over microscopy

- RDTs are simple to perform and to interpret.
- They do not require electricity, special equipment or training in microscopy.
- Health workers with minimal skill can be trained in RDT techniques in periods varying from three hours to one day.
- Since RDTs detect circulating antigens, they may detect *P. falciparum* infection even when the parasites are sequestered in the deep vascular compartment and thus undetectable by microscopic examination of a peripheral blood smear.

Disadvantages of RDTs

- RDTs are more expensive than microscopy.
- Kits cannot differentiate between *P. vivax*, *P. ovale* and *P. malariae* nor can they distinguish pure *P. falciparum* infections from mixed infections that include *P. falciparum*.
- RDTs that detect antigens produced by gametocytes (such as pLDH) can give positive results in infections where only gametocytes are present. Gametocytes do not cause any febrile condition, and those of *P. falciparum* are not affected by schizonticidal drugs. Such positive RDT results can thus lead to erroneous interpretations and unnecessary treatment.

Quantitative Buffy Coat (QBC) Test

The QBC test developed by Becton and Dickenson Inc. is a new method for identifying the malaria parasite in the peripheral blood. It involves staining of the centrifuged and compressed red cell layer with acridine orange and its examination under UV light source. It is fast, easy and claimed to be more sensitive than the traditional thick smear examination.

Method

The QBC tube is a high-precision glass hematocrit tube, pre-coated internally with acridine orange stain and potassium oxalate. It is filled with 60 µl of blood from a finger, ear or heel puncture. A clear plastic closure is then attached. A precisely made cylindrical float, designed to be suspended in the packed red blood cells, is inserted. The tube is centrifuged at 12,000 rpm for 5 minutes. The components of the buffy coat separate according to their densities, forming discrete bands (Fig. 31.3A). Because the float occupies 90% of the internal lumen of the tube, the leucocyte and the thrombocyte cell band widths and the top-most area of red cells are enlarged to 10 times normal. The QBC tube is placed on the tube holder (Fig. 31.3B) and examined using a standard white light microscope equipped with the UV microscope adapter, and epi-illuminated microscope objective. Fluorescing parasites are then observed at the red blood cell/while blood cell interface.

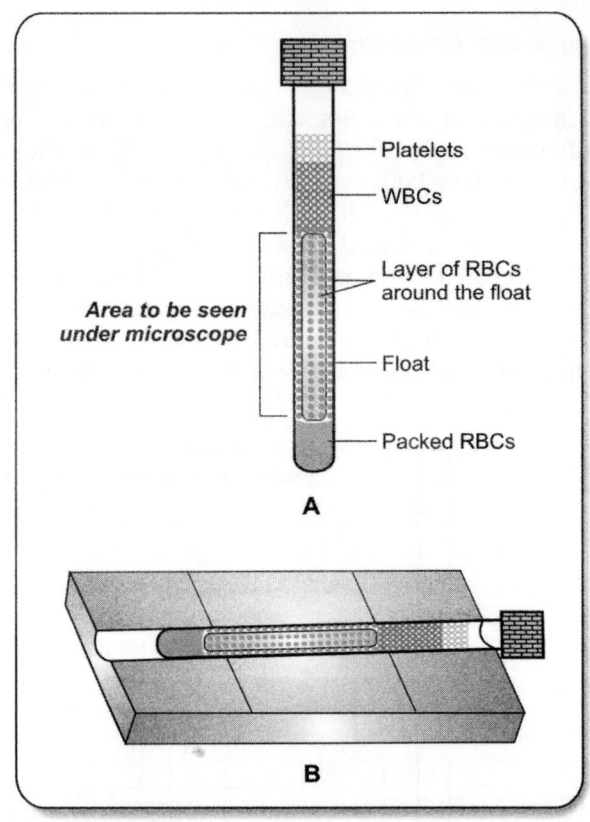

Fig. 31.3A & B. Quantitative buffy coat (QBC) test.

The key feature of method is centrifugation and thereby concentration of the red blood cells in a predictable area of the QBC tube, making detection easy and fast. Red cells containing plasmodia are less dense than normal ones and concentrate just below the leucocytes, at the top of the erythrocyte column. The float forces all the surrounding red cells into the 40 µm space between its outside circumference and the inside of the tube. Since the parasites contain DNA which takes up the acridine orange stain, they appear as bright specks of light among the non-fluorescing red as bright specks of light among the non-fluorescing red cells. Virtually all of the parasites found in the 60 µl of blood can be visualized by rotating the tube under the microscope. A negative test can be reported within one minute and positive result within minutes.

Other Techniques

Other diagnostic methods include microscopy using fluorochromes such as acridine orange, polymerase chain reaction and antibody detection by serology. However, serology only measures prior exposure and not specifically current infection.

Discussion

1. **Enumerate the parasites which can be detected in peripheral blood smear.**
   - Malaria parasites
   - *Leishmania* spp.
   - Microfilariae
   - *Babesia* spp.
   - Trypanosomes

2. **What is the advantage of wet preparation of blood sample?**

   Motile exoerythrocytic parasites, such as trypanosomes and microfilariae can be detected in a wet preparation.

3. **How do you collect blood sample for the preparation of blood films?**
   - Fresh blood collected with no anticoagulants.
   - Anticoagulated blood.
   - Sediment from the various concentration procedures.

4. **Which is the best sample for detection of haemoparasites?**

   The best sample for the detection of haemoparasites is the sample collected without the use of anticoagulants.

5. **What is the effect of anticoagulant on blood films containing malaria parasites?**

   All anticoagulants have some effect on the morphology of the red blood cells containing malaria parasites. This effect is time dependent and the severity varies with the type of anticoagulant used and morphological stage of the parasite. Generally, schizonts and gametocytes are more affected than the early morphological forms.

6. **Which anticoagulant should be used, if required, during collection of blood sample?**

   EDTA has less effect as compared to other anticoagulants. Therefore, it should be used for malaria parasites and trypanosomes, and sodium citrate should be used for microfilariae, when smears cannot be prepared directly.

7. **How do you clean the slides for preparing blood films?**

   Old slides should be cleaned first with detergent and then with 70% ethyl alcohol. New slides should be cleaned with alcohol before use.

8. **Which part of the body is preferred for collection of blood in infants?**

   Big toe/heal is used for collection of blood in infants.

9. **Why blood should not be 'milked' out from the finger after finger is pricked?**

   This will dilute the blood with tissue fluids and hence will decrease the number of parasite per field.

10. **What is the advantage of preparation of thin blood film?**

    Thin blood film is used for the definitive species identification of plasmodia and other intraerythrocytic parasites.

11. **How do you identify a well-prepared thin film?**
    - A well-prepared thin film is thick at one end and thin at the other (one layer of evenly distributed RBCs with no cell overlap).
    - The thin, feathered end should be at least 2 cm long.
    - Thin film should occupy the central area of the slide, with free margins on both sides.

12. **What problem can arise, if you use a greasy slide?**

    Blood film spreads unevenly on a greasy slide.

13. **Why should heat fixation of blood film be avoided?**

    Because heat will fix the blood, causing the RBCs to remain intact during staining; the result is stain retention and inability to identify the parasite.

14. **What is the advantage of preparation of thick blood film?**

    Thick blood films are useful in detecting malaria parasites in light infection.

15. **Why continuous stirring of blood drops is required in thick blood film preparation?**

    Continuous stirring for 30 seconds is required to prevent the formation of fibrin strands that may obscure the parasite after staining. But if anticoagulated blood is used, then stirring is not required.

16. **What problem can arise, if you use too much blood for preparing blood films?**

    In case of thin smear, separate RBCs may not be available for examination and we may miss some parasites, and in case of thick smear, too many WBCs may interfere the diagnosis (obscure the parasites).

17. **What problem can arise, if you use too little blood?**

    We may miss the infection.

18. **What is the advantage of combined thick and thin films on the same slide?**

    This method is useful in survey work.

19. **Which step is essential prior to staining of thick blood film?**

    Laking of thick smears is essential to remove haemoglobin before staining is done.

20. **What is the advantage of dehaemoglobinization of thick blood films?**

Dehaemoglobinization permits the remaining structures, including blood parasites, to be seen microscopically even when lying deep in the film.

21. **Enumerate various stains for staining of blood films.**
    - Leishman
    - Giemsa
    - Field
    - JSB (Jaswant Singh, Bhattacharjee) stain.

22. **Why should you examined the feathered end of the film more carefully?**
    - Microfilariae are commonly found at the feathered end of the film, because they are carried to these sites during the process of spreading the blood.
    - Morphology and size of infected RBCs are more clearly seen as RBCs are drawn out into one single, distinctive layer of cells at this site.
    - Malaria parasites and trypanosomes are easily seen at the edges of thin film.

23. **State major difference between Giemsa staining and Leishman staining?**

With Giemsa staining, fixation of smear is required while with Leishman staining no fixation is required.

24. **Describe the colour of the different components of blood and parasite after Giemsa staining.**

RBC	Pale red
WBC	
Cytoplasm	Pale purple
Nuclei	Purple
Malaria parasites	
Cytoplasm	Blue
Nucleus	Red to purple-red
Schüffner's dots	Red

25. **What important precautions should be taken, if the slides cannot be stained within 48 hours?**
    - Thin films should be fixed in methyl alcohol and thick films should be laked in distilled water before storage.
    - Slides should be stored at low temperature (27°C).
    - Dry films should be stored in dust-free containers.

26. **At what time blood should be collected in cases of nocturnal filarial infections?**

Blood should be collected during night, optimally between 10 pm and 2 am.

27. **Enumerate the microfilariae with sheaths.**
    - *Wuchereria bancrofti*
    - *Brugia malayi*
    - *Loa loa*

28. **Enumerate methods used for the concentration of haemoparasites.**
    - Microhaematocrit centrifugation
    - Buffy coat concentration
    - Knott concentration
    - Membrane filtration
    - Gradient centrifugation
    - Triple centrifugation

29. **In which microfilariae, tail tip is free of nuclei?**
    - *W. bancrofti*
    - *Onchocerca volvulus*
    - *Mansonella ozzardi*

30. **Which blood concentration methods are used for detection of microfilariae?**
    - Knott concentration
    - Membrane filtration
    - Gradient centrifugation

31. **What is the disadvantage of knott concentration?**

The disadvantage is that the microfilariae are killed by the formalin and are, therefore, not seen as motile organisms.

32. **What is the disadvantage of membrane filtration technique?**

This method is unsatisfactory for the isolation of *Mansonella perstans* microfilariae because of their small size.

33. **What is the major advantage of blood concentration methods?**

These are very helpful methods when the parasitaemia is low.

34. **Describe principle of rapid diagnostic tests (RDTs) for diagnosis of malaria parasites?**

RDTs are based on the detection of antigens derived from malaria patients in lysed blood, using immunochromatographic methods. Most frequently, they employ a dipstick or test strip bearing monoclonal antibodies directed against the target parasite antigens.

35. **Enumerate antigens detected by RDTs.**
    - Histidine-rich protein II (HRP-II) of *Plasmodium falciparum*.
    - Parasite lactate dehydrogenase (pLDH).

36. **Who first developed quantitative buffy coat (QBC) test?**

Becton and Dickenson.

37. **Which blood film should be examined first, if you are provided with both thick and thin blood films?**

Thin blood film should be examined first and if malaria parasite is seen, there is no need to examine thick film.

But if you examine thick film first and you find malaria parasites, then for species identification, thin film is also examined.

38. **Which species of *Plasmodium* is most pathogenic?**
    P. falciparum

39. **In India which species are commonly present?**
    P. vivax and *P. falciparum*.

40. **In which malaria parasite infection, only ring stage and gametocytes are seen in peripheral blood smear and why?**
    P. falciparum infection. Because other stages are sequestrated in the capillaries of internal organ.

41. **What is the shape of *P. falciparum* gametocytes?**
    Crescent shape.

42. **Young RBCs are infected by which malaria parasites?**
    P. vivax and *P. ovale*.

43. **The infected RBCs are enlarged due to infection by which malaria parasite?**
    P. vivax.

44. **Relapse of malaria is seen due to infection by which parasite?**
    P. vivax and *P. ovale*

45. **What are the complications of *P. falciparum* infection?**
    Pernicious malaria and black water fever.

46. **Which is the gold standard test for the detection of malaria parasites?**
    Peripheral blood smear examination.

47. **Which stage of *Leishmania* is seen in peripheral blood films?**
    Amastigote form in monocytes and less often in neutrophils.

48. **Why thick blood film is preferred for *Leishmania* parasites?**
    Owing to the small number of *Leishmania* parasites present in the peripheral blood.

49. **Which morphological form of *Trypanosoma cruzi* is seen in peripheral blood film?**
    Trypomastigote form.

Section 4

Systemic Bacteriology

- *Staphylococcus*
- *Streptococcus pyogenes, S. agalactiae* and Enterococci
- *Streptococcus pneumoniae* (Pneumococcus)
- *Neisseria*
- *Corynebacterium*
- *Mycobacterium tuberculosis*
- Diagnostic approach to anaerobes
- *Clostridium*
- *Escherichia coli*
- *Klebsiella*
- *Proteus*
- *Shigella*
- *Salmonella*
- *Pseudomonas*
- *Vibrio*
- Spirochaetes
- Bacteriological examination of water

Staphylococcus

Introduction

Genus *Staphylococcus* contains more than 45 defined species, 20 of which are known to be associated with colonization and/or infection of man and animals. Of the 20 species, one (*Staphylococcus aureus*) is coagulase-positive and 19 are coagulase-negative.

Staphylococcus aureus

Morphology

They are Gram-positive, spherical cocci about 0.8–1.0 μm in diameter, arranged characteristically in grape-like clusters (Fig. 32.1). They are non-motile, non-sporing and with the exception of rare strains, non-capsulated.

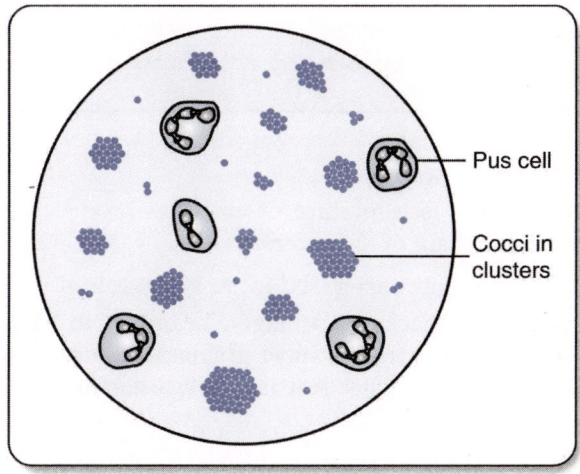

Pus cell

Cocci in clusters

Fig. 32.1. Staphylococci in Gram-stained smear of pus.

Cultural characteristics

They are aerobes and facultative anaerobes. Optimum temperature for growth is 37°C, range being 12–44°C. Optimum pH is 7.5. They can grow well on ordinary media.

Nutrient agar

After overnight incubation at 37°C, colonies are 1–2 mm in diameter with a smooth glistening surface. They are opaque and easily emulsifiable. Most strains produce golden-yellow (aureus) pigment, though some strains may form white colonies.

Blood agar

Colonies are similar to those on nutrient agar, but may be surrounded by a zone of β-haemolysis (Colour Plate VI, Fig. 27), especially when the medium contains sheep, ox, or rabbit blood and it is incubated in an atmosphere of 20% CO_2. Haemolysis is weak on horse blood agar.

MacConkey agar

Colonies are smaller and pink due to lactose fermentation.

Mannitol salt agar

This is both selective and indicator medium. Colonies are similar to those on nutrient agar, but they are surrounded by yellow zones due to fermentation of mannitol by most strains of *S. aureus*.

Phenolphthalein phosphate agar

This is an indicator medium. This assists in the identification of *S. aureus* in mixed cultures. Colonies are similar to those on nutrient agar. All strains of *S. aureus* produce phosphatase which liberates phenolphthalein from sodium phenolphthalein diphosphate. To detect it, 0.1 ml of ammonia solution is placed in the lid and the culture plate, with the culture, is inverted over it. Colonies of *S. aureus* become bright pink in a minute or so, because phenolphthalein is pink in alkaline pH.

Biochemical reactions

Catalase	+
Oxidase	–
Indole	–

Systemic Bacteriology

MR	+
VP	+
Urease	+
Nitrate reduction	+

Acid from

Glucose	+
Maltose	+
Lactose	+
Sucrose	+
Mannitol	+

Tests to detect the production of coagulase

1. Slide coagulase test

This test detects clumping factor (bound coagulase) which is a cell-wall component that causes the organisms to clump when mixed with plasma. This factor reacts directly with fibrinogen in plasma, causing rapid cell clumping. It can be detected by emulsifying a few colonies of bacteria in a drop of normal saline on a clean glass slide and mixing it with a drop of rabbit plasma. Prompt clumping of the organisms indicates the presence of clumping factor. Positive and negative controls are also set up.

2. Tube coagulase test

This test detects an extracellular enzyme called coagulase. It activates a coagulase-reacting factor (CRF) normally present in plasma, causing the plasma to clot by conversion of fibrinogen to fibrin. To perform this test, 0.1 ml of an overnight broth culture is mixed with 0.5 ml of a 1 in 10 dilution of human or rabbit plasma. The mixture is incubated in a water-bath at 37°C for three to six hours. If positive, the plasma clots and does not flow when the tube is inverted. Continued incubation is not recommended as the clot may be lysed by fibrinolysin produced by some strains. Controls with plasma alone, and known coagulase-positive and coagulase-negative cultures must be set up with each batch of tests.

Coagulase-Negative Staphylococci

Coagulase-negative staphylococci (CoNS) form part of the normal flora of the skin but may cause opportunistic infection in immunocompromised patients. Their colonies are non-pigmented (white) (Colour Plate VI, Fig. 28), and in contrast to *S. aureus*, they are clumping factor, coagulase test and deoxyribonuclease negative. Majority (70–80%) of infections with CoNS, in humans, are caused by *S. epidermidis* followed by *S. saprophyticus*, *S. haemolyticus*, *S. hominis* and *S. warneri*.

Discussion

1. **What is the chemical nature of pigment produced by** *S. aureus*?

   The pigment is believed to be a lipoprotein allied to carotene.

2. **Name methods of enhancement of pigment production by** *S. aureus*.

   Pigment production is enhanced by following methods:
   - Addition of 1% glycerol monoacetate to nutrient agar
   - Using milk agar plate
   - Using fatty media such as Tween agar
   - Prolonged incubation
   - Leaving plates at room temperature

3. **Does pigment of** *S. aureus* **diffuse into the medium?**

   No.

4. **How can this pigment production be decreased?**

   Pigment production can be decreased by repeated sub-cultures.

5. **What do you mean by term** *Staphylococcus*?

   Staphyle in Greek means bunch of grapes, and *kokkos* means a berry.

6. **What are the important differences between** *Staphylococcus* **and** *Micrococcus*?

   Important differences between *Staphylococcus* and *Micrococcus* are given in Table 32.1.

Table 32.1. Important differences between *Staphylococcus* and *Micrococcus*

	Staphylococcus	*Micrococcus*
Growth	Facultative anaerobe	Obligate aerobe
Oxidase	–	+
Sensitivity to		
Lysostaphin	Sensitive	Resistant
Bacitracin (0.04U disc)	Resistant	Sensitive

7. **What is lysostaphin?**

   Lysostaphin is a mixture of enzymes produced by a particular strain of *S. epidermidis*.

8. **Why micrococci are resistant to lysostaphin?**

   Lysostaphin attacks the pentaglycine bridges in *S. aureus* but micrococci do not have glycine residues in their peptide bridges, hence resistant to lysostaphin.

9. **Why salt agar is used as selective medium for isolation of staphylococci?**

   Salt agar is used as selective medium because staphylococci can grow in the presence of 10% or more of sodium chloride, while many other bacteria are inhibited at this concentration.

10. **How much salt concentration is tolerated by plano-cocci?**

    Planococci are associated with marine environment, therefore, they can tolerate salt concentration up to 12%.

11. Name indicator media of *S. aureus*.

- Phenolphthalein phosphate agar
- Mannitol salt agar

12. Enumerate characteristic features of pathogenic strains of *S. aureus*.

Pathogenic strains of *S. aureus* usually exhibit the following features:

- Coagulase-positive
- Ferment mannitol
- Produce golden-yellow pigment
- Liquefy gelatin
- Produce phosphatase
- β-haemolysis on blood agar medium.

13. Why staphylococci are arranged characteristically in grape-like clusters?

Cluster formation is due to cell division occurring in more than one plane with daughter cells remaining close together.

14. What is protein A?

Protein A is a cell wall component which binds to Fc region of IgG molecules leaving specific Fab sites free to combine with specific antigen. It is involved in coagglutination test.

15. What do you mean by term clumping factor?

Clumping factor (bound coagulase) is a surface component that causes the organisms to clump when mixed with plasma. This factor reacts directly with fibrinogen in plasma, causing rapid cell clumping. Here, fibrinogen is not converted into fibrin.

16. Do all strains of *S. aureus* produce clumping factor?

No, 12% of coagulase-producing strains may not produce clumping factor.

17. What is the principle of tube coagulase test?

S. aureus produces an extracellular enzyme called coagulase. It activates a coagulase-reacting factor (CRF) normally present in plasma, causing plasma to clot by the conversion of fibrinogen to fibrin.

18. Why guinea pig plasma cannot be used for tube coagulase test?

Plasma of guinea pig lacks CRF. Therefore, it cannot be used for detecting free coagulase.

19. At which phase of growth coagulase is produced?

Coagulase is produced during the logarithmic phase of growth.

20. What is the role of coagulase in pathogenesis?

Coagulase may act to coat the bacterial cell with fibrin, rendering them resistant to opsonization and phagocytosis.

21. Why citrated plasma should not be used for conducting tube coagulase test?

Citrated plasma should not be used because contaminating Gram-negative bacilli may utilize the citrate and produce false positive reaction.

22. Enumerate the pathogenic lesions produced by *S. aureus*.

- *Cutaneous infections:* Boils, furuncles, carbuncles, styes, etc.
- *Deep infections:* Osteomyelitis, tonsillitis, bronchopneumonia, meningitis, etc.
- *Exfoliative disease:* Ritter's disease or staphylococcal scalded skin syndrome
- Food poisoning
- Toxic shock syndrome

23. Which toxins of *S. aureus* are recognized as superantigens?

- Toxic shock syndrome toxin-1 (TSST-1)
- Enterotoxins

24. How much time after consuming contaminated food patient develops staphylococcal food poisoning?

Within 2–6 hours.

25. What are the characteristic features of enterotoxins produced by *S. aureus*?

They are:

- Heat stable
- Not destroyed by gut enzymes
- And they act directly on autonomic nervous system to cause the illness, rather than on GIT mucosa.

26. How many antigenic types of enterotoxins have been identified?

Nine antigenic types (A, B, C_1, C_2, C_3, D, E, H and I)

27. Why human blood should not be used for preparing blood agar plate?

Human blood should not be used because of following reasons:

- Human blood may contain antibodies or other inhibitors.
- Activity of α-lysin and β-lysin is weak on human red blood cells.

28. Which haemolysin is known as hot-cold haemolysin?

β-lysin

29. Which species of coagulase-negative staphylococci is associated with urinary tract infection in young healthy sexually active women?

S. saprophyticus.

30. Name one important test to differentiate *S. saprophyticus* from *S. aureus* and *S. epidermidis*.

Novobiocin resistance test. *S. saprophyticus* is resistant to novobiocin while *S. aureus* and *S. epidermidis* are sensitive.

31. Differentiate between *S. aureus* and *S. epidermidis*.

Differences between *S. aureus* and *S. epidermidis* are given in Table 32.2.

Table 32.2. Differences between *S. aureus* and *S. epidermidis*

	S. aureus	*S. epidermidis*
Production of		
Coagulase	+	–
DNase	+	–
a toxin	+	–
Phosphatase	+	–\weak +
Protein A in cell wall	+	–
Mannitol fermentation	+	–

32. What is the characteristic appearance of confluent growth of *S. aureus* on nutrient agar plate?

'Oil-paint' appearance.

33. Which staphylococcal haemolysin does not possess leucocidal activity?

β-haemolysin

34. Enumerate organisms producing black colonies on blood tellurite agar medium.

- *Corynebacterium diphtheriae*
- *S. aureus*
- Enterococci

35. What are the mechanisms of resistance to β-lactam drugs in *S. aureus*?

- Production of β-lactamase
- Changes in bacterial surface receptors, reducing binding of β-lactam antibiotics to the bacterial cells.
- Development of tolerance

36. Why capsulated strains of *S. aureus* may show negative clumping factor (slide coagulase) test?

Capsulated strains may sometimes show a negative test because the clumping factor may be enveloped by the capsular polysaccharide.

37. Differentiate between bound coagulase (clumping factor) and free coagulase of *S. aureus*.

Differences between bound coagulase (clumping factor) and free coagulase of *S. aureus* are given in Table 32.3.

Table 32.3. Differences between bound coagulase (clumping factor) and free coagulase of *S. aureus*

Bound coagulase	Free coagulase
Cell wall component	Extracellular enzyme
Only one antigen type is known	Eight antigenic types have been identified
Does not require participation of coagulase-reacting factor for its action	Requires the participation of coagulase-reacting factor for its action
Detected by slide coagulase test	Detected by tube coagulase test

38. Which toxin is known as Panton-Valentine toxin?

Leucocidin

39. What is the advantage of serological test in diagnosis of *S. aureus* infections?

They are helpful in the diagnosis of hidden deep infections.

40. Name one test which can differentiate genus *Staphylococcus* from genus *Streptococcus*.

Catalase test is positive in *Staphylococcus* but negative in *Streptococcus*.

41. Name the gene involved in methicillin resistance of *S. aureus*.

MeCA.

42. Which method is used for typing *S. aureus*?

Bacteriophage typing.

43. What is the use of bacteriophage typing method?

It is useful for epidemiological purpose especially to identify the source of infection in epidemics of food poisoning.

Streptococcus pyogenes, S. agalactiae and Enterococci

Introduction

On the basis of group-specific carbohydrate antigen in the cell wall, β-haemolytic streptococci are divided into 20 serological groups. These are known as Lancefield groups. Group A β-haemolytic strains, which are responsible for many important human infections, are given the species name *Streptococcus pyogenes*.

Streptococcus pyogenes

Morphology

They are Gram-positive, spherical cocci about 0.6–1.0 μm in diameter. They occur in chains of varying length (Fig. 33.1). They are non-motile, non-sporing and some strains produce a capsule of hyaluronic acid.

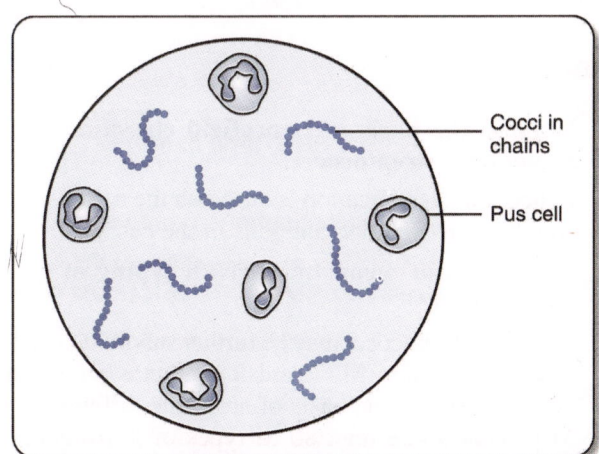

Cocci in chains

Pus cell

Fig. 33.1. Streptococci in Gram-stained smear of pus.

Cultural characteristics

They are aerobes and facultative anaerobes. Temperature range is 22–40°C, optimum temperature being 37°C. They are exacting in nutritive requirements, growth occurring only in media containing fermentable carbohydrates or enriched with blood or serum.

Blood agar

After 24-hour incubation, colonies are small (0.5–1 mm), semitransparent, grey-white with a matt or glossy surface. The colonies are surrounded by a wide zone of β-haemolysis (Colour Plate VI, Fig. 29). Mucoid colonies are formed by strains which produce large capsule. On ageing and drying, mucoid colonies turn into flatter, rougher, matt colonies. Growth and haemolysis are promoted by 10% CO_2.

Crystal violet blood agar

This is a selective medium for isolation of *S. pyogenes*. The addition of 0.0002% crystal violet to blood agar inhibits the growth of some bacteria, notably staphylococci, while permitting the growth of streptococci.

PNF medium

PNF medium (horse blood agar containing polymyxin B sulphate, neomycin sulphate and fusidic acid 17 units/ml, 4.25 μg/ml and 0.50 μg/ml, respectively) is a selective medium for β-haemolytic streptococci. It inhibits the growth of staphylococci and coliform species.

Glucose broth or serum broth

These are liquid media used for isolation of streptococci. Growth occurs as granular turbidity with a powdery deposit. No pellicle is formed.

Biochemical reactions

Catalase	–
Acid from	
Sorbitol	+
Lactose	+
Maltose	+
Mannitol	+

Systemic Bacteriology

4

Solubility in 10% bile   –
Sensitivity to
  Bacitracin disc (0.04 µg)   +
  Trimethoprim/sulphamethoxazole   –
  (1.2 µg/23.8 µg)

Group B Streptococci (*Streptococcus agalactiae*)

Morphology

They are chain forming Gram-positive cocci. They are non-motile and non-sporing.

Cultural characteristics

Blood agar

On blood agar, they produce β-haemolysis, though the zones are usually narrow. Sometime they may produce α-haemolysis and occasionally they produce no haemolysis at all. Colonies are grey, mucoid and larger (about 2 mm) than those of other streptococci.

Columbia agar or starch/serum agar

They form orange-coloured colonies on anaerobic incubation at 37°C for 18 hours.

Islam medium

Pigment production is more intense on this medium.

Tests for presumptive identification of group B streptococci

Hydrolysis of sodium hippurate

S. agalactiae possesses the enzyme hippuricase, which hydrolyses sodium hippurate to form sodium benzoate and glycine. This hydrolysis can be detected by adding ninhydrin, which reacts with the α-amino groups to form a purple colour. All group B streptococci hydrolyse hippurate.

CAMP test

This test detects the production of CAMP factor produced by group B streptococci. CAMP factor enhances the β-lysin produced by *Staphylococcus*.

    To perform this test, streak a β-lysin-producing *Staphylococcus aureus* strain (NCTC 1803) on a sheep blood agar plate. Then make a single streak of the streptococcal test strain perpendicular to the staphylococcal streak. Leave about 1 cm space between the two inoculation lines. Incubate the inoculated plate at 37°C for 24 hours in air or in air with 10% CO_2. CAMP factor enhances the β-lysin produced by *Staphylococcus* and an increased area of lysis appears at the junction of the two organisms which assume the shape of an arrowhead (Fig. 33.2).

Enterococcus

They are Gram-positive cocci occurring in pairs or short

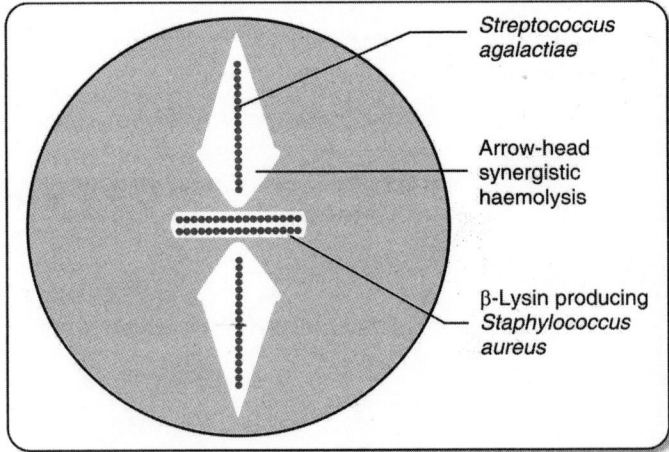

Fig. 33.2. CAMP test.

Labels: Streptococcus agalactiae; Arrow-head synergistic haemolysis; β-Lysin producing Staphylococcus aureus

chains. They are non-motile and non-capsulated. They are normal flora of lower GIT and vagina. They may be α-haemolytic, β-haemolytic or nonhaemolytic on sheep blood agar. They produce tiny, deep pink colonies on MacConkey agar.

Important characteristics of enterococci

- They can grow in the presence of 40% bile and hydrolyse aesculin to aesculetin and glucose.
- They can grow in the presence of 6.5% NaCl, at pH 9.6, and at 10°C and 45°C.
- They are positive for PYRase test.
- They can tolerate heat at 60°C for 30 minutes.
- They are resistant to penicillin.

Discussion

1. **What is the basis of Lancefield classification of β-haemolytic streptococci?**

   Lancefield classification is based on the nature of group-specific carbohydrate antigens in the cell wall.

2. **What do you mean by Griffith typing of group A streptococci?**

   Group A streptococci may be further subdivided into types based on protein (M, T and R) antigens present on the cell surface. On the basis of antigenic differences in the M protein, more than 80 M types of *S. pyogenes* have been recognized so far (types 1, 2, 3 and so on). This is known as Griffith typing.

3. **Why there is chain formation in streptococci?**

   Chain formation is due to the cocci dividing in one plane only and the daughter cells failing to separate completely.

4. **Name longest chain forming *Streptococcus*.**

   S. salivarius.

5. **What is the chemical nature of the capsule of streptococci?**

   Some strains of *S. pyogenes* and some group C strains have capsule composed of hyaluronic acid, while strains of groups B and D have polysaccharide capsules.

6. **What is the characteristic of colonies produced by virulent strains of *S. pyogenes*?**

   Virulent strains of *S. pyogenes*, on fresh isolation, produce 'matt' colonies.

7. **How many types of haemolysis are seen in streptococci?**

   Three types of haemolysis are seen:
   - Alpha
   - Beta
   - Gamma (nonhaemolytic)

8. **Enumerate important β-haemolytic streptococci.**
   - Group A streptococci: *S. pyogenes*
   - Group B streptococci: *S. agalactiae*
   - Group C streptococci: *S. equisimilis*

9. **What is the colour of the colonies of *Enterococcus* spp. on MacConkey agar medium?**

   Deep pink.

10. **Which toxin of streptococci acts as superantigen?**

    Erythrogenic toxin (streptococcal pyrogenic toxin).

11. **Enumerate non-suppurative complications of *S. pyogenes*.**
    - Acute rheumatic fever
    - Acute glomerulonephritis
    - Erythema nodosum

12. **Name the transport medium used for the isolation of streptococci.**

    Pike's medium (blood agar containing 1 in 100,000 crystal violet and 1 in 16,000 sodium azide distributed as for stab cultures in tubes).

13. **Why sheep blood agar is recommended for primary isolation of β-haemolytic streptococci?**

    Sheep blood agar is recommended for primary isolation of β-haemolytic streptococci because it is inhibitory to *Haemophilus haemolyticus*, colonies of which may be confused with those of β-haemolytic streptococci.

14. **Enumerate pathogenic lesions produced by group B streptococci.**

    In neonates
    - Early-onset type meningitis
    - Late-onset type meningitis

    In adults
    - Puerperal sepsis
    - Endocarditis
    - Meningitis, and
    - Occasionally pneumonia, empyema, arthritis and osteomyelitis

15. **Name presumptive tests for identification of group B streptococci.**
    - Hydrolysis of sodium hippurate
    - CAMP test
    - Pigment production

16. **Who first described the CAMP test?**

    CAMP test was first described in 1944 by Christie, Atkins and Munch-Peterson.

17. **Name streptococci responsible for dental caries.**

    Viridans streptococci, chiefly *S. mutans* and to a lesser extent *S. sanguis*, are involved in the production of dental caries.

18. **Describe in brief the mechanism of dental caries.**

    Viridans streptococci, chiefly *S. mutans* and to a lesser extent *S. sanguis* break down dietary sucrose, producing acid and a tough adhesive dextran. The acid damages dentin and the dextran binds together food debris, epithelial cells, mucus and bacteria to form dental plaques which lead to dental caries.

19. **Enumerate viridans streptococci associated with infective endocarditis.**
    - *S. salivarius*
    - *S. sanguis*
    - *S. mutans*
    - *S. mitior*
    - *S. milleri*

20. **What is the typical arrangement of enterococci?**

    Enterococci typically appear as pairs of oval cocci, the cells in a pair are arranged at an angle to each other.

21. **Why culture plate for CAMP factor production should not be incubated anaerobically?**

    The culture plate for CAMP factor production should not be incubated anaerobically because some group A streptococci produce a positive reaction in the absence of oxygen.

22. **Name streptococci other than group A (with percentage) sensitive to bacitracin.**
    - Group B streptococci (6%)
    - Groups C and G β-haemolytic streptococci (7.5%)
    - α-haemolytic streptococci (7.5%)

23. **Name one presumptive test for identification of *S. pyogenes* in throat swab.**

    A blood agar plate is inoculated with a pure culture of β-haemolytic *Streptococcus*, a 0.04 units bacitracin disc is placed in the area of inoculation and the plate is incubated at 37°C for 24 hours. The inhibition of growth around the disc is seen with *S. pyogenes*, but not with other streptococci. However, bacitracin-susceptible strepto-cocci may belong to groups other than group A (see Sr. No. 22 above).

24. **What is the therapeutic role of streptokinase and streptodornase (deoxyribonuclease) produced by streptococci?**

    Mixtures of streptokinase and streptodornase have been used therapeutically for breaking down blood clots, thick pus and fibrinous exudates in closed spaces such as joints or pleural cavity.

25. **Which enzymes of group A streptococci are responsible for serous character of pus?**

    Deoxyribonucleases

26. **Enumerate structural components of *S. pyogenes* which cross react with human tissues.**

    Structural components of *S. pyogenes* which cross react with human tissues are given in Table 33.1.

27. **Why viridans streptococci (α-haemolytic streptococci) are not included in Lancefield classification?**

    Viridans streptococci are not included in Lancefield classification because they do not have group-specific carbohydrate antigen in the cell wall.

28. **Enumerate enzymes of streptococci responsible for spreading character of streptococcal infections.**

Table 33.1. Structural components of *S. pyogenes* which cross react with human tissues

Structural component of *S. pyogenes*	Human tissue with which it cross reacts
Capsular hyaluronic acid	Synovial fluid
Cell wall protein	Myocardium
Cell wall carbohydrate	Cardiac valves
Cytoplasmic membrane	Vascular intima
Peptidoglycan	Skin antigens

- Hyaluronidase (spreading factor)
- Streptokinase
- Deoxyribonuclease

29. **Which test can differentiate streptococci from staphylococci?**

    Catalase test, the former are negative and the later are positive.

30. **Which *Streptococcus* is strict anaerobe?**

    Peptostreptococcus.

31. **What is the major difference between lesions produced by staphylococci and streptococci?**

    Staphylococci produce localized lesions while strepto-cocci produce spreading lesions.

Streptococcus pneumoniae (Pneumococcus)

Morphology

Pneumococci are small (1 μm), slightly elongated Gram-positive cocci, with one end broad or rounded and the other pointed, presenting a flame-shaped or lanceolate appearance. They occur in pairs with rounded ends adjacent to each other. They are capsulated. The capsule encloses each pair and it is best seen in the material taken directly from the exudates and may be lost on repeated cultivation (Fig. 34.1). They are non-sporing and non-motile.

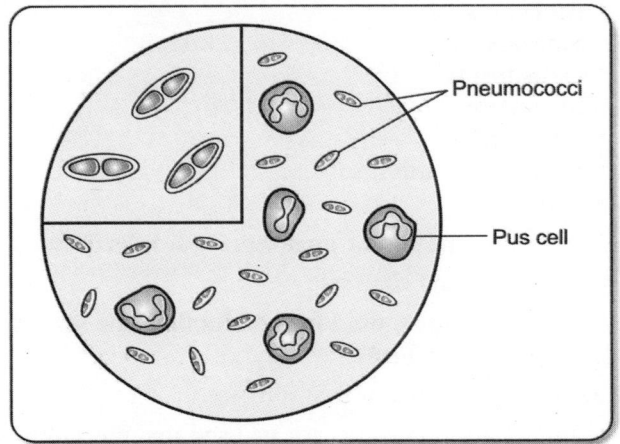

Fig. 34.1. Pneumococci in pus. Inset: Enlarged view.

Cultural Characteristics

They are aerobes and facultative anaerobes, the optimum temperature being 37°C (range 25–40°C) and pH 7.8 (range 6.5–8.3). They grow only in enriched media and growth is improved by 5–10% CO_2.

Blood agar

Virulent strains with abundant capsular polysaccharide produce small (0.5–1 mm in diameter), moist, mucoid, transparent colonies after 18–24-hour incubation at 37°C.

Poorly capsulated strains produce small, round, translucent colonies. The colonies are surrounded by a 2–3 mm zone of α-haemolysis (Colour Plate VI, Fig. 30). On further incubation, the colonies develop a central depression because of autolysis with raised rim (draughtsman colony). Under anaerobic incubation, β-haemolysis is seen due to the liberation of oxygen-labile pneumolysin.

Biochemical Reactions

Catalase	–
Acid from	
Glucose	+
Sucrose	+
Lactose	+
Inulin	+
Bile solubility	+

Fermentation reactions are tested in Hiss's serum sugar media.

Tests for Identification of Pneumococci

1. Optochin sensitivity

Optochin (ethyl hydrocuprein hydrochloride) is a quinine derivative that inhibits the growth of pneumococci. For testing, a filter paper disc (5 μg) of optochin is applied to the surface of a blood agar plate streaked with a lawn of pure culture. Plate is incubated at 37°C in air with 5–10% CO_2. Pneumococcus shows a zone of inhibition of 14 mm or more around the 6 mm optochin disc or 16 mm or more if 10 mm disc is used. This test is also used for distinguishing pneumococci from viridans streptococci, both of which produce α-haemolysis on blood agar. Viridans streptococci are resistant to optochin.

2. Bile solubility

For bile solubility test, inoculate the test organism in 5 ml serum digest broth or infusion broth, incubate it at 37°C for 18 hours. While still warm, add 0.5 ml of 10% sodium deoxycholate solution and reincubate at 37°C. Within 15 minutes initially turbid culture becomes clear and transparent due to the lysis of pneumococci. Alternatively, touch a suspected pneumococcal colony on blood agar plate with a loopful of 2% sodium deoxycholate solution at pH 7. Incubate the plate at 37°C for 30 minutes. The colony disappears, leaving an area of α-haemolysis.

Discussion

1. **What is the chemical nature of capsule produced by pneumococci?**

   Polysaccharide.

2. **Enumerate methods for the demonstration of capsule of pneumococci.**

   * A clear halo around the organism in India ink preparation.
   * By direct special staining techniques.
   * It can also be seen and typed by treatment with homologous type-specific antibody which combines with the capsular polysaccharide and renders it refractile – Quellung reaction.

3. **Why is it difficult to preserve pneumococci on blood agar or chocolate agar medium for long time?**

   Because they undergo autolysis in cultures due to the activity of intracellular autolytic enzymes.

4. **Enumerate agents enhancing autolysis of pneumococci.**

   * Bile salts
   * Sodium lauryl sulphate

5. **What is the basis of bile solubility test of pneumococci?**

   The bile solubility test is based on the presence in the pneumococci of an autolytic amidase that cleaves the bond between alanine and muramic acid in the peptidoglycan. The amidase is activated by bile salts, resulting in lysis of the organisms.

6. **What is the historical importance of pneumococci?**

   Research work with pneumococcal transformations provided the initial proof that DNA alone is the carrier of genetic information.

7. **Which type of haemolysis is seen in pneumococci?**

   α-haemolysis

8. **How do you differentiate S. pneumoniae from viridans streptococci?**

   Differences between S. pneumoniae and viridans streptococci are given in Table 34.1.

Table 34.1. Differences between S. pneumoniae and viridans streptococci

	S. pneumoniae	Viridans streptococci
Morphology	Flame-shaped cocci in pairs	Oval or round cocci in chains
Capsule	Present	Absent
Bile solubility	+	–
Inulin fermentation	+	–
Optochin sensitivity	+	–
Animal pathogenicity (intraperitoneal inoculation in mice)	Fatal, death of mice in 1–3 days	Nonpathogenic

9. **What name is given to the colonies of S. pneumoniae?**

   Draughtsman colonies or colonies with carrom coin appearance. The colonies are flat with raised edges and central umbonation.

10. **Enumerate pathogenic lesions produced by S. pneumoniae.**

    * Pneumonia, either a lobar pneumonia or a bronchopneumonia
    * Bronchitis
    * Sinusitis
    * Otitis media
    * Meningitis
    * Endocarditis
    * Suppurative arthritis
    * Peritonitis

11. **Name the commonest pneumococcal infections.**

    Otitis media and sinusitis

12. **Which medium is used for conducting bile solubility test of pneumococci?**

    Serum digest broth or infusion broth.

13. **Which medium should not be used for bile solubility test of pneumococci?**

    A glucose-containing medium should not be used as the reaction of the culture must not become more acid than pH 6.8.

14. **Which antigen of S. pneumoniae is known as specific soluble substance?**

    Capsular polysaccharide antigen.

15. **How do you detect pneumococcal antigen in cerebrospinal fluid?**

    * Coagglutination test
    * Latex agglutination test
    * Countercurrent immunoelectrophoresis (CIE)

Neisseria

Introduction

The genus *Neisseria* has Gram-negative cocci with adjacent sides flattened. Important species of the genus *Neisseria* are *N. meningitidis*, *N. gonorrhoeae*, *N. flavescens*, *N. subflava*, *N. sicca*, *N. mucosa* and *N. lactamica*. They are saccharolytic, catalase-positive and oxidase-positive. *N. gonorrhoeae* and *N. meningitidis* are the primary human pathogens of the genus. Other species are commonly found as commensals in the upper respiratory tract.

Neisseria meningitidis (Meningococcus)

Morphology

They are Gram-negative cocci, 0.6–1.0 μm in diameter. They usually occur in pairs with adjacent sides flattened or concave and long axes parallel. They are typically seen in large numbers inside polymorphonuclear leucocytes (Fig. 35.1). Fresh isolates of most *N. meningitidis* serogroups are encapsulated. They are non-sporing and non-motile.

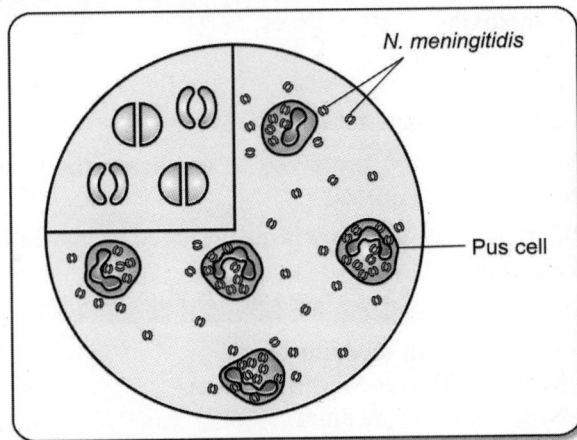

Fig. 35.1. *Neisseria meningitidis* in CSF. Inset: Enlarged view showing adjacent sides flattened or concave and long axes parallel.

Cultural characteristics

Meningococci have exacting growth requirements and do not grow on ordinary media. Growth occurs on media enriched with blood or serum. However, they grow well on trypticase-soy agar and Mueller-Hinton medium without the addition of blood or serum. They are strict aerobes, no growth occurring anaerobically. The growth is facilitated by 5–10% CO_2 and high humidity. The optimum temperature and pH for the growth of meningococci are 35–36°C and 7.0–7.4, respectively.

Blood agar

On blood agar, after 24-hour incubation, the colonies of meningococci are small about 1 mm in diameter, round, convex, grey, nonhaemolytic and translucent. After 48-hour incubation, colonies are larger with an opaque raised centre and thin transparent margins which may be crenated.

Chocolate agar

Colonies of meningococci are slightly larger than those on blood agar.

Thayer-Martin medium

This is a selective medium for the isolation of gonococci and meningococci. This medium is used for the culture of materials expected to yield a mixture of organisms. Vancomycin, colistin and nystatin, which are present in this medium, inhibit Gram-positive bacteria, Gram-negative bacteria and yeast contaminants, respectively, while allowing the growth of pathogenic *Neisseria*.

Biochemical reactions

Catalase	+
Oxidase	+
Acid from	
Glucose	+
Maltose	+

Neisseria gonorrhoeae (Gonococcus)

Morphology and staining characteristics

These are similar to those of *N. meningitidis*.

Cultural characteristics

Gonococci are more difficult to grow than meningococci. They are aerobes, but may grow anaerobically. Addition of 5–10% CO_2 is essential for primary isolation. Growth occurs best at pH 7.0–7.4 and at a temperature of 35–36°C. They can be isolated on media enriched with blood, either partially lysed by heat (chocolate agar) or completely lysed by saponin.

Heated blood agar

On heated blood agar, after 24-hour incubation, colonies are small about 1 mm in diameter, grey, convex and translucent. After 48-hour incubation, colonies are larger 1.5–2.5 mm in diameter with an opaque raised centre and thin transparent margins which may be crenated.

Thayer-Martin medium

This is a selective medium for the isolation of gonococci. This is prepared by addition of vancomycin 3 mg/litre, colistin 7.5 mg/litre and nystatin 12,500 units/litre to heated blood agar. This selective medium is valuable in isolating gonococci from heavily contaminated specimens. On Thayer-Martin medium, growth is slower, although, colonies are similar to those on heated blood agar (Colour Plate VI, Fig. 31).

Modified Thayer-Martin medium

Trimethoprim lactate (5 mg/litre) may be added to Thayer-Martin medium to inhibit swarming *Proteus* species that are occasionally present in cervicovaginal and rectal specimens. The chocolate agar medium containing vancomycin, colistin, nystatin and trimethoprim is known as modified Thayer-Martin medium.

New York City medium

This is a transparent peptone-corn starch agar-based medium containing yeast dialysate, citrated horse plasma, lysed horse erythrocytes, vancomycin (2 mg /litre), colistin (5.5 mg/litre), amphotericin B (1.2 mg/litre) and trimethoprim (5 mg/litre). This medium has added advantage of supporting the growth of the possible urogenital pathogens—*Mycoplasma hominis* and *Ureaplasma urealyticum*. Colonies on this medium are similar to those on heated blood agar.

Biochemical reactions

Catalase	+
Oxidase	+
Acid from	
Glucose	+
Maltose	–

Discussion

1. **Why blood or serum is added to the medium for culture of meningococci?**

   They promote growth of meningococci by neutralizing certain inhibitory substances found in culture media rather than by providing additional nutrients.

2. **Enumerate important bacteria causing meningitis.**
   - Meningococci
   - Pneumococci
   - *Haemophilus influenzae* type b
   - Group B streptococci
   - *Listeria monocytogenes*

3. **Name transport medium for *Neisseria meningitidis*.**

   Stuart's transport medium.

4. **Which site acts as a reservoir of meningococci?**

   The human nasopharynx is the only reservoir of meningococci.

5. **What is the carriage rate of meningococci in human nasopharynx?**

   Five to ten per cent of healthy individuals carry meningococci in nasopharynx.

6. **Name oxidase-positive organisms.**
   - *Neisseria* spp.
   - *Alcaligenes faecalis*
   - *Aeromonas* spp.
   - *Vibrio* spp.
   - *Campylobacter* spp.
   - *Pseudomonas* spp.

7. **Enumerate virulence factors of meningococci.**
   - Capsular polysaccharide
   - Endotoxins
   - IgA1 protease
   - Pili
   - Outer membrane proteins

8. **Which drugs are preferred to eradicate the carrier state of meningococci?**

   Rifampicin or ciprofloxacin are preferred to eradicate the carrier state.

9. **Name selective media for isolation of gonococci.**
   - Thayer-Martin medium.
   - Modified Thayer-Martin medium.
   - New York City medium

10. **Which species of *Neisseria* is strict aerobe?**

    Neisseria meningitidis.

11. **What is the advantage of New York City medium?**

    This medium has added advantage of supporting the

growth of possible urogenital pathogens—*Mycoplasma hominis* and *Ureaplasma urealyticum* in addition to *N. gonorrhoeae*.

12. **Which organ is the primary site of gonococcal infection in women?**

   In women, endocervix is the primary site of infection.

13. **Enumerate organisms causing non-gonococcal urethritis (NGU).**

   - *Chlamydia trachomatis*
   - *Ureaplasma urealyticum*
   - *Candida albicans*
   - *Mycoplasma genitalium*
   - *Gardnerella vaginalis*
   - *Mycoplasma hominis*
   - *Trichomonas vaginalis*

14. **How do you diagnose a case of non-gonococcal urethritis (NGU) microscopically?**

A Gram-stained smear with more than five polymorphonuclear neutrophils per oil-immersion field suggests NGU.

15. **How many serogroups of *N. meningitidis* are there?**
   Thirteen.

16. **Enumerate pathogenic lesions caused by *N. meningitidis*.**

   - Meningitis
   - Septicaemia or meningococcaemia
   - Waterhouse-Friderichsen syndrome

17. **Why vaginal mucosa of adult females is not infected by gonococci?**

   The vaginal mucosa is usually not infected in adult females because of the following reasons:

   - Stratified squamous epithelium is resistant to infection by the gonococci.
   - Acidic pH of vaginal secretions.

Corynebacterium

Corynebacteria are pleomorphic, Gram-positive bacilli arranged in V forms or palisades. They frequently show club-shaped swellings—hence the name *Corynebacterium* (from *coryne*, meaning club). The most important member of the genus is *C. diphtheriae*, the causative agent of diphtheria.

Corynebacterium diphtheriae

Morphology

They are thin, slender, non-sporing, non-capsulated, non-motile, non-acid-fast, Gram-positive bacilli of varying lengths with an average size of 3×0.3 μm. They frequently possess club-shaped swellings at one or both ends. When dividing, the bacilli snap and bend abruptly and appear as angled pairs or parallel rows of 3–4 bacilli (palisades) which resemble Chinese letters (Fig. 36.1).

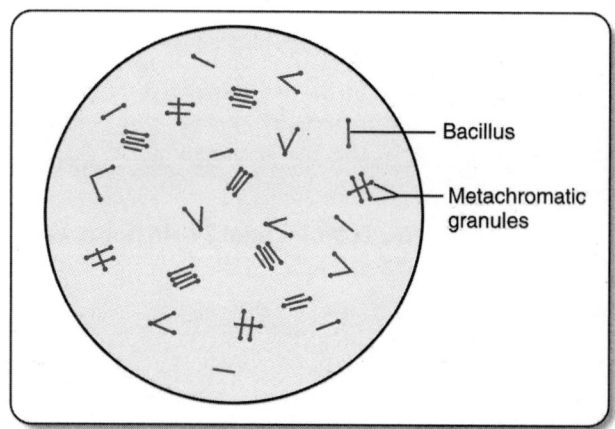

Fig. 36.1. *Corynebacterium diphtheriae* showing metachromatic granules and Chinese letter arrangement.

Although Gram-positive, *C. diphtheriae* is readily decolourised. Another characteristic of this organism is its granular and uneven staining. When stained with methylene blue or toluidine blue, the granules in the cell stain metachromatically reddish-purple. Most cells contain 2 or 3 of these, and they tend to be on the poles. With Albert's stain, the granules stain bluish-black and the cytoplasm green.

Cultural characteristics

They are aerobes and facultative anaerobes. Optimum temperature for growth is 37°C (range 15–40°C). They can grow on ordinary nutrient agar, but their growth is improved by the presence of animal proteins such as serum or blood (Colour Plate VI, Fig. 32).

Loeffler's serum slope

Diphtheria bacilli grow rapidly on Loeffler's serum slope and colonies can be seen in 6–8 hours, long before other bacteria grow. The colonies are at first small, white, opaque discs, but on continued incubation increase in size and may acquire a yellow tint.

Blood tellurite agar (BTA)

The addition of 0.03–0.04% potassium tellurite to blood agar makes the medium selective for corynebacteria by inhibiting most other pathogenic and commensal bacteria. On this medium, colonies of *C. diphtheriae* become grey to black (Colour Plate VI, Fig. 33) because tellurite or tellurous ions are able to diffuse through the cell wall and membrane and are reduced to tellurium metal, which is precipitated inside the cell. On the basis of colonial morphology on BTA, diphtheria bacilli can be divided into three biotypes—mitis, intermedius and gravis.

- *Mitis:* Colonies are grey, opaque, 1.5–2.0 mm in diameter with regular margins and glossy smooth surface. On further incubation, the colonies become flat with central elevation and regular margins—'**poached egg**' colony.
- *Intermedius:* Small (0.5–0.75 mm in diameter), grey colony with darker centre and a shining surface—'**frog's egg**'

colony. There is little change in size after 48-hour incubation.

- *Gravis:* Colonies are dull greyish-black, opaque, 1.5–2.5 mm in diameter. In 2–3 days, 3–5 mm in diameter flat colony with raised dark centre, radially striated periphery and crenated edge—**'daisy-head'** colony.

Biochemical reactions

Catalase	+
Acid from	
Glucose	+
Maltose	+
H_2S production	+
Nitrate reduction	+

The fermentation tests are usually done by culture for 24 hours at 37°C in Hiss serum sugar media.

Virulence tests of C. diphtheriae

These are of two types:

1. *In vitro*
   - Elek's gel precipitation test
2. *In vivo* (*in guinea pig or rabbit*)
   - Subcutaneous
   - Intradermal

Elek's gel precipitation test

This is a gel precipitation test. Pipette 10 ml of nutrient agar that has been cooled to 55°C in a water bath and 2 ml sterile calf serum in a petri dish and rotate 20 times to mix. Before the medium solidifies, place a 8 × 1 cm filter paper strip that has been soaked in the diphtheria antitoxin 500–1,000 units/ml across the middle of the plate on the surface of the agar. Allow the medium to solidify and then place the plate in the incubator with the lid ajar to allow the surface moisture to evaporate. Inoculate the plate within 2 hours after drying by streaking a heavy inoculum of the culture to be tested across the plate at right angles to the antitoxin strip. Parallel to this streak, at a distance of about 15 mm from it, streak a known toxigenic strain of *C. diphtheriae* on one side of the test strain and streak a non-toxigenic strain on the other side.

Incubate the plate at 37°C and examine after 24 and 48 hours. Look for white lines of precipitation a few mm from the paper strip, that extend out from the line of bacterial growth, forming an angle of about 45°. These white precipitin lines form where the toxin from pathogenic strains of *C. diphtheriae* combines with antitoxin in an optimum concentration from the paper strip, thus identifying the strains of *C. diphtheriae* that produce toxin. Look for continuity between the lines from unknown culture and that from the known toxigenic culture (Fig. 36.2).

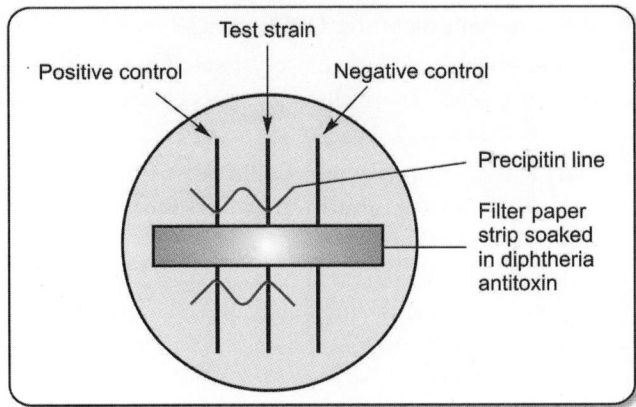

Fig. 36.2. Elek's test.

Discussion

1. **Which medium is used to obtain early growth of C. diphtheriae?**

   Loeffler's serum slope (LSS).

2. **Enumerate various advantages of Loeffler's serum slope.**
   - Growth of *C. diphtheriae* on LSS is obtained within 6–8 hours.
   - It is used for rich production of metachromatic granules.
   - It is used for growth of pure culture of *C. diphtheriae* for conducting toxigenicity test of *C. diphtheriae*.

3. **Name selective medium for C. diphtheriae.**

   Blood tellurite agar (BTA).

4. **Why does C. diphtheriae produce grey to black colonies on BTA?**

   On this medium, colonies of *C. diphtheriae* become grey to black because tellurite or tellurous ions are able to diffuse through the cell wall and membrane and are reduced to tellurium metal, which is precipitated inside the cell.

5. **Why C. diphtheriae colonies take 24–48 hours to grow on BTA medium?**

   Potassium tellurite may retard the growth even of corynebacteria, so that colonies may be very small after 24 hours, therefore, incubation should be continued for 48 hours.

6. **How many biotypes of C. diphtheriae are there?**

   Three biotypes—mitis, intermedius and gravis.

7. **Which biotype of C. diphtheriae ferments starch and glycogen?**

   Gravis.

8. **Which biotype of C. diphtheriae produces β-haemolysis on sheep or rabbit blood agar plate?**

   Mitis

9. **What do you mean by CMN group?**

The corynebacteria are closely related to mycobacteria and nocardiae. These three groups collectively may be referred to as the CMN group.

10. **Why calf or rabbit serum should be used in Hiss serum sugar media for conducting fermentation test of *C. diphtheriae*?**

Calf or rabbit serum should be used in the Hiss serum sugar media because some batches of ox and sheep sera contain a saccharolytic enzyme that gives rise to false positive results.

11. **Why does *C. diphtheriae* show Chinese letter arrangement?**

When dividing, the diphtheria bacilli snap and bend abruptly and appear as angled pairs or parallel rows of 3–4 bacilli which resemble Chinese letters. This arrangement is due to the incomplete separation of daughter cells after binary fission.

12. **What is the characteristic name given to colony of 'mitis' biotype on BTA?**

'Poached egg' colony.

13. **What is the mechanism of the necrotic and neurotoxic effects of diphtheria toxin?**

Inhibition of protein synthesis.

14. **Which strain of *C. diphtheriae* is used as a source of toxin for preparation of diphtheria toxoid?**

Park-William strain (PW8) of *C. diphtheriae* isolated in 1896, is used as a source of toxin for preparation of toxoid.

15. **What is the incubation period of *C. diphtheriae*?**

Three to four days, however, it may be as short as one day.

16. **What are the constituents of pseudomembrane produced by *C. diphtheriae*?**

Necrotic cellular material, erythrocytes, fibrin, epithelial cells, leucocytes and bacteria.

17. **Enumerate complications of diphtheria.**

- Asphyxia due to mechanical obstruction of the respiratory passage by the pseudomembrane.
- Acute circulatory failure.
- Postdiphtheritic paralysis.

18. **What are the advantages of intradermal virulence test over subcutaneous test of *C. diphtheriae*?**

The advantages of intradermal virulence test over subcutaneous are:

- Animals do not die.
- As many as 5 strains can be tested at a time on each animal (guinea pig or rabbit).

19. **Name the sources of infection of *C. diphtheriae*.**

Carriers and symptomatic patients are the sources of infection. But carriers are more important than symptomatic patients.

20. **Name tissues for which diphtheria toxin has special affinity.**

- Heart muscles
- Nerve endings
- Adrenal glands

21. **Which is the most common non-respiratory site of infection of *C. diphtheriae*?**

Skin is the most common nonrespiratory site of infection.

22. **What is the principle of Schick test?**

Toxin-antitoxin neutralization *in vivo*.

23. **What is the immunization schedule of DPT?**

DPT (diphtheria toxoid in combination with tetanus toxoid and killed suspension of pertussis bacilli) is given at the age of 6 weeks, 10 weeks, 14 weeks and 16–24 months followed by DT at the age of 5–6 years.

24. **What is the advantage of combined preparation of DPT (triple vaccine)?**

- It minimizes the number of injections.
- It also improves immune response because the pertussis vaccine acts as an adjuvant for the toxoids.

25. **What is the role of antimicrobial agents in treatment of diphtheria?**

Antimicrobial agents kill diphtheria bacilli and prevent further toxin production.

26. **Name common diphtheroids.**

Corynebacterium pseudodiphtheriticum and *C. xerosis* are common diphtheroids.

27. **How do diphtheroids differ from *Corynebacterium diphtheriae* on Gram's staining?**

Diphtheroids are strongly Gram-positive, short and thick bacilli with palisade arrangement. *C. diphtheriae* are weakly Gram-positive thin bacilli with Chinese letter arrangement.

28. **What are the constituents of LSS medium?**

Nutrient broth, glucose and calf or rabbit serum.

29. **Name one bacterium, other than corynebacteria, which produces black colonies on potassium tellurite medium.**

Staphylococcus aureus.

30. **What is the use of Hiss serum sugar media?**

Hiss serum sugar media are used for testing fermentation reactions of sugars by *Corynebacterium diphtheriae*.

31. **What type of toxin is produced by *Corynebacterium diphtheriae*?**

Exotoxin

32. **How does *Corynebacterium diphtheriae* acquire the property of toxin production?**

Only those strains of *C. diphtheriae* which are lysogenic for β phage or related temperate phages, that contain the structural gene (*tox* gene), produce diphtheria toxin. Non-toxigenic strain may be rendered toxigenic by infecting it with β phage.

33. **Why is it necessary to demonstrate exotoxin in *Corynebacterium diphtheriae*?**

It is necessary, because virulence of *C. diphtheriae* depends on the production of exotoxin.

34. **Why the disease caused by *Corynebacterium diphtheriae* is called diphtheria?**

It is named diphtheria because of leathery pseudo-membrane produced in the disease (*diphtheros* means leather).

35. **What is a Schick test?**

This is an intradermal test to demonstrate circulating diphtheria antitoxin. This test demonstrates immunity or susceptibility of a person against diphtheria.

Mycobacterium tuberculosis

Morphology

Tubercle bacilli are slender, straight or slightly curved rods with rounded ends. They measure $1-4 \times 0.2-0.8$ µm (average 3×0.3 µm) in size. In sputum and other clinical specimens, they may occur singly or in small clumps. True branching is occasionally seen in old cultures and in smears from caseous lymph nodes. They are non-motile, non-sporing, non-capsulated and acid-fast. The Ziehl-Neelsen acid-fast stain is useful in staining organisms from cultures or from clinical material. With this stain, the tubercle bacilli stain bright red, while the tissue cells and other organisms are stained blue (Colour Plate I, Fig. 3). Organisms in tissue and sputum smears often stain irregularly and have a beaded or barred appearance, presumably because of their vacuoles and poly-phosphate content. Tubercle bacilli are Gram-positive but it is difficult to stain them with the Gram stain. This is because of the failure of the dye to penetrate the cell wall.

Cultural Characteristics

Mycobacterium tuberculosis is an obligate aerobe. Optimum temperature for growth is 37°C and optimum pH is 7.0. Tubercle bacilli can grow on a wide range of enriched culture media but Lowenstein-Jensen (LJ) medium is most widely used. This medium consists of whole egg, asparagine, some mineral salts, malachite green and glycerol or sodium pyruvate and solidified by heating (inspissation). Lowenstein-Jensen glycerol medium is recommended for the isolation of human tubercle bacillus whose growth is enhanced by 0.75% glycerol, but glycerol at this concentration is inhibitory to *M. bovis*, therefore, it may fail to grow on this medium. However, when the concentration of glycerol is reduced to 0.5%, it still improves the growth of *M. tuberculosis* but, generally, does not inhibit the growth of *M. bovis*. Sodium pyruvate improves the growth of both *M. tuberculosis* and *M. bovis*. LJ medium may be made selective by addition of cycloheximide (400 µg/ml), lincomycin (2 µg/ml) and nalidixic acid (35 µg/ml)

in addition to malachite green (0.025 g/ml) to suppress bacterial and fungal contaminants.

LJ medium

M. tuberculosis grows well on LJ medium (eugonic growth). It produces visible growth on LJ glycerol medium, incubated at 37°C, in about 2 weeks, although on primary isolation from clinical material, colonies may take up to 8 weeks to appear. It grows as rough, tough and buff colonies—rough due to dry, irregular growth, tough due to difficulty in lifting the colony from the surface, and buff due to the pale yellow colour (Colour Plate VI, Fig. 34).

Glycerol broth

In glycerol broth, the hydrophobic properties of the organism's cell surface result in a whitish wrinkled pellicle and granular deposit.

Biochemical Reactions

1. Niacin accumulation

Niacin is formed as a metabolic byproduct by all myco-bacteria, but most species possess an enzyme that converts free niacin to niacin ribonucleotide. *M. tuberculosis* lacks this enzyme and accumulates niacin as a water-soluble byproduct in the culture medium.

2. Neutral red test

This test detects the ability of a strain to bind neutral red in an alkaline buffer solution. Positive tests are obtained with *M. tuberculosis*, *M. bovis* and *M. ulcerans*.

3. Catalase activity

M. tuberculosis is weakly catalase-positive. The test for myco-bacterial catalase differs from that used to detect catalase in other types of bacteria by using 30% hydrogen peroxide in a strong detergent solution (10% Tween 80) instead of the usual 3% hydrogen peroxide solution.

4. Susceptibility to pyrazinamide

M. tuberculosis is sensitive to 50 µg/ml pyrazinamide.

5. Amidase test

M. tuberculosis produces nicotinamidase and pyrazinamidase.

6. Nitrate reduction test

M. tuberculosis produces enzyme nitroreductase. Therefore, it reduces nitrate to nitrite. The test organism is suspended in a buffer solution containing nitrate and incubated at 37°C for 2 hours. Then sulphanilamide and *n*-naphthylethylenediamine dihydrochloride solution is added. Positive reaction is indicated by development of pink or red colour within 30–60 seconds.

7. Tween 80 hydrolysis

Certain mycobacteria possess a lipase that splits Tween 80 into oleic acid and polyoxyethylated sorbitol which modifies the optical characteristics of the test solution from a straw-yellow to pink. *M. tuberculosis* gives variable result.

Discussion

1. **Who first isolated the mammalian tubercle bacilli and proved its causative role in tuberculosis?**
   Robert Koch (1882).

2. **Name organisms causing tuberculosis in humans.**
   - *M. tuberculosis*
   - *M. bovis*
   - *M. africanun*

3. **Name saprophytic mycobacteria.**
   - *M. butyricum*
   - *M. phlei*
   - *M. stercoris*
   - *M. smegmatis*

4. **Why does *M. tuberculosis* often stain irregularly and have beaded or barred appearance?**
   This is due to their vacuoles and polyphosphate content.

5. **What are Much's granules?**
   These are Gram-positive and non-acid-fast form of tubercle bacilli. Much (1907) demonstrated the presence of granules in cold abscess pus where there was no evidence of acid-fast bacilli.

6. **What is the role of malachite green in LJ medium?**
   Malachite green inhibits the growth of organisms other than mycobacteria and provides a colour contrast against which colonies of mycobacteria can be easily seen.

7. **Why prolonged incubation of LJ medium is required to culture *M. tuberculosis*?**

The average generation time of tubercle bacilli is about 14–15 hours, prolonged incubation is, therefore, necessary.

8. **Describe the colonies of *M. tuberculosis* on LJ medium.**
   Colonies of *M. tuberculosis* on LJ medium are rough, tough and buff.

9. **What is the effect of sodium pyruvate in LJ medium on the growth of mycobacteria?**
   Sodium pyruvate improves the growth of both *M. tuberculosis* and *M. bovis*.

10. **What is the effect of glycerol (in LJ medium) on the growth of mycobacteria?**
    Growth of human tubercle bacillus is enhanced by 0.75% glycerol, but glycerol at this concentration is inhibitory to *M. bovis*. However, 0.5% glycerol still improves the growth of *M. tuberculosis* but generally does not inhibit the growth of *M. bovis*.

11. **Which reagent is used to demonstrate catalase activity of mycobacteria?**
    Thirty per cent hydrogen peroxide in a strong detergent solution (10% Tween 80).

12. **What is the role of detergent solution in catalase test?**
    The detergent helps to disperse the hydrophobic, tightly clumped mycobacteria from large aggregates to individual bacilli, so that catalase can be detected easily.

13. **Name disinfectants which can destroy tubercle bacilli.**
    Tincture of iodine and 80% ethanol.

14. **How do you interpret positive Mantoux test?**
    0.1 ml of purified protein derivative (PPD) containing 5 IU is injected intradermally into the skin of the volar aspect of the forearm. The site of inoculation is palpated 72 hours later. The development of an area of palpable, firm induration 10 mm or more in diameter is recorded as positive.

15. **Enumerate conditions in which tuberculin test is false negative.**
    - Early tuberculosis
    - Miliary/advanced tuberculosis
    - Measles
    - Sarcoidosis
    - Lymphoreticular malignancy
    - Defective CMI

16. **Enumerate conditions in which BCG vaccination is contraindicated.**
    - Tuberculosis
    - AIDS
    - Measles
    - Pertussis
    - Eczema

- Tuberculin positive individuals
- Patients on steroids

17. Name mycobacteria causing skin ulcers.
- *M. ulcerans*
- *M. marinum*

18. How many tubercle bacilli can be detected by culture on LJ medium?
It can detect as few as 10–100 bacilli per ml.

19. What happens when CSF is taken from a case of tuberculous meningitis and allowed to stand?
CSF from tuberculous meningitis often develops a spider web clot on standing.

20. What do you mean by positive tuberculin test?
A positive tuberculin test indicates hypersensitivity to tuberculoprotein denoting clinical or subclinical infection with tubercle bacillus, or BCG immunization.

21. Name biochemical tests to differentiate between *M. tuberculosis* and *M. bovis*.
Biochemical tests for differentiation of *M. tuberculosis* and *M. bovis* are given in Table 37.1.

Table 37.1. Differences between *M. tuberculosis* and *M. bovis*

	M. tuberculosis	*M. bovis*
Nitrate reduction	+	–
Niacin production	+	–
Tween 80 hydrolysis	Variable	–

22. How many phage types of *M. tuberculosis* are there?
There are 4 phage types of *M. tuberculosis*, i.e. A, B, C and I. Type A is the commonest type and has a worldwide distribution.

23. Name liquid media used for the growth of *M. tuberculosis*.
- Glycerol broth
- Dubos and Davis liquid medium.

24. What are the advantages of growing *M. tuberculosis* in liquid medium?
Liquid media are useful for:
- Biochemical reactions
- Preparation of antigens
- Preparation of vaccine
- Sensitivity testing.

25. Which *Mycobacterium* has not been cultured *in vitro*?
Mycobacterium leprae

26. Which *Mycobacterium* causes swimming pool granuloma?
M. marinum.

27. What do you mean by the term 'MOTT'?
Mycobacteria other than tubercle bacilli that normally exist as saprophytes of soil and water and occasionally cause opportunistic disease in man resembling tuberculosis are known as nontuberculous, environmental, opportunistic tuberculoid mycobacteria or mycobacteria other than typical tubercle (MOTT) bacilli.

28. Name the most commonly used medium for the isolation of *Mycobacterium tuberculosis*.
Lowenstein-Jensen (LJ) medium.

29. Name the solid media used for the isolation of *Mycobacterium tuberculosis*.
- Lowenstein-Jensen medium ⎫ Egg-based
- Dorset egg medium ⎭
- Middlebrook 7-H-10 medium ⎫ Agar-based
- Middlebrook 7-H-11 medium ⎭

30. Name the solidifying agent used in Lowenstein-Jensen medium.
Egg acts as solidifying agent.

31. Name the method used to sterilize Lowenstein-Jensen medium.
Inspissation.

32. Why Lowenstein-Jensen medium is prepared in universal container and not in petri dish?
Mycobacterium tuberculosis takes 2–8 weeks to grow; therefore, the medium in petri dish will get dry due to such long period of incubation.

33. How does the growth of *Mycobacterium bovis* differ from that of *M. tuberculosis* on Lowenstein-Jensen medium?
M. bovis grows poorly on LJ medium (dysgonic growth) forming small, moist, smooth, flat and white colonies which easily break up when touched. *M. tuberculosis*, on the other hand, grows well on LJ medium (eugonic growth) forming 'rough, tough and buff' colonies.

34. Name the specimen to be collected for laboratory diagnosis of renal tuberculosis.
In case of renal tuberculosis, three morning specimens of urine should be collected. 24-hour collection is unsatisfactory due to increased bacterial contamination and lower recovery rate as compared to a single voided specimen. Each specimen should consist of 50–100 ml.

35. What are the advantages of concentration of the specimens for the diagnosis of tuberculosis?
The specimens are homogenized, decontaminated and concentrated into a small volume without inactivation.

36. Name the various concentration methods used in laboratory diagnosis of tuberculosis.

- Petroff's method by using 4% sodium hydroxide.
- Dilute acids (5% oxalic acid, 3% hydrochloric acid or 6% sulphuric acid).
- N-acetyl-L-cystine with sodium hydroxide and pancreatin.

37. How is *Mycobacterium tuberculosis* differentiated from *M. bovis* on animal inoculation?

M. tuberculosis is highly pathogenic for guinea pig and virtually nonpathogenic for rabbit, while *M. bovis* is highly pathogenic for both guinea pig and rabbit.

38. Name the methods used for sensitivity testing of *Mycobacterium tuberculosis*.

- Resistance ratio method
- Absolute concentration method
- Proportion method
- BACTEC radiometric method
- Non-radiometric method
- GeneXpert system—Xpert MTB/Rif test.

39. Enumerate conditions in which tuberculin test is false positive.

False positive tuberculin test may be seen in patients infected with nontuberculous mycobacteria. These are usually low grade reactions and can be differentiated by testing with tuberculin prepared from these mycobacteria.

40. Enumerate conditions in which tuberculin test is false negative.

- Early tuberculosis
- Advanced tuberculosis
- Miliary tuberculosis
- In patients with measles and other exanthematous reactions

41. What is the full form of BCG?

Bacille Calmette-Guérin.

42. What type of vaccine is BCG?

Live-attenuated vaccine.

43. Which strain is used for preparation of BCG vaccine?

A strain of *M. bovis*.

44. What is the protective efficacy of BCG vaccine?

The protective efficacy of BCG has been determined in a number of vaccine trials. The results have varied from 80% to a total absence of protection. The consensus of opinion, at present, is that BCG does protect from tuberculosis.

45. Who classified nontuberculous mycobacteria into four groups?

Runyon.

46. Which nontuberculous *Mycobacterium* produces AIDS-related disseminated disease?

Mycobacterium avium-intracellulare.

47. What is ICRC bacillus?

Indian Cancer Research Centre, Mumbai (1962) isolated an acid-fast bacillus from a leprosy patient employing human foetal spinal ganglion cell culture. This is named as ICRC bacillus. It has been adapted for growth on Lowenstein-Jensen medium and taxonomical studies suggest that this organism is not *Mycobacterium leprae* and belongs to *Mycobacterium avium-intracellulare* group.

48. Which type of leprosy is highly infectious and why?

Lepromatous leprosy is highly infectious because lepra bacilli are numerous in the lesions.

Diagnostic Approach to Anaerobes

Anaerobes are organisms that do not require oxygen for life and reproduction. In addition, oxygen's direct toxic effect may prohibit the growth of these organisms in environment in which oxygen is present. Anaerobes outnumber aerobes at mucosal surfaces. These heavily colonized surfaces are the usual portals of entry into the tissues and bloodstream for endogenous anaerobes. Factors that commonly predispose the human body to anaerobic infections include trauma of mucous membranes or skin, vascular stasis, tissue necrosis, and decrease in the redox potential of tissue. Certain hints suggest that a given specimen is likely to contain anaerobic bacteria:

- Foul odour
- Gas in specimen
- Black discolouration of blood containing exudates. These exudates may fluoresce red under ultraviolet light involving pigmented *Bacteroides*.
- Presence of 'sulphur granules' in discharges (actino-mycosis).
- Infection secondary to human or animal bite.
- Location of infection in proximity to mucosal surface.
- Infection persists despite aminoglycoside therapy.

Specimen Collection

Collection of specimens with swab should be discouraged because they dry out and also because they expose anaerobes, if present, to ambient oxygen. Specimens collected with needle and syringe are better for anaerobic bacteriology than those collected with swab. Since anaerobes normally inhabit the skin and mucous membranes as part of the normal indigenous flora, the following specimens are always unacceptable for anaerobic culture:

- Throat swabs
- Nasopharyngeal swabs
- Gingival swabs
- Expectorated sputum or bronchoscopic specimens
- Gastric contents
- Small bowel contents
- Large bowel contents and faeces; except for *Clostridium difficile*, *C. botulinum*
- Voided or catheterized urine
- Ileostomy or colostomy effluents
- Vaginal, cervical or urethral swabs

The specimens acceptable for anaerobic culture and the collection methods that avoid contamination with normal flora are listed in Table 38.1.

Table 38.1. Acceptable specimens for anaerobic bacteriology

Source	Recommended methods of collection
Localized abscesses	Needle and syringe aspiration of closed abscesses
Sinus tracts or draining wounds	Aspiration with syringe and small plastic catheter introduced as deeply as possible through decontaminated skin orifice
Deep tissue or bone	Specimens obtained during surgery from depth of wound or underlying bone lesion
Central nervous system	Cerebrospinal fluid, aspirated abscess material, tissue from biopsy or autopsy
Dental/ENT specimens	Aspirated abscess material, biopsied tissue
Pulmonary	Percutaneous transtracheal aspiration or direct lung puncture, biopsied tissue, 'sulphur granules' from draining fistula
Pleural fluid	Thoracocentesis
Intra-abdominal	Aspirate from abscess, ascitic fluid, biopsied tissue
Urinary tract	Suprapubic bladder aspiration
Female genital tract	Culdocentesis specimen
Others	Blood, bone marrow, aspirated synovial fluid

Specimen Transport

Regardless of the type of specimen submitted for anaerobic bacteriology, it must be transported and processed as rapidly as possible and with minimum exposure to oxygen. Transporting specimens within a needle and syringe assembly is no longer acceptable because of the hazard of accidental skin puncture. The aspirate should be injected into some type of oxygen-free transport tube or vial, preferably one containing a prereduced anaerobically sterilized (PRAS) transport medium such as the Hungate tube.

Tissue specimens collected by biopsy or at autopsy from usually sterile sites are acceptable specimens for anaerobic culture. Small pieces of tissue can be placed in oxygen-free transport tubes or vials containing PRAS medium to keep the tissue moist. Larger tissues may be transported in bags or pouches containing an oxygen-free atmosphere to prevent exposure to oxygen en route to the laboratory.

Processing of Specimens

Ideally, once a specimen arrives in the laboratory, it is placed immediately in an anaerobic chamber to prevent further exposure of specimens to oxygen. All anaerobic chambers contain a catalyst, desiccant, H_2 gas (5–10%), CO_2 gas (5–10%), N_2 gas (80–90%) and an indicator. Anaerobic chambers may be fitted with airtight rubber gloves to insert hands and manipulate specimens, plates, tubes or they may be gloveless where airtight rubber sleeves fit tightly against user's bare forearms. The specimens should be processed as soon as possible in the following manner:

* Macroscopic examination of the specimen.
* Microscopic examination of the specimen.
* Inoculation of non-selective, selective, enriched and liquid media.
* Anaerobic incubation of inoculated media.

Macroscopic examination of specimen

The specimen is inspected for characteristics that include:

* Foul odour
* Black discharge or black necrotic tissue
* Sulphur granules
* Brick red fluorescence

Microscopic examination of specimen

This examination always includes a Gram stain. This helps in preliminary identification of organisms and initiation of appropriate antibiotic therapy. This also helps in selection of the media to be inoculated.

Inoculation of solid and liquid media

The ideal media for use in the culture of anaerobes are those that have been freshly prepared or stored under anaerobic conditions from the time they were made. Anaerobes have special nutritional requirements for vitamin K, haemin and yeast extract, and all primary isolation media for anaerobes should contain these three ingredients. Liquid media soon become aerobic unless a reducing agent is added. Liquid media should be prereduced by holding in a boiling water bath for 10 minutes to drive off dissolved oxygen, then quickly cooled to 37°C just before use. Different media are inoculated depending upon the organisms suspected (Table 38.2).

Table 38.2. Culture media for isolation of various anaerobes

Medium	Organisms
Brucella blood agar	All obligate and facultative anaerobes
Bacteroides bile esculin agar	*Bacteroides* and some strains of *Fusobacterium mortiferum*
Kanamycin-vancomycin-laked blood agar	*Bacteroides* and *Prevotella* spp.
Phenylethyl alcohol (PEA) agar	All obligate anaerobes and Gram-positive facultative anaerobes
Egg yolk agar	*Clostridium* spp.
Thioglycollate or cooked meat broth	All types of bacteria

Anaerobic incubation of inoculated media

Inoculated plates are incubated anaerobically at 37°C for at least 48 hours, and reincubated for another 2–4 days to allow slow-growing organisms to form colonies. The most common choices for anaerobic incubation systems are anaerobic chambers, anaerobic jars, and anaerobic bags or pouches.

Anaerobic chamber

This is an ideal anaerobic incubation system, which provides oxygen-free environment for inoculating media and incubating cultures. Identification and susceptibility tests can also be performed in anaerobic chambers.

Anaerobic jars

The most widely used anaerobic jar is the McIntosh and Fildes' anaerobic jar. Inoculated culture plates are placed inside the jar after creating anaerobic condition. The GasPak is now the method of choice for preparing anaerobic jar. The GasPak is commercially available as disposable envelope containing chemicals which generate hydrogen and carbon dioxide on the addition of water. After the inoculated plates are kept in the jar, the GasPak envelope with water added, is placed inside and the lid screwed tight. Hydrogen and carbon dioxide are liberated and the presence of a cold catalyst in the envelope permits the combination of hydrogen and oxygen to produce an anaerobic environment. Methylene blue indicator is used for verifying the anaerobic conditions in the jar. When it is placed in an anaerobic environment it is reduced from its coloured oxidized form to a colourless reduced leuco-compound.

Anaerobic bags or pouches

These bags are available commercially and one or two inoculated plates are placed into a bag and an oxygen removal system is activated and the bag is sealed and incubated. Plates can be examined for growth without removing the plates from bag, thus, without exposing the colonies to oxygen. But as with anaerobic jar, plates must be removed from the bags in order to work with the colonies at the bench. These bags are also useful for the transportation of biopsy specimens for anaerobic cultures.

Procedures for Identifying Anaerobic Isolates

Examination of culture plates

- Foul odour
- Colony morphotype on selective and non-selective anaerobic blood agar plate.
- Gram stain reaction of anaerobic isolates.

Subculture of isolates suspected of being anaerobe on following media

- Blood agar plate to be incubated anaerobically with appropriate discs—kanamycin (1 mg), colistin (10 µg), vancomycin (5 µg). A sodium polyanethol sulfonate (SPS) disc and nitrate disc may be applied for rapid identification.
- Chocolate agar plate to be incubated in CO_2 for aero-tolerance testing.
- Egg yolk agar plate for suspected lipase and lecithinase producers.

  Definitive identification of anaerobes is made by following techniques:
- Gas-liquid chromatographic analysis of metabolic end products.
- Biochemical-based and pre-existing enzyme-based mini-systems.

Discussion

1. **Define obligate or strict anaerobes.**

   Obligate anaerobes may be defined as microorganisms that cannot multiply in the presence of more than 0.5% O_2 and are killed by exposure to air within a few minutes.

2. **Define moderate anaerobes.**

   Moderate anaerobes may be defined as microorganisms that cannot tolerate an atmosphere containing more than 2–8% O_2.

3. **Define aerotolerant anaerobes.**

   Aerotolerant anaerobes may be defined as micro-organisms that are capable of growing in atmosphere containing molecular oxygen but grow best in an anaerobic environment.

4. **Classify nonsporing anaerobes.**

   (i) **Cocci**
   Gram-positive
   - *Peptococcus*
   - *Peptostreptococcus*
   Gram-negative
   - *Veillonella*

   (ii) **Bacilli**
   Gram-positive
   - *Lactobacillus*
   - *Bifidobacterium*
   - *Propionibacterium*
   - *Actinomyces*
   Gram-negative
   - *Bacteroides*
   - *Fusobacterium*
   - *Leptotrichia*

   (iii) **Spirochaetes**
   - *Treponema*
   - *Borellia*

5. **Enumerate conditions that predispose a patient to anaerobic infections.**
   - Human or animal bite
   - Road-side accidents
   - Aspiration of oral contents into the lungs after vomiting
   - Tooth extraction or oral surgery
   - Gastrointestinal or genital tract surgery

6. **Why anaerobic infection persists despite aminoglycoside therapy?**

   Because aminoglycosides are ineffective against most anaerobes.

7. **Enumerate anaerobes which produce foul-smelling end products.**
   - *Porphyromonas*
   - *Fusobacterium* spp.

8. **Enumerate reducing agents incorporated in culture media used for isolation of anaerobes.**
   - Particles of meat
   - Glucose (0.5–1.0%)
   - Ascorbic acid (0.1%)
   - Cysteine (0.1%)
   - Sodium thioglycollate (0.1%)

9. **Name three ingredients essential for growth of anaerobes.**

   Vitamin K, haemin and yeast extract.

10. **What are the advantages of GasPak system?**
    - The operation of the jar is very quick and simple.

- This system does away the need for a vacuum pump and cylinders of compressed gas.

11. What is major drawback of GasPak system?

The standard GasPak jar is not evacuated before use. Therefore, a relatively large volume of water is collected which is formed during catalysis.

12. Which catalyst is used in McIntosh and Fildes' anaerobic jar?

Alumina pellets coated with palladium.

13. What is the role of catalyst in anaerobic jar?

It converts hydrogen and oxygen into water.

14. Enumerate chemical and biological indicators for the anaerobic jar.

- *Chemical indicator:* Methylene blue
- *Biological indicator:* A strict anaerobe such as *Clostridium tetani* or *Bacteroides fragilis*, and a strict aerobe such as *Pseudomonas aeruginosa*.

15. What is the major disadvantage of any anaerobic jar system?

Culture plates have to be removed from the jar for examination. This exposes the colonies to oxygen, which is especially hazardous to the anaerobes during their first 48 hours of growth.

16. What are the advantages of anaerobic bags or pouches?

- Plates can be examined for growth without removing the plates from the bags, thus, without exposing the colonies to oxygen.
- These bags are useful for the transportation of biopsy specimens for anaerobic culture.

17. Which anaerobe fluoresces brick-red in ultraviolet light?

Bacteroides melaninogenicus.

18. Which is the commonest anaerobic coccus associated with puerperal infection?

Peptostreptococcus anaerobius.

19. What is the ratio of anaerobic and aerobic bacteria in the gut?

1000 : 1.

20. Which anaerobes are responsible for the highly acidic pH of the vagina?

Lactobacilli/Doderlin's bacilli.

21. How do you fix the smear carrying anaerobes for Gram staining and why?

Direct smears for Gram staining are methanol-fixed rather than heat-fixed. Methanol fixation preserves the morphology of bacteria and leucocytes better than heat fixation.

22. Which counterstain should be used for Gram staining of anaerobes?

Basic fuchsin. Gram-negative anaerobes frequently stain a very pale pink when safranin is used and, thus, are easily overlooked in Gram-stained smears of the specimens.

23. What is the role of laked blood in kanamycin-vancomycin-laked blood (KVLB) agar plate?

Laked blood accelerates production of brown-black pigmented colonies by certain *Prevotella* spp.

24. Why SPS disc is added to the anaerobic blood agar subculture plate?

The SPS disc is used to presumptively identify *Peptostreptococcus anaerobius*, which is susceptible to SPS.

25. Name antibiotic discs placed on the anaerobic blood agar subculture plate for identification of anaerobic isolates.

- Kanamycin (1 mg)
- Vancomycin (5 µg)
- Colistin (10 µg)

26. What is the role of bile disc in identification of anaerobes?

Bile disc is used to determine an organism's ability to grow in the presence of relatively high concentration of bile (20%), e.g., *Bacteroides fragilis*.

Clostridium

Introduction

Clostridia are anaerobic, Gram-positive, spore-bearing bacilli. Spores are refractile, oval or spherical. They may be terminal, subterminal or central in the cell. Most clostridia possess flagella and are motile except *C. perfringens*.

Clostridium perfringens (Clostridium welchii)

Morphology

They are large, Gram-positive, spore-bearing bacilli measuring 4–6 × 1 μm with straight parallel sides and truncated or slightly rounded ends. They occur singly, in pairs or in small bundles. They are non-motile and form capsule in animal body. Spores are oval, subterminal or central and non-bulging (Fig. 39.1A). They are formed under natural conditions, e.g., in the bowel. They are only rarely seen in direct smears from wounds or cultures but can be demonstrated on growth in special media such as Ellner's medium.

Cultural characteristics

It is an anaerobe, but can grow under microaerophilic conditions. Optimum temperature for growth is 37°C. It grows best on media containing carbohydrate such as glucose blood agar and forms two main types of colonies. One is round, 2–4 mm in diameter, smooth, regular, convex, amorphous, greyish-yellow and slightly opaque. Other is umbonate with an opaque brownish centre and a lighter, translucent, radially striated periphery with a crenated edge. On horse blood agar, colonies are usually surrounded by a zone of β-haemolysis and commonly also by an outer wider zone of incomplete haemolysis owing to the action of θ and α toxins, respectively (double zone haemolysis) (Colour Plate VI, Fig. 35).

Biochemical reactions

It is actively saccharolytic. When grown in cooked meat broth (CMB), they rapidly produce acid and gas but they do not

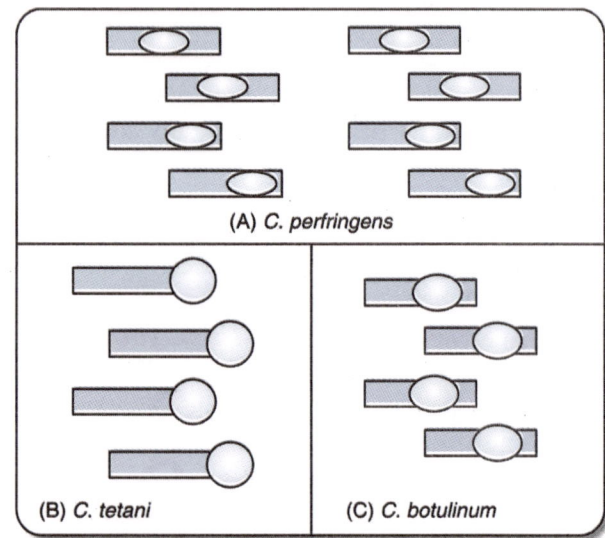

Fig. 39.1. (A) *Clostridium perfringens*, (B) *Clostridium tetani*, (C) *Clostridium botulinum*.

digest the meat. The culture may have a slightly sour smell and the meat is often reddened. It ferments glucose, maltose, sucrose, lactose and starch with the production of acid and gas. In litmus milk medium, it ferments lactose and produces acid and gas. The acid clots the milk and gas breaks up the clot resulting in *stormy clot reaction*. Production of acid is also indicated by change in the colour of the litmus from blue to red. The culture has sour butyric acid odour. It is indole negative, MR positive, VP negative and H_2S positive.

Gelatin is liquefied but coagulated serum is usually not liquefied. It produces phospholipase (lecithinase-C) which gives opalescence around the colonies on egg yolk containing medium.

Nagler's reaction

This is a useful test for the rapid detection of *C. perfringens* in clinical specimens. Several clostridia like *C. perfringens*,

C. novyi, C. bifermentans and some vibrios, produce phospholipase enzyme that gives rise to opalescence in both human serum and egg yolk containing media. The reaction produced by *C. perfringens* is specifically neutralized by *C. perfringens* antitoxin, but serologically related phospholipases of *C. bifermentans* and *C. sordellii* and some other phospholipases are also inhibited.

For rapid detection of *C. perfringens*, a culture plate containing 6% agar, 5% peptic digest of sheep blood and 20% human serum or 5% egg yolk is prepared. The plate is dried. On one-half of the plate, 2–3 drops of *C. perfringens* antitoxin are spread and allowed to dry. The plate is then inoculated with the test organisms or the exudates under study and incubated anaerobically at 37°C for 18 hours. On the section containing no antitoxin, *C. perfringens* colonies show surrounding zone of opalescence, i.e., Nagler's reaction, whereas colonies of the remainder half of the plate show no change (Fig. 39.2). Neomycin sulphate may be added to this medium to inhibit aerobic spore-forming organisms and coliforms.

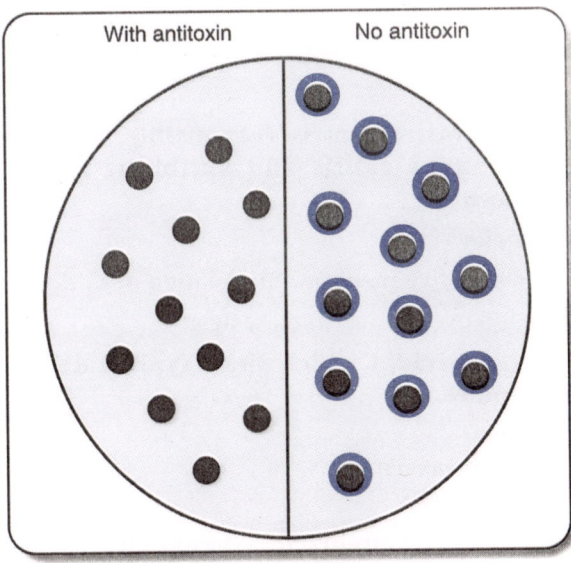

Fig. 39.2. Nagler's reaction.

Clostridium tetani

Morphology

C. tetani is a slender, Gram-positive bacillus, 2–5 × 0.4–0.5 μm with rounded ends. It tends to be pleomorphic and filamentous. It is non-capsulated and motile by peritrichate flagella. The spores are spherical, terminal and twice the diameter of vegetative cells giving them typical drumstick appearance (Fig. 39.1B). The spores do not take up the Gram stain and appear as colourless round structures.

Cultural characteristics

C. tetani is an obligate anaerobe. The optimum temperature and pH for its growth are 37°C and 7.4, respectively. It can grow well on ordinary media, but its growth is improved by the addition of blood or serum. Colonies on solid media are irregularly round, 2–5 mm in diameter with fine branching projections. Some strains form colonies with thicker, translucent, yellow brown centre and thin, colourless periphery. Isolated colonies of *C. tetani* may not be obtained because of the tendency of the organism to swarm over the surface of the medium. However, non-motile variants may produce isolated colonies.

Horse blood agar

On this medium, the colonies of *C. tetani* are surrounded by a zone of α-haemolysis, which subsequently develops into β-haemolysis owing to the production of an oxygen labile haemolysin known as tetanolysin.

Egg yolk agar

On this medium, it does not produce opalescence or pearly layer.

Cooked meat broth (CMB)

It grows well in CMB. The meat is not digested but shows slight blackening on prolonged incubation (slightly proteolyic)

Biochemical reactions

It has no saccharolytic activity.

Indole	+
MR	–
VP	–
H_2S	–
Nitrate reduction	–
Gelatin	Slowly liquefied

Clostridium botulinum

Morphology

C. botulinum is a straight or slightly curved Gram-positive bacillus with rounded ends. It measures about 5 × 1 μm in size. It is non-capsulated and motile by peritrichate flagella. It produces heat-resistant spores that are oval, subterminal and bulging (Fig. 39.1C).

Cultural characteristics

It is an obligate anaerobe. Optimum temperature for growth is 35°C, but some strains can grow and produce toxin at 1–5°C. It can grow well on routine culture media. Surface colonies are large, irregular, smooth and semitransparent with fimbriate border. On horse blood agar, all strains except those of type G are β-haemolytic. All types except G produce opalescence and a pearly effect on egg yolk agar.

Biochemical reactions

Indole	–
Gelatinase	+
Lecithinase-C activity	–

All strains except G (A, B, C$_1$, C$_2$, D, E and F) have lipase activity and ferment glucose, maltose and sucrose with the production of acid. They do not ferment lactose.

Discussion

1. **Name clostridia which are non-motile.**
   - *C. perfringens*
   - *C. tetani* type VI

2. **Which type of motility is seen in clostridia?**
   The motility is slow and has been described as 'stately'.

3. **Enumerate predominantly saccharolytic clostridia.**
   - *C. perfringens*
   - *C. septicum*
   - *C. novyi*

4. **Enumerate predominantly proteolytic clostridia.**
   - *C. sporogenes*
   - *C. histolyticum*
   - *C. bifermentans*

5. **Name one *Clostridium* which is slightly proteolytic in action.**
   C. tetani

6. **Enumerate clostridia which are obligate anaerobes.**
   - *C. tetani*
   - *C. septicum*
   - *C. novyi*

7. **Why *C. perfringens* is also called as *C. welchii*?**
   This is after the name of scientist, Welch, who first described this bacterium in detail.

8. **Which *Clostridium* produces 'stormy clot reaction' in litmus milk medium?**
   C. perfringens

9. **What do you mean by double zone haemolysis or target haemolysis?**
   After overnight incubation on horse blood agar, colonies of *C. perfringens* are surrounded by a zone of β-haemolysis due to theta (θ) toxin and also by an outer wider zone of incomplete haemolysis due to alpha (α) toxin. This is known as double zone haemolysis.

10. **Enumerate organisms which produce phospholipase enzyme and hence Nagler's reaction.**
    - *C. perfringens*
    - *C. novyi*
    - *C. bifermentans*
    - Some vibrios
    - Some aerobic spore-formers

11. **Enumerate clostridia whose phospholipase enzymes are serologically related to *C. perfringens*.**
    - *C. bifermentans*
    - *C. sordellii*

12. **Enumerate properties of alpha (α) toxin.**
    - It is lethal, dermonecrotic and haemolytic.
    - It is hot-cold haemolysin.
    - It is Ca^{++} or Mg^{++} dependent phospholipase (lecithinase-C).
    - It is thermostable.
    - It is responsible for the profound toxaemia of gas gangrene.

13. **Enumerate clostridia causing gas gangrene.**
    - *C. perfringens*
    - *C. novyi*
    - *C. septicum*
    - *C. histolyticum*
    - *C. sordellii*

14. **Name clostridia which produce swarming on solid media.**
    - *C. tetani*
    - *C. septicum*

15. **Which *Clostridium* is responsible for pseudo-membranous colitis and antibiotic-associated diarrhoea?**
    C. difficile

16. **Name selective medium for isolation of *C. difficile*.**
    Cefoxitin cycloserine fructose agar

17. **Name clostridia which show typical drumstick appearance.**
    - *C. tetani*
    - *C. tetanomorphum*
    - *C. sphenoides*

18. **Which toxin is considered as the most toxic substance known to mankind?**
    Botulinum toxin

19. **Which *Clostridium* is responsible for floppy child syndrome?**
    C. botulinum

20. **Does the food poisoning caused by *C. botulinum* lead to diarrhoea or constipation?**
    Constipation.

21. **What is the mechanism of action of botulinum toxin?**
    It is a neurotoxin which apparently acts by inhibiting the release of acetylcholine from the motor nerve endings of the parasympathetic system.

22. **Enumerate capsulated clostridia.**

- *C. perfringens*
- *C. butyricum*

23. **Why tetanus patients are isolated in the hospital?**

The reason for isolation is to protect them from noise and light which may provoke the convulsions. Tetanus patients are hardly ever infectious, and person-to-person transmission does not occur at all.

24. **Does an attack of tetanus confer immunity?**

No, an attack of tetanus does not confer immunity. Second attacks of tetanus have been recorded.

25. **What is the role of human tetanus immunoglobulin (HTIG) in patients of tetanus?**

HTIG can inactivate the unbound toxin and any further toxin that may be produced.

26. **What is the therapeutic role of botulinum toxin?**

Botulinum toxin is given as intramuscular injection to treat strabismus.

27. **How many *C. perfringens* are carried in faeces of healthy individuals?**

10^3–10^4 organisms per gram of faeces are carried in healthy individuals.

28. **Which medium is used to induce spore formation in *C. perfringens*?**

Ellner's medium.

29. **Name selective medium for the isolation of *Clostridium perfringens*.**

Willis and Hobbs medium

30. **What is the immunization schedule for individuals who have not been immunized for tetanus in infancy?**

The immunization should be carried out with 3 spaced intramuscular injections. The intervals recommended are 6–8 weeks between the first and second injections and 4–6 months between the second and third and booster doses every 10 years.

Escherichia coli

Morphology

It is a Gram-negative, non-capsulated bacillus measuring 1–3 × 0.4–0.7 µm in size. Most (about 80%) strains are motile by peritrichous flagella. The fimbriae are present on 80% of the strains. In most of the strains, these are of type I, i.e. haemagglutinating and mannose-sensitive and are found in both motile and non-motile strains. A few strains, especially those from extraintestinal infections, possess polysaccharide capsule and many other form abundant loose slime when grown on sugar-containing medium at 15–20°C.

Cultural Characteristic

It is an aerobe and facultative anaerobe. Optimum temperature for its growth is 37°C (range 10–45°C). It can grow on ordinary media like nutrient agar.

Nutrient agar

Colonies are large (2–3 mm in diameter), circular, low convex, colourless, opaque or partially translucent after 18-hour incubation at 37°C.

MacConkey agar

Colonies are red or pink in colour due to lactose fermentation (Colour Plate VII, Fig. 36).

Deoxycholate citrate agar (DCA)

The growth is partially or totally inhibited by sodium citrate and sodium thiosulphate. Colonies that form are small, pink and opaque.

Blood agar

Colonies of some strains of *Escherichia coli* are surrounded by a complete zone of haemolysis.

Biochemical Reactions

Indole	+
MR	+
VP	−
Citrate utilization	−
Urease test	−
H_2S production	−
Phenylalanine deaminase test	−
Gelatin liquefaction	−
Malonate utilization	−

Acid and gas from

Glucose	+	
Mannitol	+	
Maltose	+	Acid and gas
Lactose	+	
Sucrose	+	

Indole production and fermentation of sugars takes place both at 37°C and 44°C. Variants of *E. coli* that utilize citrate have been isolated. The citrate-utilizing ability has been shown to be controlled by a transmissible plasmid. Similarly, H_2S positive variants of *E. coli* have also been described in which the ability to produce H_2S is controlled by a transmissible plasmid.

Discussion

1. **Who first isolated *Escherichia coli*?**

   Escherich (1885) first isolated it from the faeces of an infant.

2. **Name various agents which inhibit the growth of *E. coli*.**

   * Sodium selenite
   * Sodium tetrathionate
   * Brilliant green
   * 7% sodium chloride

3. **Enumerate various toxins produced by *E. coli*.**

Systemic Bacteriology

- Enterotoxins
  - Heat-labile toxin (LT)
  - Heat-stable toxin (ST)
- Haemolysin
- Verocytotoxin

4. Which organism is the commonest cause of urinary tract infection (UTI)?

E. coli

5. Define urinary tract infection.

Urinary tract infection may be defined as the presence of bacteria undergoing multiplication in urine within the urinary drainage system.

6. What do you mean by Kass concept of significant bacteriuria?

Kass gave a criterion of active bacterial infection of urinary tract according to which a count exceeding 10^5 organisms/ml denotes significant bacteriuria and indicates active UTI.

7. Why urinary tract infection occurs more often in females?

UTI occurs more often in females than in males. This is due to short urethra, pregnancy, infrequent voiding and sexual intercourse which may lead to **'honey-moon' cystitis.** Shorter and wider female urethra appears to be less effective in preventing access of the bacteria to the bladder. The high incidence of UTI in pregnant women can be attributed to impairment of urine flow due to pressure on the urinary tract and due to hormonal changes.

8. Why there is relative infrequency of UTI in males?

Relative infrequency of UTI in males is due to following factors:

- Long urethra
- Bactericidal activity of prostatic fluid.

9. Which enterotoxin of *E. coli* is antigenically related to cholera toxin?

Heat-labile toxin-I (LT-I) is antigenically related to cholera toxin.

10. Which toxin of *E. coli* is identical to Shiga toxin?

Verocytotoxin 1 (VT1) (phage-encoded cytotoxin) is identical to the Shiga toxin.

11. Enumerate various pathogenic lesions produced by *E. coli*.

- Urinary tract infection
- Diarrhoea and dysentery
- Pyogenic infections
- Septicaemia

12. Enumerate various groups of *E. coli* causing diarrhoeal diseases.

- Enteropathogenic *E. coli* (EPEC)
- Enterotoxigenic *E. coli* (ETEC)
- Enteroinvasive *E. coli* (EIEC)
- Enteroaggregative *E. coli* (EAEC)
- Verocytotoxigenic *E. coli* (VTEC)
- Diffusely adherent *E. coli* (DAEC)

13. Which strains of *E. coli* are responsible for traveller's diarrhoea?

Enterotoxigenic *E. coli*

14. What do you mean by Sereny test?

Sereny test is used to detect enteroinvasive *E. coli* (EIEC). The organism is instilled into the conjunctival sac of guinea pig and examined after 72 hours for the production of keratoconjunctivitis.

15. What is haemolytic uraemic syndrome (HUS)?

HUS is characterized by acute renal failure, microangiopathic haemolytic anaemia and thrombocytopenia.

16. Which strains of *E. coli* are responsible for HUS?

Verocytotoxigenic *E. coli* (VTEC)

17. How do you interpret significant pyuria in a wet film of urine?

Number larger than one leucocyte per seven high power fields in a wet film of uncentrifuged urine, which corresponds with 10^4 leucocytes per ml, indicates significant pyuria.

18. Enumerate conditions in which low bacterial counts in urine may be significant.

- Patients on antibacterial drugs or diuretic drugs.
- *Staphylococcus aureus* infection.
- *M. tuberculosis* infection.

19. What type of flagella is present in *Escherichia coli*?

Peritrichous flagella.

20. Which antigens are involved in serotyping of *Escherichia coli*?

Somatic (O) antigen, capsular (K) antigen and flagellar (H) antigen.

21. What is the method of counting the bacteria in urine specimen?

A standard calibrated loop is used to culture a fixed volume of uncentrifuged urine on blood agar and MacConkey agar. The number of colonies is counted and total count per ml is calculated.

22. Define family Enterobacteriaceae.

They are aerobes and facultative anaerobes, noncapsulated, non-sporing, Gram-negative bacilli, motile by peritrichous flagella or are nonmotile. They grow readily on ordinary media, ferment glucose with production of acid or acid and gas, reduce nitrates to nitrites, oxidase-negative and catalase-positive, except *S. dysenteriae* type I which is catalase-negative.

Klebsiella

Morphology

They are Gram-negative, non-sporing, non-motile bacilli, 1–2 μm long and 0.5–0.8 μm wide with parallel or bulging sides and slightly pointed or rounded ends. They occur either in end-to-end pairs or are arranged singly. Freshly isolated strains possess a well-defined polysaccharide capsule. In the Gram-stained smears, capsule appears as an empty halo around the bacterium. Some extracellular polysaccharide is also secreted from the bacteria as loose soluble slime, accumulation of which gives mucoid appearance to the colonies. Non-capsulated and non-slime forming mutants appear from time-to-time. They form small and non-mucoid colonies.

Cultural Characteristics

Klebsiellae grow well on ordinary media in a temperature range of 12–43°C with optimum growth at 37°C. On MacConkey agar, the colonies typically appear large, mucoid and red (Colour Plate VII, Fig. 37). However, some strains are not mucoid.

Biochemical Reactions

Biochemical reactions of different subspecies of *Klebsiella pneumoniae*, and *K. oxytoca* are given in Table 41.1.

Discussion

1. **Enumerate various subspecies of *K. pneumoniae*.**
   * *Ozaenae*
   * *Pneumoniae*
   * *Rhinoscleromatis*

2. **Name indole positive species of *Klebsiella*.**
   K. oxytoca

3. **Serotyping of *Klebsiella* is based on which antigen?**
   This is on the basis of capsular (K) antigen.

Table 41.1. Differentiation of species and subspecies of *Klebsiella*

	K. pneumoniae subspecies			*K. oxytoca*
	pneu-moniae	*ozaenae*	*rhino-scleromatis*	
Indole	–	–	–	+
MR	+	+	+	v
VP	–	–	–	v
Citrate	+	v	–	+
Urease	+	–	–	+
Lactose (acid production)	+	+	–	+
ONPG	+	+	–	+

4. **How many serotypes of *Klebsiella* are there?**
   Klebsiella has been differentiated into 80 (1–80) serotypes.

5. **Which serotypes are most frequently associated with human respiratory tract infection?**
   Serotypes 1–6.

6. **Enumerate pathogenic lesions caused by *Klebsiella pneumoniae* subsp. *pneumoniae*.**
   * Hospital-associated (nosocomial) urinary tract infection
   * Wound and burn infection
   * Bronchopneumonia
   * Septicaemia
   * Meningitis
   * Diarrhoea

7. **Which *Klebsiella pneumoniae* subsp. is associated with atrophic rhinitis?**
   K. pneumoniae subsp. *ozaenae*

8. **What is the other name given to *K. pneumoniae*?**
   Friedlander's bacillus.

9. **Why colonies of *Klebsiella* spp. are mucoid?**

   Mucoid colonies are due to the presence of slime layer produced by the bacteria.

10. **What are klebosins?**

   These are bacteriocins produced by *Klebsiella* spp.

11. **Name Gram-negative bacilli, which are nonmotile.**

   - *Klebsiella pneumoniae*
   - *Shigella* spp.
   - *Burkholderia mallei*
   - *Gardnerella vaginalis*

Proteus

Tribe Proteeae, in the family Enterobacteriaceae, comprises three genera – *Proteus*, *Morganella* and *Providencia*. The tribe has a unique ability to oxidatively deaminate amino acids to the corresponding keto acids and ammonia. It is tested by growing the organism in a medium containing phenylalanine, from which phenylpyruvic acid is formed (PPA test). Genus *Proteus* has four species – *P. mirabilis*, *P. vulgaris*, *P. myxofaciens* and *P. penneri*.

Morphology

They are Gram-negative coccobacilli, 1–3 μm long and 0.6 μm wide. In young cultures, most of them are long (up to 80 μm) curved and filamentous. They may be arranged singly, in pairs or in short chains. They are actively motile by peritrichous flagella. However, non-flagellate and non-motile variants are also encountered. They also possess more than one type of fimbriae.

Cultural Characteristics

They can grow on ordinary media like nutrient agar and culture emits characteristic putrefactive (fishy or seminal) odour. *P. mirabilis* and *P. vulgaris* possess the ability to swarm (spread) on solid media (Colour Plate VII, Fig. 38). Swarming of *Proteus* appears to be due to vigorous motility of the organism. Non-motile variants do not swarm. Swarming does not occur on MacConkey agar on which smooth, colourless colonies are formed.

Dienes phenomenon

When two identical strains of *Proteus* are inoculated at different points of the same culture plate, without any swarming inhibiting substance, the resulting swarms of growth coalesce without signs of demarcation. When, however, two different strains of *Proteus* species are inoculated, the spreading films of growth fail to coalesce and remain separated by a narrow but easily visible furrow. This is known as Dienes phenomenon. It has been used to determine the identity or non-identity of various strains of *Proteus*.

Biochemical Reactions

All species of *Proteus* produce acid from glucose and no acid from lactose, mannose, mannitol, inositol, sorbitol and arabinose. They do not utilize malonate and are positive for nitrate reduction test. Differentiation of four species of *Proteus* is given in Table 42.1.

Table 42.1. Differentiation of four species of *Proteus*

	Proteus			
	mirabilis	*vulgaris*	*penneri*	*myxofaciens*
Swarming on solid media	+	+	–	–
Indole	–	+	–	–
MR	+	+	+	+
VP	v	–	–	+
Citrate utilization	v	v	–	v
Phenylalanine deaminase test	+	+	+	+
Urease production	+	+	+	+
H₂S production	+	+	–	+

Discussion

1. **Briefly describe the types of swarming exhibited by *Proteus*.**
   - *Continuous swarming:* Swarming growth on a culture plate appears as a uniform film of growth extending over the whole plate.
   - *Discontinuous swarming:* Swarming growth on a culture plate appears as a series of concentric circles of growth around the point of inoculation.

2. **Enumerate various agents which can inhibit swarming of *Proteus*.**

- Increasing the concentration of agar in the medium from 1–2% to 6%.
- Incorporating chloral hydrate (1 in 500), sodium azide (1 in 500), alcohol (5–6%) or boric acid (1 in 100) in the medium.
- Addition of bile salts in the medium.

3. **Name one unique test for tribe Proteeae.**

Phenylalanine deaminase (PPA) test.

4. **Enumerate four species of genus *Proteus*.**

- *P. mirabilis*
- *P. vulgaris*
- *P. myxofaciens*
- *P. penneri*

5. **Which species of *Proteus* is indole positive?**

Proteus vulgaris.

6. **Which species of *Proteus* shows swarming on solid nutrient media?**

- *P. vulgaris*
- *P. mirabilis*

7. **What is the characteristic odour of *Proteus* culture?**

Fishy or seminal odour.

8. **What is the use of Dienes phenomenon?**

Dienes phenomenon is used to determine the identity or non-identity of various strains of *Proteus*.

9. **Which species of *Proteus* is most frequently isolated from clinical specimens?**

P. mirabilis.

10. **Why urinary tract infection caused by *Proteus* is more serious than that caused by coliform bacteria?**

Proteus produces urease which liberates ammonia from urea. Ammonia inactivates complement, damages renal epithelium and makes the urine alkaline. The alkaline conditions lead to the precipitation of phosphates and the formation of calculi in the urinary tract. It may also lead to hyperammonaemic encephalopathy and coma.

11. **What do you understand by the term *Proteus*?**

Proteus means pleomorphism and the name is after the Greek God *Proteus* who could assume any shape.

12. **Name nonmotile strains of *Proteus*.**

- *Proteus vulgaris* OX2 strain
- *Proteus vulgaris* OX19 strain
- *Proteus mirabilis* OXK strain.

13. **What is the use of nonmotile strains of *Proteus*?**

These strains are employed as the antigens for Weil-Felix reaction.

14. **Name the three genera of the tribe Proteeae.**

Proteus, *Morganella* and *Providencia*.

15. **What is the colour of positive PPA test?**

Green.

16. **Which species of *Proteus* is ornithine decarboxylase positive?**

Proteus mirabilis.

Shigella

The genus *Shigella* is closely related to the genus *Escherichia* and belongs to the tribe Escherichieae. *Shigella* species, however, are not members of the normal gastrointestinal flora, and all *Shigella* species can cause bacillary dysentery. Genus *Shigella* has four species—*Shigella dysenteriae*, *Shigella flexneri*, *Shigella sonnei* and *Shigella boydii*.

Morphology

Shigellae are non-motile, non-flagellate, non-sporing, non-capsulate, Gram-negative bacilli measuring $2-4 \times 0.6$ μm. *S. flexneri*, with the exception of serotype 6 and some strains of other serotypes, possess fimbriae of type 1. Other species of *Shigella* do not possess fimbriae.

Cultural Characteristics

They are aerobes and facultative anaerobes, growing within a temperature range of 10–40°C and pH of 7.4. They can grow on ordinary media.

Nutrient agar

On nutrient agar or blood agar, colonies are 2–3 mm in diameter, circular, convex, smooth, greyish or colourless and translucent. Colonies of *S. sonnei* are slightly larger and more opaque than those of other shigellae.

MacConkey agar

Colonies on this medium are colourless due to the absence of lactose fermentation. However, colonies of *S. sonnei*, a late lactose-fermenter, become pink when incubation is prolonged beyond 24 hours.

Deoxycholate citrate agar (DCA)

This is a selective medium for isolation of shigellae from faeces. Colonies on this medium are smaller (1–1.5 mm in diameter) and do not form a black centre. On prolonged incubation, colonies of *S. sonnei* form pink papillae due to late lactose-fermentation.

Xylose lysine deoxycholate (XLD) agar

This is a better selective medium than DCA because it is less inhibitory to *S. dysenteriae* and *S. flexneri* than DCA. On this medium, colonies of *Shigella* are red and unlike those of most salmonellae, without black centres (Colour Plate VII, Fig. 39).

Salmonella-Shigella (SS) agar

This is a highly selective medium for the isolation of *Shigella* and *Salmonella*. Colonies of *Shigella* on this medium are colourless with no blackening (Colour Plate VII, Fig. 40).

Hektoen enteric (HE) agar

This is a useful direct plating medium for faecal specimens for the isolation of *Shigella* and *Salmonella*. This medium contains peptone, yeast extract, bile salt, lactose, sucrose, salicin, sodium chloride, sodium thiosulphate, ferric ammonium citrate, acid fuchsin, thymol blue and agar in distilled water. Acid produced from the carbohydrates and acid fuchsin reacting with thymol blue produces a yellow colour when pH is lowered. Colonies of *Shigella* on this medium are green in colour (Colour Plate VII, Fig. 39).

Enrichment media

- **Selenite F broth:** Sodium selenite in this medium inhibits coliform bacilli while permitting shigellae and salmonellae to grow. Therefore, it is recommended for the isolation of these organisms from faeces.
- **Gram-negative (GN) broth:** Enrichment of faecal specimens in GN broth for 4–6 hours and then subculturing on HE or XLD agar is an optimal technique for recovery of *Shigella* species in suspected cases of bacillary dysentery. Sodium deoxycholate and sodium citrate inhibit Gram-positive bacteria. This medium also contains 0.1% glucose and 0.2% D-mannitol. The increased concentration of mannitol over glucose limits the growth of *Proteus* species and encourages growth of *Salmonella* and *Shigella* species because both these species, with the exception of *S. dysenteriae*, can ferment mannitol.

Biochemical Reactions

Indole	v
MR	+
VP	–
Citrate utilization	–
Urease	–
H$_2$S production	–
Malonate utilization	–
Lysine decarboxylation	–
Phenylalanine deamination	–

All shigellae produce acid from glucose and with the exception of *S. dysenteriae*, from mannitol. *S. dysenteriae* serotype 1, *S. flexneri* serotype 6 and *S. sonnei* are always indole negative. *S. sonnei* is a late lactose-fermenter and forms ornithine decarboxylase. With the exception of *S. dysenteriae* serotype 1, many strains of *S. dysenteriae* serotypes 3, 4, 6 and 9, *S. flexneri* serotype 4a, and *S. boydii* serotype 13; shigellae produce catalase.

Discussion

1. **Who isolated the first member of the genus *Shigella*?**

   Japanese microbiologist Kiyoshi Shiga isolated the first member of the genus. It was then called *S. shigae* and is now known as *S. dysenteriae* serotype 1.

2. **Enumerate four species of *Shigella*.**

   * *S. dysenteriae*
   * *S. flexneri*
   * *S. sonnei*
   * *S. boydii*

3. **Which species of *Shigella* is most resistant to adverse environmental conditions as compared to other species?**

   S. sonnei

4. **What is the infective dose of shigellae?**

   The infective dose is small between 10 and 100 organisms.

5. **Which *Shigella* species is most pathogenic?**

   S. dysenteriae

6. **Enumerate toxins produced by *S. dysenteriae* serotype 1.**

   * Exotoxin (acts as enterotoxin and neurotoxin)
   * Verocytotoxin—VT1 and VT2
   * Endotoxin

7. **Which is the most predominant species of *Shigella* in India?**

   S. flexneri

8. **Which is the most prevalent species of *Shigella* in the United States of America?**

   S. sonnei.

9. **Which species of *Shigella* produces mild infection?**

   S. sonnei.

10. **Enumerate complications produced by *S. dysenteriae* serotype 1.**

    * Haemolytic uraemic syndrome
    * Intussusception
    * Parotitis
    * Toxic neuritis
    * Arthritis

11. **How will you differentiate ulcers of *Shigella* dysentery from those of amoebic ulcers?**

    The ulcers of the bacillary dysentery are much shallower than amoebic ulcers. The intervening mucosa is inflamed and oedematous in bacillary dysentery. Thus, there is diffuse involvement, unlike the amoebic dysentery in which the mucosa in between the ulcerative lesions is healthy.

12. **What is the incubation period of *Shigella* dysentery?**

    It is usually 2–3 days, but may be as short as 12 hours.

13. **Which test is used to detect *Shigella* endotoxin in the blood in toxaemia?**

    Limulus test.

14. **How many biotypes of *S. flexneri* serotype 6 are there?**

    There are three biotypes of *S. flexneri* serotype 6—Boyd 88, Manchester and Newcastle.

15. **Enumerate indole negative shigellae.**

    * *S. sonnei*
    * *S. dysenteriae* serotype 1
    * *S. flexneri* serotype 6

16. **Name the *Shigella* species which may possess fimbriae.**

    S. flexneri

17. **Which serotype of *S. dysenteriae* is most virulent?**

    S. dysenteriae serotype 1

18. **The extrachromosomal (plasmid) mechanism of drug resistance was first reported in which organism?**

    Shigella.

19. **Why shigellae tend to die in faeces within a few hours?**

    They die due to the acidity produced by the growth of coliforms.

20. **Name lactose fermenting species of *Shigella*.**

    S. sonnei is a late lactose-fermenting species of genus *Shigella*.

21. **Which serotypes of *Shigella* were first named as *S. shigae* and *S. schmitzi*?**

    S. dysenteriae serotype 1 was first named as *S. shigae*, and *S. dysenteriae* serotype 2 as *S. schmitzi*.

22. **Name the shigellae which produce acid and gas on fermentation of carbohydrates.**

    S. flexneri serotype 6, biotypes Manchester and Newcastle.

Salmonella

Morphology

Salmonellae are Gram-negative, non-sporing, non-acid-fast, non-capsulated bacilli measuring $2-4 \times 0.6$ µm. Most strains are motile by means of peritrichous flagella except *S.* serotype Gallinarun and *S.* serotype Pullorum which are non-motile. Most strains of most serotypes produce type 1 fimbriae. Most strains of *S.* serotype Paratyphi A and a few strains of *S.* serotype Paratyphi B, *S.* serotype Typhi and *S.* serotype Typhimurium fail to produce fimbriae.

Cultural Characteristics

Salmonellae are aerobes and facultative anaerobes, growing within a temperature range of 15–45°C (optimum temperature 37°C). They can grow on ordinary media.

Nutrient agar or blood agar

Colonies on this medium are 2–3 mm in diameter, greyish-white, circular, moist, convex and translucent. Rough (R) strains form opaque and granular colonies with irregular surface. They have a hydrophobic surface and tend to autoagglutinate. Due to the production of loose polysaccharide slime, many strains of *S.* serotype Paratyphi B and a few of other serotypes form large mucoid colonies.

MacConkey agar

Colonies are 1–3 mm in diameter and pale yellow or colourless due to absence of lactose fermentation (Colour Plate VII, Fig. 41).

Brilliant green MacConkey agar

This is a selective medium for the isolation of salmonellae from faeces. Salmonellae produce pale green translucent colonies. However, *S.* serotype Typhi does not grow well on this medium.

Deoxycholate citrate agar

Colonies are similar to or slightly smaller in size than those on MacConkey agar. After 48-hour incubation, the colonies may develop a black centre.

Wilson and Blair's brilliant-green bismuth sulphite agar medium

On this medium, *S.* serotype Typhi and *S.* serotype Paratyphi B form small (about 1 mm in diameter) black colonies (Colour Plate VII, Fig. 42). This is due to the reduction of sulphite to sulphide. Due to the production of hydrogen sulphide, the colonies of *S.* serotype Typhi are surrounded by a metallic sheen. Brilliant green inhibits the growth of *Escherichia coli*, *Proteus* and other commensal enterobacteria.

Xylose lysine deoxycholate agar

Most strains of *Salmonella* produce red colonies with black centres (Colour Plate VII, Fig. 42) and H_2S negative serotypes of *Salmonella* produce red colonies without black centres.

Salmonella-Shigella agar

Colonies of *Salmonella* are colourless with black centres (Colour Plate VII, Fig. 43).

Hektoen enteric agar

Colonies of *Salmonella* are blue green with black centres due to H_2S production (Colour Plate VII, Fig. 43).

Enrichment media

- **Tetrathionate broth:** It enriches salmonellae and sometimes shigellae, but permits the growth of *Proteus*.
- **Brilliant green tetrathionate broth:** Brilliant green in tetrathionate broth inhibits the growth of *Proteus*, thus makes it more selective for the growth of salmonellae. But it is also inhibitory, to some extent, to *S.* serotype Typhi and shigellae
- **Selenite F broth:** It is an excellent enrichment medium for the isolation of *S.* serotype Typhi and *S.* serotype Dublin,

but some salmonellae, e.g., *S.* serotype Paratyphi A and *S.* serotype Choleraesuis and some shigellae may fail to grow in this medium.

Biochemical Reactions

Indole	–
MR	+
VP	–
Citrate	+ (except *S.* serotype Typhi and *S.* serotype Paratyphi A)
H₂S production	+ (except strain of *S.* serotype Paratyphi A and *S.* serotype Choleraesuis)
Urease	–
Phenylalanine deaminase test	–

Acid and gas from

Glucose	+	
Maltose	+	*S.* serotype Typhi and *S.* serotype Gallinarum form acid only
Mannitol	+	
Sorbitol	+	
Lactose	–	
Sucrose	–	

Decarboxylation of

Lysine	+
Ornithine	+
Arginine	+

Discussion

1. **How many serotypes of *Salmonella* are there?**

   The genus *Salmonella* is very complex, with more than 2,500 serotypes currently, described in Kauffmann-White scheme.

2. **Name non-motile serotypes of *Salmonella*?**

   S. serotype Gallinarum and *S.* serotype Pullorum.

3. **Name selective media for isolation of *Salmonella*.**

   Wilson and Blair's brilliant-green bismuth sulphite agar, deoxycholate citrate agar, xylose lysine deoxycholate agar and *Salmonella-Shigella* agar.

4. **What is the role of selenite in selenite F broth?**

   Sodium selenite inhibits coliform bacilli while permitting salmonellae and many shigellae to grow.

5. **Name citrate negative serotypes of *Salmonella*.**

   S. serotype Typhi and *S.* serotype Paratyphi A

6. **Name H₂S negative serotypes of *Salmonella*.**

   Strains of *S.* serotype Paratyphi A and *S.* serotype Choleraesuis.

7. **Name anaerogenic salmonellae.**

   S. serotype Typhi and *S.* serotype Gallinarum.

8. **Which salmonellae do not decarboxylate ornithine and lysine?**

   S. serotype Typhi and *S.* serotype Paratyphi A.

9. **Name monophasic serotypes of *Salmonella*.**

   S. serotype Typhi, *S.* serotype Paratyphi A and *S.* serotype Enteritidis.

10. **Which serotype of *Salmonella* produces loose polysaccharide slime layer?**

    S. serotype Paratyphi B.

11. **Enumerate pathogenic lesions produced by *Salmonella*.**

    - Enteric fever (typhoid fever and paratyphoid fever)
    - Gastroenteritis
    - Septicaemia

12. **What are the complications of typhoid fever?**

    - Intestinal perforation
    - Haemorrhage
    - Circulatory collapse
    - Other complications include cholecystitis, arthritis, haemolytic anaemia, peripheral neuritis and rarely osteomyelitis.

13. **What do you mean by rose spots?**

    Rose spots are often found on the front of the chest during the second or third week of typhoid fever. These are 2–4 mm in diameter, slightly raised discrete irregular macules. They are seldom noticeable in dark-skinned patients.

14. **When should you perform faecal culture for isolation of salmonellae in a patient of typhoid fever?**

    Faecal culture should be done between third to fifth week of illness.

15. **What is the advantage of clot culture over blood culture in diagnosis of typhoid fever?**

    - Clot culture yields a higher rate of isolation than blood culture as the bactericidal action of the serum is obviated.
    - Sample of serum also becomes available for Widal test.

16. **When can you demonstrate circulating antigen of salmonellae in typhoid fever?**

    Typhoid bacillus antigens are consistently present in the blood and urine of the patient. They can be detected in the first week of illness by coagglutination test.

17. **Name oral vaccine for typhoid fever.**

    S. serotype Typhi (Ty 21a)

18. **Which serotype of *Salmonella* is associated with septicaemia?**

    Salmonella septicaemia is commonly caused by *S.* serotype Choleraesuis.

19. **Enumerate common serotypes of *Salmonella* causing gastroenteritis.**

S. serotype Typhimurium, *S.* serotype Enteritidis, *S.* serotype Newport and *S.* serotype Dublin.

20. Who first reported chloramphenicol resistance in *S.* serotype Typhi?

Agarwal (1962), for the first time reported chloramphenicol resistance in *S.* serotype Typhi.

21. Who first reported multidrug resistant *S.* serotype Typhi (MDRST)?

Paniker and Vimla in Calicut (India) in 1972.

22. Name killed vaccine of *Salmonella*.

TAB vaccine

23. Enumerate serotypes of Salmonella and other organism possessing Vi antigen.

S. serotype Typhi, *S.* serotype Paratyphi C, *S.* serotype Dublin and some strains of *Escherichia* and *Citrobacter*

24. What do you mean by Kauffmann-White scheme?

This scheme classifies salmonellae into different O serogroups, each of which contains a number of serotypes possessing a common O antigen not found in other O serogroups. Within each O serogroup, the different serotypes are distinguished by their particular H antigen or combination of H antigens.

25. How do you express antigenic formula of a *Salmonella* serotype?

The antigenic formula has three parts describing the O antigens, the phase 1 H antigens and phase 2 H antigens in that order. The three parts are separated by colons and the component antigens in each part by commas.

26. Which specimen is most appropriate for culture of *Salmonella* in first week of enteric fever?

Blood.

27. Which medium is used for blood culture in case of enteric fever?

Bile broth.

28. Which specimens are important for detection of carriers of *Salmonella*?

Faeces and bile.

29. For determining the serotype of infecting organism, detection of which agglutinin is more important in Widal test?

'H' agglutinin.

30. What are the typical clinical features of typhoid fever?

The typical clinical features of typhoid fever are stepladder pyrexia, with relative bradycardia and toxaemia.

31. What do you mean by term 'Typhoid Mary'?

Mary Mallon (Typhoid Mary) was a typhoid carrier, a New York cook, who, over a period of 15 years, caused at least seven outbreaks affecting over 200 persons.

32. What is the advantage of faecal culture in typhoid fever?

Faecal culture is particularly valuable in patients on antibiotics as the drug does not eliminate the bacilli from the gut as rapidly as it does form the blood. A positive faecal culture may detect patients as well as carriers.

33. Why urine culture is less useful than blood or faeces culture?

Urine culture is less useful because salmonellae are shed in the urine irregularly and infrequently.

34. What is anamnestic reaction?

Persons who had enteric infection in the past or who have been vaccinated with TAB vaccine may develop anamnestic response during an unrelated fever like malaria, influenza, etc. The anamnestic response shows only a transient rise of agglutinins, whereas the rise is sustained in enteric fever.

35. Which typing method is used to type *Salmonella* spp.?

Bacteriophage typing.

Pseudomonas

The genus *Pseudomonas* belongs to the family Pseudo-monadaceae which contains over 200 species. Majority of them are free-living, occurring as saprophytes in soil and water. Human disease has been caused by *P. aeruginosa*, *P. fluorescens*, *P. putida* and *P. stutzeri*.

Pseudomonas aeruginosa

Morphology

It is a slender, Gram-negative bacillus, 1.5–3.0 × 0.5 μm, arranged singly, in pairs or short chains. It is non-sporing, non-capsulate, though mucoid strains may sometime occur and usually motile by one or two polar flagella.

Cultural characteristics

It is strict aerobe and grows well on ordinary media. It can grow over a temperature range of 5–42°C, the optimum temperature being 37°C.

Nutrient agar

After aerobic incubation on nutrient agar at 37°C for 24 hours, the colonies are large, 2–3 mm in diameter, smooth, translucent, irregularly round (Colour Plate VII, Fig. 44) and emit a characteristic fruity odour. Mucoid strains often produce copious amounts of an extracellular polysaccharide on agar culture.

MacConkey agar

It produces non-lactose-fermenting colonies.

Blood agar

Many strains are haemolytic on blood agar.

P. aeruginosa produces at least 4 distinct pigments:

1. *Pyocyanin:* It is bluish-green phenazine pigment soluble in chloroform and water. It diffuses into the surrounding medium. This pigment is not produced by other species of this genus, therefore, its detection is diagnostic of *P. aeruginosa*.
2. *Pyoverdin (fluorescein):* It is soluble in water but not in chloroform. It imparts a yellowish tinge to the cultures.
3. *Pyorubin:* It is bright red water soluble pigment. It is a phenazine pigment that is insoluble in chloroform.
4. *Pyomelanin:* It is brown to black pigment and its production is uncommon.

Biochemical reactions

The metabolism of *P. aeruginosa* is oxidative and non-fermentative.

Catalase	+
Oxidase	+
Indole	–
MR	–
VP	–
H_2S production	–
Nitrate reduction to N_2 gas	+
Arginine dihydrolase	+
Gelatinase	+

Discussion

1. **Why culture of *Pseudomonas aeruginosa* emits a characteristic fruity odour?**

   This is due to the production of aminoacetophenone from tryptophan.

2. **Enumerate pigments produced by *P. aeruginosa*.**
   - Pyocyanin
   - Pyoverdin
   - Pyorubin
   - Pyomelanin

Systemic Bacteriology

4

3. **What is the chemical nature of pyocyanin produced by *P. aeruginosa*?**

It is a phenazine pigment.

4. **Does pigment produced by *P. aeruginosa* diffuse into the medium.**

Yes

5. **Which pigment produced by *P. aeruginosa* is soluble in chloroform?**

Pyocyanin

6. **Name the pigment which is produced only by *P. aeruginosa*.**

Pyocyanin

7. **Name one disinfectant to which *Pseudomonas* is sensitive.**

It is sensitive to 2% aqueous alkaline solution of glutaraldehyde (*cidex*).

8. **Name virulence factors of *P. aeruginosa*.**

- Proteases (general protease, alkaline protease and elastase)
- Haemolysins
- Exotoxin
- Endotoxin

9. **Name selective medium used for isolation of *P. aeruginosa*.**

Cetrimide agar.

10. **Enumerate common infections caused by *P. aeruginosa*.**

- Urinary tract infection
- Meningitis
- Necrotizing pneumonia
- Septicaemia
- Wound and burn infection
- Chronic otitis media and otitis externa.

11. **Why *P. aeruginosa* is dominant bacterium in mixed infections?**

P. aeruginosa produces pyocyanin pigment, which inhibits the growth of many other bacteria.

12. **Why *P. aeruginosa* is frequently responsible for nosocomial infections?**

P. aeruginosa is important causative agent of nosocomial infections due to following reasons:

- It is resistant to commonly used antibiotics and antiseptics.
- It can survive and multiply even with minimal nutrients, if moisture is available.
- It can contaminate equipment such as respirators, endoscopes and articles such as bed pans and medicines such as lotions, ointments and eye drops.

13. **Which medium is used for detection of oxidative metabolism of *P. aeruginosa*?**

An ammonium salt medium in which the sugar is the only carbon source is used for oxidative metabolism of *Pseudomonas*.

14. **How does pyocyanin act as virulence factor?**

Pyocyanin inhibits mitochondrial enzymes in mammalian tissue and causes disruption and cessation of ciliary beat on ciliated nasal epithelium. This favours colonization of the organism in the nasal mucosa by avoiding clearance from respiratory mucosa by primary host defences.

15. **Name one species of *Pseudomonas* which can grow at 42°C.**

P. aeruginosa.

16. **What are important tests to identify non-pigment producing *P. aeruginosa*.**

- Oxidative metabolism of sugars.
- Positive oxidase test.
- Ability to reduce nitrate to nitrogen gas.
- Growth at 42°C.

17. **Enumerate epidemiological typing methods of *P. aeruginosa*.**

- Bacteriocin (pyocin) typing
- Serotyping
- Restriction endonuclease typing

18. **Name pigments enhancing media of *Pseudomonas*.**

- *Pseudomonas* isolation agar.
- King's medium (A and B)

19. **Name non-fermenting organisms other than *Pseudomonas*.**

- *Alcaligenes faecalis*
- *Acinetobacter* spp.
- *Eikenella corodens*
- *Flavobacterium meningosepticum*

20. **Name a member of family pseudomonadaceae which is oxidase-negative.**

Stenotrophomonas maltophilia.

21. **Name a member of family Pseudomonadaceae which is nonmotile.**

Burkholderia mallei.

22. **Which type of flagellum/flagella is/are present in *Pseudomonas aeruginosa*.**

One or two polar flagella.

23. **Why is surface pellicle formed by *Pseudomonas aeruginosa* in liquid medium?**

Pseudomonas, being a strict aerobe, tends to collect on the surface for more oxygen.

24. Name non-lactose fermenting organisms other than *Pseudomonas* **spp.**

- *Proteus* spp.
- *Morganella morganii*
- *Providencia* spp.
- *Vibrio cholerae*
- *Stenotrophomonas maltophilia*
- *Salmonella* spp.
- *Shigella* spp.
- *Burkholderia* spp.

Vibrio

The genus *Vibrio* belongs to the family Vibrionaceae. Genus *Vibrio* has more than 110 species. The most important pathogens of man are *V. cholerae*, *V. parahaemolyticus* and *V. vulnificus*.

Vibrio cholerae

Morphology

These are short, curved or comma-shaped rods with rounded or pointed ends and 1.5–2.5 × 0.5–0.8 µm in size. S forms or spirals may be seen due to two or more cells lying end-to-end (Fig. 46.1). In old cultures, they are frequently highly pleomorphic. They show vigorous darting motility which is mediated by a single polar flagellum. They are Gram-negative, non-sporing, non-capsulated and non-acid-fast.

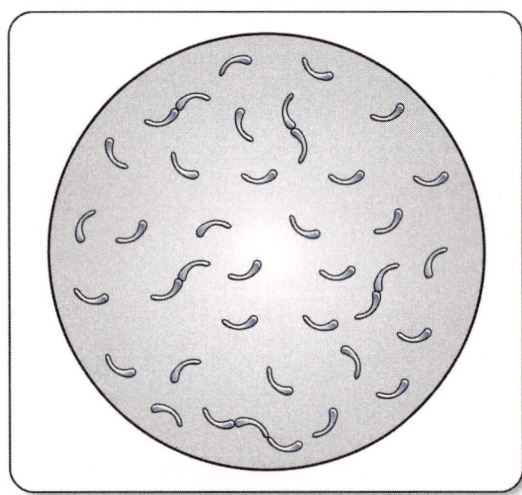

Fig. 46.1. *Vibrio cholerae.*

Cultural characteristics

V. cholerae is aerobe and facultative anaerobe, but under anaerobic conditions only scanty and slow growth is obtained.

It grows within a temperature range of 16–40°C (optimum temperature 37°C). Growth occurs freely between pH 7.4 and 9.6 (optimum pH 8.2). *V. cholerae* is a non-halophilic vibrio. It cannot grow in media with a concentration of sodium chloride more than 5%. However, it can grow in media without any sodium chloride. On the other hand, halophilic vibrios like *V. parahaemolyticus* can grow in media containing 7–10% sodium chloride and cannot grow in media lacking it.

On nutrient agar, after overnight incubation at 37°C, the colonies are glistening translucent discs, 1–2 mm in diameter with bluish or greenish tinge in transmitted light. On MacConkey agar, they are smaller than those on nutrient agar and are colourless, but become reddish on prolonged incubation due to the late fermentation of lactose. On horse blood agar, classical biotype does not produce haemolysis although some strains produce greenish discolouration around individual colonies which later becomes clear due to haemodigestion. However, colonies of El Tor biotype are haemolytic.

In a gelatin stab, at first a white line of growth appears along the track of the inoculating wire. Liquefaction of gelatin begins at the top which spreads downwards in a funnel-shaped form (infundibuliform appearance) in 3 days at 22°C. In peptone water, this organism grows as a surface pellicle because of its affinity for oxygen. The surface pellicle becomes visible in 6–9 hours.

Special media

A number of special culture media have been employed for the cultivation of *V. cholerae*. They may be classified as under:

Transport (holding) media

Venkataraman-Ramakrishnan (VR) medium: It is prepared by dissolving 20 g common salt and 5 g peptone in 1 litre of distilled water and pH is adjusted to 8.6–8.8. It is dispensed in screw-capped bottles in 10–15 ml amounts. About 1–3 g of stool is added to each bottle. *V. cholerae* does not multiply but remain viable for several weeks. Moreover, it prevents overgrowth by other organisms.

Cary-Blair medium

This medium is buffered solution of disodium hydrogen phosphate, sodium thioglycollate, sodium chloride and calcium chloride at pH 8.4.

Enrichment media

- *Alkaline peptone water (APW):* This medium contains 1% each of peptone and sodium chloride at pH 8.6. This is also an excellent transport medium. About 1 g of the stool or a rectal swab should be placed into 10 ml of APW in a screw-capped bottle and transported to the laboratory. Subcultures on plating media should be done within 3–6 hours because other organisms can begin to overgrow after prolonged incubation
- *Monsur's taurocholate tellurite peptone water:* In 1 litre distilled water, dissolve peptone, sodium chloride and sodium taurocholate in amounts of 10 g, 10 g and 5 g respectively. Adjust pH at 9.0, distribute in 20 ml amounts and autoclave at 121°C for 15 minutes. To make the medium more selective for vibrios, add sterile potassium tellurite solution to the autoclaved medium to give a final concentration of 1 in 200,000. Place about 1 g stool or a rectal swab in the medium and transport to the laboratory. Subculture a loopful onto a selective plating medium within 6–8 hours at ambient temperature. Also, incubate it overnight at 37°C and subculture again on a plating medium next day.

Plating media

- *Alkaline bile salt agar (BSA) pH 8.2:* This is modified nutrient agar medium containing 0.5% sodium taurocholate (bile salt). The colonies on BSA are similar to those on nutrient agar medium.
- *Monsur's gelatin taurocholate trypticase tellurite agar (GTTA) medium:* This medium is useful for the isolation of cholera and other vibrios from faeces. High pH and potassium tellurite, in this medium are inhibitory to most enterobacteria (except *Proteus*) and Gram-positive bacteria. After 24-hour incubation, vibrios produce small (1–2 mm) translucent colonies with greyish-black centre and a turbid halo, due to hydrolysis and denaturation of gelatin. After 48-hour incubation, colonies increase in size to 3–4 mm.
- *Thiosulphate citrate bile sucrose (TCBS) agar:* This is most commonly used selective plating medium for vibrios. This medium resembles DCA except that it contains sucrose instead of lactose. Sucrose-fermenting vibrios such as *V. cholerae* form yellow colonies and non-sucrose-fermenters such as *V. parahaemolyticus* blue green ones (Colour Plate VIII, Fig. 45).

Biochemical reactions

Catalase	+
Oxidase	+
Indole	+
MR test	–
VP test	+ (El Tor biotype)
Nitrate reduction test	+
Acid from	
Glucose	+
Sucrose	+
Mannitol	+
Maltose	+
Mannose	+
Lactose	Late lactose fermenter
Gelatin liquefaction	+
Decarboxylation of	
Lysine	+
Ornithine	+

Cholera red reaction

V. cholerae is strongly indole positive and reduces nitrates to nitrites. These two properties contribute to the 'cholera red reaction', the development of a red colour when concentrated sulphuric acid is added to a 4-day-old culture at 37°C in peptone water. It is due to the formation of nitrosoindole which is red in colour.

Discussion

1. **Enumerate species of genus *Vibrio* which are pathogenic to man.**
   - *V. cholerae*
   - *V. parahaemolyticus*
   - *V. vulnificus*

2. **What is the characteristic motility of *V. cholerae*?**
   Darting motility

3. **How much sodium chloride concentration is tolerated by *V. cholerae*?**
   V. cholerae can tolerate sodium chloride concentration up to 5%.

4. **What do you mean by term 'halophilic vibrios'?**
   Halophilic vibrios can grow in media containing 7–10% sodium chloride, and cannot grow in media lacking it.

5. **Enumerate halophilic vibrios.**
   - *V. parahaemolyticus*
   - *V. vulnificus*
   - *V. alginolyticus*

6. **Which type of colonies are produced by *V. cholerae* on MacConkey agar.**

Colonies are colourless after 24-hour incubation, but become reddish on prolonged incubation due to late fermentation of lactose.

7. **Name late lactose fermenting organisms.**
   - *V. cholerae*
   - *Shigella sonnei*

8. **Which biotype of *V. cholerae* produces haemolysis on blood agar plate?**

   El Tor biotype.

9. **Enumerate transport media of *V. cholerae*.**
   - Venkataraman-Ramakrishnan (VR) medium.
   - Cary-Blair medium

10. **Why there is need of transport media for *V. cholerae*?**

    V. cholerae is quite sensitive to drying, exposure to sunlight and extreme changes in pH. It is also inhibited by normal intestinal flora. So if the cultures cannot be put up immediately, then the stool samples should be transported in transport media.

11. **What alternative can be used, if transport medium is not available?**

    If a transport medium is not available, a 5 × 1.5 cm strip of thick blotting paper can be soaked in the faecal matter, then placed in a sealed plastic bag, and sent to the laboratory.

12. **What should be the pH of alkaline peptone water (APW).**

    The pH of APW should be 8.6.

13. **What is the advantage of high pH of APW?**

    High pH of the medium suppresses the growth of many commensal intestinal bacteria while permitting uninhibited growth of *V. cholerae*.

14. **Which organism shows cholera red reaction?**

    V. cholerae.

15. **How many biotypes of *V. cholerae* are there?**

    Two biotypes—classical and El Tor.

16. **Differentiate between classical and El Tor biotypes of *V. cholerae*.**

    Differences between classical and El Tor biotypes of *V. cholerae* are given in Table 46.1.

17. **Why vibrios do not survive in grossly contaminated water, such as the Ganges water in India?**

    This is perhaps due to the presence of a large number of vibriophages in this water.

18. **Which biotype of *V. cholerae* is hardier?**

    El Tor.

19. **How many serogroups of *V. cholerae* are there?**

    There are 139 serogroups or serovars which depend upon 139 different 'O' antigens.

Table 46.1. Differences between classical and El Tor biotypes of *V. cholerae*

Property	Biotype	
	Classical	El Tor
Voges-Proskauer test	–	+
Agglutination of fowl RBCs	–	+
Haemolysis of sheep RBCs	–	+
Sensitivity to:		
Polymyxin B	+	–
Mukerjee's group IV phage	+	–
Basu and Mukerjee's group V phage	–	+

20. **Name choleragenic serogroups of *V. cholerae*.**

    Two recognized choleragenic serogroups of *V. cholerae* are serogroups O1 and O139.

21. **What do you mean by non-O1, non-O139 vibrios?**

    The serogroups (O2–O138) are referred to as non-O1, non-O139, vibrios. Serogroups O2–O138 are known as non-cholera vibrios or non-agglutinable (NAC) vibrios as they are not agglutinated by O1 antiserum.

22. **How many subtypes of O1 serogroup of *V. cholerae* are there?**

    O1 serogroup can be further subdivided into three subtypes—Ogawa, Inaba and Hikojima.

23. **What is the characteristic of stool in *V. cholerae* infection?**

    The cholera stool is typically a colourless watery fluid with flecks of mucus and hence called rice water stool.

24. **Which serogroups of *V. cholerae* show positive CAMP test?**

    V. cholerae O1 and O139.

25. **Enumerate sucrose-fermenting vibrios.**
    - *V. cholerae*
    - *V. alginolyticus*

26. **Enumerate vaccines for prophylaxis of cholera disease.**
    - Killed cholera vaccine
    - Live vaccine
    - B subunit toxoid vaccine.

27. **Describe the mechanism of action of cholera toxin.**

    It consists of subunit A and B. The A is active subunit and B is binding subunit. The subunit A stimulates cell bound adenylate cyclase. This, in turn, converts ATP to cyclic adenosine monophosphate (CAMP) in the gut epithelial cells (enterocytes). This causes an irreversible hypersecretion of electrolytes and water out of the cell and into the lumen of the intestine.

28. **Which species of *Vibrio* shows positive 'string test'?**

    V. cholerae.

29. **Which biotype of *V. cholerae* was responsible for seventh pandemic of cholera?**

    El Tor.

30. **Which biotype of *V. cholerae* is responsible for mild and asymptomatic infections.**

    El Tor

31. **Which species of *Vibrio* is responsible for food poisoning?**

    V. parahaemolyticus

32. **What do you mean by Kanagawa phenomenon?**

    Strains of *V. parahaemolyticus* associated with gastro-enteritis lyse human erythrocytes in Wagatsuma's agar, a special high salt mannitol medium. This haemolysis is known as Kanagawa phenomenon and is due to a heat-stable haemolysin.

Spirochaetes

Treponema

Treponemes are slender spirochaetes with fine spirals and pointed ends. Some of them are pathogenic for man, while others occur as commensals in mouth and genitalia. *Treponema* species pathogenic for man include the causative agents of venereal syphilis (*T. pallidum*), and non-venereal treponematoses—yaws (*T. pertenue*), endemic syphilis (*T. endemicum*) and pinta (*T. carateum*).

Treponema pallidum

Morphology

It is a thin, delicate, long, motile, flexible organism which is twisted spirally around its long axis. It is 6–14 μm long. Its width is 0.13 μm in dried state, but is about 0.2 μm in the wet living state, which is just great enough for resolution with the light microscope. It has 6–12 coils which are remarkably evenly disposed at 1 μm intervals and the amplitude of spirals is 1–1.5 μm. They have tapering ends. It is actively motile exhibiting flexion and extension, translatory and corkscrew-like motility. As the spirochaete moves across the dark-field of the microscope, it often displays a characteristic tendency to bend at right angle near its midpoint. These secondary curves appear and disappear but its primary spirals remain unchanged.

T. pallidum cannot be seen under the light microscope in wet films. Its morphology and motility can be seen under the dark ground microscope (Fig. 47.1). It cannot be stained by simple aniline dyes or by Gram's method. By prolonged Giemsa staining, it stains pale pink. It can be stained by silver impregnation methods. Fontana's method is useful for staining films, and Levaditi's method for tissue section. By immuno-fluorescence method, treponemes can be detected in tissues and body fluids.

Ultrastructurally, *T. pallidum* possesses usually three but occasionally four endoflagella attached subterminally at each

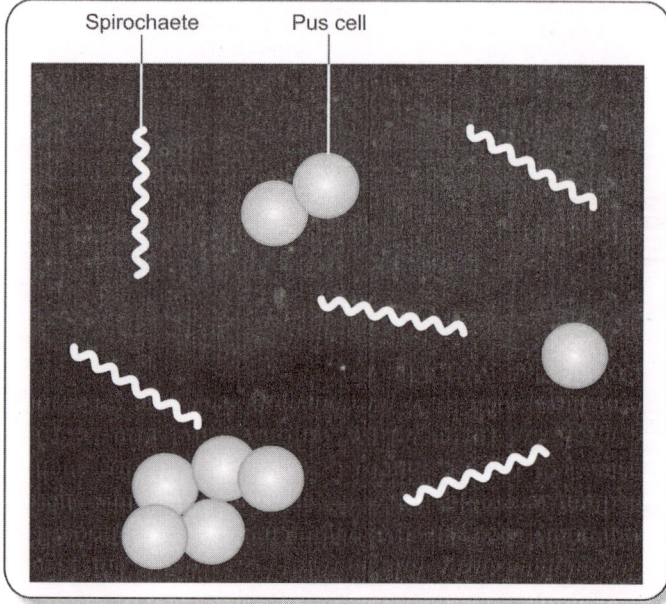

Fig. 47.1. Dark-ground illumination preparation of serous exudate from primary syphilitic chancre.

end of the cell and extend towards the opposite pole between outer membrane and peptidoglycan layer of cell wall.

Cultivation

Pathogenic treponemes cannot be cultivated in artificial media and are maintained by subculture in susceptible animals. Nichols strain of *T. pallidum* has been maintained, in rabbit testis, for several decades by serial testicular passages since it was isolated in 1913 from CSF of a patient with neuro-syphilis. Cultivable treponemes such as *T. phagedenis* (Reiter treponeme) and *T. refringens* are nonpathogenic. They can be grown under strictly anaerobic conditions in Smith-Noguchi medium or in digest broth enriched with serum.

Discussion

1. **How many endoflagella per cell are present in genus *Treponema*?**

   Three but occasionally four.

2. **Which type of motility is seen in *Treponema pallidum*?**

   T. pallidum is actively motile exhibiting flexion and extension, translatory and corkscrew-like motility. As the spirochaete moves across the dark-field of the microscope, it often displays a characteristic tendency to bend at right angle near its midpoint. The secondary curves appear and disappear but its primary spirals remain unchanged.

3. **What is the method of cultivation of pathogenic treponemes?**

   Pathogenic treponemes cannot be cultivated in artificial media and are maintained by subculture in susceptible animals.

4. **What is the method of cultivation of nonpathogenic treponemes?**

   Nonpathogenic treponemes can be cultivated in Smith-Noguchi medium or in digest broth enriched with serum under strict anaerobic conditions.

5. **Which disease is caused by *T. pallidum*?**

   T. pallidum causes syphilis.

6. **What is the incubation period of syphilis?**

   It is about a month (range 10–90 days).

7. **Can you preserve *T. pallidum* by lyophilization?**

   No, lyophilization (freeze-drying) kills the *T. pallidum*.

8. **How can you prevent transfusion syphilis?**

   Transfusion syphilis can be prevented by storing blood for at least 5 days in the refrigerator before transfusion.

9. **Name specific antigens of *T. pallidum*.**

   There are two types of specific antigens:

   - Group-specific antigen.
   - Species-specific antigen.

10. **Enumerate routes of transmission of syphilis?**

    - Sexual intercourse.
    - Blood transfusion.
    - Congenital (mother to foetus)

11. **How many stages of syphilis are there?**

    There are four stages of syphilis:

    - Primary syphilis
    - Secondary syphilis
    - Latent syphilis
    - Tertiary syphilis

12. **Which type of chancre is produced in primary syphilis?**

    Hard chancre. It is also known as Hunterian chancre, after John Hunter who produced the lesion on himself experimentally.

13. **What are the characteristic features of regional lymph nodes in primary syphilis?**

    The lymph nodes are swollen, discrete, rubbery and non-tender.

14. **Name the organs involved in tertiary syphilis.**

    Tertiary syphilis involve following sites:

    - Heart and aorta
    - Joints
    - Central nervous system
    - Skin and mucous membrane.

15. **What important precautions should be taken in the collection of serum which exudes from lesions of primary syphilis?**

    Following precautions should be taken:

    - The surface of the lesion should be cleansed with a gauze swab soaked in warm normal saline.
    - Serum which exudes should be free from blood.

Bacteriological Examination of Water

Introduction

Water is one of the chief vehicles of gastrointestinal diseases. Water is said to be contaminated or polluted when it contains infective and parasitic agents, poisonous chemical substances, industrial or other wastes or sewage. Therefore, water for human consumption must be free from chemical substances and microorganisms which may cause disease in man.

Collection of Water Samples

Water sample should be collected in heat-sterilized glass bottle of 230 ml with ground glass stopper. To neutralize the bactericidal effect of chlorine in water, it should contain 0.23 ml of a fresh 1.8% aqueous solution of sodium thiosulphate. To collect sample from a tap, clean the tap from outside. Turn on the tap at maximum flow rate and let the water flow for 2–3 minutes. Then open the stopper, fill the bottle, replace the stopper and wrap the bottle in a craft paper. The water sample should be properly labelled with full details of the source, time and date of collection and it should be delivered to the laboratory as quickly as possible, at least within 6 hours, in a cool container and protected from light.

Bacteriological Examination

Total coliform (presumptive coliform) count

This test is called presumptive coliform count because the reaction observed may occasionally be due to the presence of some other organisms.

Double strength and single strength MacConkey broth containing bromocresol purple indicator in bottles or tubes containing inverted Durham's tubes for indication of gas production is used. Measured amount of water sample is added by sterile graduated pipettes as under:

1. One, 50 ml volume of water to 50 ml double strength medium.
2. Five, 10 ml volumes of water each to 10 ml double strength medium.
3. Five, 1 ml volumes of water each to 5 ml single strength medium.
4. Five, 0.1 ml volumes of water each to 5 ml single strength medium.

The inoculated tubes/bottles are incubated at 37°C for 48 hours. The presumptive coliform count per 100 ml is determined from the tubes/bottles showing acid and gas production using the probability table. The probability table with one 50 ml and five each of 10 ml and 1 ml of water is given in Table 48.1.

The presumptive coliform count of water is interpreted as:

Presumptive coliform count/100 ml	Quality of water for human consumption
0	Excellent
1–3	Satisfactory
4–10	Suspicious
> 10	Unsatisfactory

Faecal Coliform and Confirmed Escherichia coli Count

Eijkman test

Some spore-bearing bacteria give false positive reactions in the presumptive coliform tests. Therefore, it is necessary to confirm the presence of true (faecal) coliform bacilli. After the usual presumptive test, subcultures are made from all the tubes/bottles showing acid and gas to fresh tubes of single

Quantity of water	50 ml	10 ml	1 ml	
No. of samples of each quantity tested	1	5	5	
	0	0	0	0
	0	0	1	1
	0	0	2	2
	0	1	0	1
	0	1	1	2
	0	1	2	3
	0	2	0	2
	0	2	1	3
	0	2	2	4
	0	3	0	3
	0	3	1	5
	0	4	0	5
	1	0	0	1
	1	0	1	3
	1	0	2	4
	1	0	3	6
	1	1	0	3
	1	1	1	5
	1	1	2	7
	1	1	3	9
	1	2	0	5
	1	2	1	7
	1	2	2	10
	1	2	3	12
	1	3	0	8
	1	3	1	11
	1	3	2	14
	1	3	3	18
	1	3	4	20
	1	4	0	13
	1	4	1	17
	1	4	2	20
	1	4	3	30
	1	4	4	35
	1	4	5	40
	1	5	0	25
	1	5	1	35
	1	5	2	50
	1	5	3	90
	1	5	4	160
	1	5	5	180 +

Table 48.1. McCrady probability table

Left column label (vertical): Number giving positive reaction (acid and gas)

Right column label (vertical): Probable number of coliform bacilli in 100 ml of water

strength MacConkey broth warmed to 44°C in thermostatically, controlled water bath and examined after 24 hours. Those tubes showing gas in Durham's tube contain *Escherichia coli*. It can be further confirmed by plating on solid media and testing for indole production and citrate utilization.

Discussion

1. **Enumerate characteristic features of water for human consumption.**
   - Water for human consumption must be free from chemical substances and microorganisms.
   - Water should be pleasant to drink; i.e. cool, clear, colourless and devoid of disagreeable taste or smell.

2. **Enumerate water-borne pathogens.**
   - **Viruses:** Hepatitis A virus, hepatitis E virus, poliovirus and rotavirus.
   - **Bacteria:** *Vibrio cholerae, Salmonella typhi, S. paratyphi* A, B and C, *E. coli, Campylobacter, Shigella* spp., *Yersinia enterocolitica.*
   - **Protozoa:** *Entamoeba histolytica, Giardia lamblia, Balantidium coli, Cryptosporidium parvum, Cytoisospora belli.*
   - **Helminths:** *Ascaris lumbricoides, Enterobius vermicularis, Trichuris trichiura, Echinococcus granulosus.*
   - **Pathogens borne by aquatic hosts:** *Dracunculus medinensis* and *Diphylobothrium latum* through Cyclops, and schistosomes through snail.

3. **Enumerate indicator organisms of faecal contamination of water.**
   - Coliforms (presumptive coliforms)
   - Faecal or thermotolerant coliforms
   - Faecal *Escherichia coli*
   - Faecal streptococci
   - Sulphite-reducing clostridia
   - *Pseudomonas aeruginosa*

4. **Enumerate characteristic features of indicator organisms of faecal contamination of water.**
   - These organisms should be present in the faeces in large number.
   - They should be unable to grow in water.
   - They should be more resistant than pathogens to stresses of aquatic environment and chlorination.

5. **What is the aim of bacteriological examination of water?**

   The aim of bacteriological examination of water is to detect whether pollution by pathogenic organisms has taken place or not. But it is impracticable to detect the presence of all the different kinds of water-borne pathogens, any of which may be present only intermittently. Therefore, indicator organisms of human/animal faecal pollution are used.

6. **Which indicator is added in MacConkey broth?**

   Bromocresol purple.

7. **Enumerate standard tests usually employed for water bacteriology.**

- Multiple tube test
  - Total coliform (presumptive coliform) count
  - Eijkman test
  - Count of faecal streptococci
  - Count of *Clostridium perfringens*
- Membrane filtration test

8. **How do you isolate specific pathogens from water?**

Specific pathogens may be isolated from water by employing enrichment and selective media. For example, for isolation of *S. typhi*, equal volume of water is added to double strength selenite broth followed by incubation and subculture on Wilson and Blair's medium. For isolation of *V. cholerae*, alkaline peptone water (10×) is mixed with nine times its volume of water, incubated and subcultured on bile salt agar. Pathogenic organisms may also be isolated by membrane filtration method.

9. **Which presumptive coliform count of water is satisfactory for human consumption?**

1–3 coliform bacilli in 100 ml of water.

10. **What is the temperature of incubation in Eijkman test?**

44°C.

Section
5

Mycology

- Laboratory diagnosis of mycoses
- *Candida albicans*
- *Cryptococcus neoformans*
- *Aspergillus*
- Mucoraceae
- Dermatophytes

Laboratory Diagnosis of Mycoses

Introduction

Fungi are a group of non-motile eukaryotic organisms which are saprophytes, parasites or commensals. Infection caused by fungus is known as mycosis. Successful laboratory diagnosis of mycoses is dependent not only upon the mycologic expertise of the clinical laboratory workers but also heavily upon the quality of the specimens provided for laboratory analysis. Specimens for the diagnosis of mycoses include:

- *Superficial mycoses*—skin, nail, hair, wet swabs or scrapings from mucous membrane.
- *Subcutaneous mycoses*—pus, exudates, grains and biopsies.
- *Systemic mycoses*—tissue biopsy, blood, sputum, cerebrospinal fluid, bone marrow aspirate, fluids and urine.

Causative agents of mycoses can be identified by following methods.

Direct Microscopic Examination of Specimens

Although the Gram stain performed in the routine microbiology laboratory often gives the first evidence of infection with yeasts, other direct stains give more specific information concerning a mold infection. The types of direct examination used in identification of fungal infection include wet preparation such as KOH preparation, KOH with calcofluor white, India ink, and tissue stains such as periodic acid-Schiff (PAS) stain, Gomori methenamine silver nitrate (GMS) stain, Giemsa stain and haematoxylin and eosin (H&E) stain.

KOH preparation

A 10–20% solution of KOH is useful for detecting fungal elements in skin, hair, nails and tissues. In this procedure, KOH is mixed in equal proportions with the specimen on a slide and the specimen material is teased with two inoculating needles. A coverslip is placed over it and heated gently. Preparation with KOH clears the tissue and cellular debris from all types of clinical specimens without damaging the fungal cells. This clearing process requires only 5–10 minutes, after which one can observe the fungal morphology as well as the pigment of the fungal cell wall under a phase-contrast or bright-field microscope, using low-power followed by high-power objectives.

KOH with calcofluor white

A drop of 0.1% calcofluor white solution can be added to the KOH preparation prior to placing coverslip over it. Calcofluor white binds to polysaccharide present in the chitin of the fungus or to cellulose. Fungal elements fluoresce apple green or blue-white, depending on the combination of filters used. The actual fungal structure must be seen before a positive preparation is reported.

India ink

India ink preparations may be used for detecting encapsulated yeast *Cryptococcus neoformans* in cerebrospinal fluid (CSF). A drop of India ink is mixed with a drop of centrifuged deposit of CSF, and the preparation is examined under high power. With this negative stain, budding yeast surrounded by a large clear area against a dark background is presumptive evidence of *C. neoformans* (Colour Plate I, Fig. 7). White blood cells and other artifacts may resemble encapsulated organisms; therefore, careful examination is necessary.

Tissue stains

The diagnosis of fungal disease should preferably be established on the basis of histopathologic evidence combined with cultural evidence, because detection of fungi in tissue and confirmation of tissue invasion are required in diagnosing many opportunistic fungal infection. For example, isolation of common fungi such as *Aspergillus*, *Penicillium*, and *Rhizopus* species from sputum does not establish pulmonary infection by these fungi unless there is also histopathological

Mycology

5

evidence. Moreover, fixed histopathologic specimens often may be the only available material for diagnosis, and certain mycoses, e.g., rhinosporidiosis, lobomycosis and *Pneumocystis jirovecii* infections can only be diagnosed by histologic studies since growth conditions of the fungi causing these infections have not been defined.

Haematoxylin and eosin (H&E) stain used routinely in the pathology laboratory is often not adequate for detecting fungal elements. Many fungi stain poorly and some fungi do not stain at all with H&E. However, with this stain, the tissue response can be demonstrated better than with any special stain and the innate colour of the fungal elements, whether dematiaceous or hyaline, can be determined. Special stains used in the histologic section for detection of fungal elements are Gomori methenamine silver (GMS), Gridley fungus (GF), periodic acid-Schiff (PAS), Giemsa, Mayer's mucicarmine and alcian blue stains. The GMS staining procedure provides better contrast between the fungi and background tissue. This procedure results in the brownish black colouration of all forms of viable and non-viable fungal cells. The GMS is the best fungal stain for screening and H&E is the best stain for studying the tissue response to etiological agents.

The GF stain colours fungal cells purplish-red with a yellow background. Muscle and elastic tissues are also stained purplish-red. Non-viable fungi at the time of fixation may not be stained. The PAS stain is one of the most widely used stains for fungal histopathology. Aldehydes produced by the oxidation of fungal polysaccharide react with periodic acid and colour the fungi pinkish-red. In old caseous foci of histoplasmosis, yeast cells may be stained by GMS but not by PAS. Giemsa stain is used primarily to detect *Histoplasma capsulatum* in blood or bone marrow. Mayer's mucicarmine and alcian blue procedures stain the mucopolysaccharide capsule of *Cryptococcus* species red and blue, respectively.

Culture

Relatively, few types of standard media are needed for primary isolation of fungi. These include Sabouraud dextrose agar (SDA), SDA with antibiotics, and brain heart infusion (BHI) agar with blood and antibiotics. The pH of Emmons modification of SDA is close to neutral and is more efficient for primary isolation than the original formulation. The antimicrobials usually included in SDA with antibiotics are chloramphenicol to inhibit bacterial growth and cycloheximide to inhibit saprophytic fungi. Special media may be used for isolation and to help rapid identification when the identity of a particular fungus is strongly suspected, for example, *C. neoformans* develops black colonies on bird seed agar.

Specimens for the isolation of fungi are inoculated onto slants or agar plates. When slants are used, the culture tube should be large enough (15×2 cm) to provide a wide surface area for growth. The screw caps should be left loosened during incubation to permit an adequate supply of oxygen. The optimum temperature for the recovery of most pathogenic fungi from clinical specimens is 25–30°C (room temperature). Fungi grow optimally at this temperature, but bacteria have a slower growth rate. If the etiologic agent suspected is a dimorphic fungus, culture should also be incubated at 37°C. Cultures are generally maintained for 4–6 weeks and should be examined weekly or twice a week for growth. Growth of *Candida*, *Aspergillus*, *Mucor* and *Rhizopus* species appears within 24–72 hours. Therefore, culture should be examined for growth daily for the first week.

Once an organism has grown, it is examined for characteristic gross and microscopic structures, so that identification can be made. Pigment on the reverse side of the colony or in aerial mycelium is noted. For microscopic examination, slide mounts should be made in lactophenol cotton blue (LCB). On occasion, a slide culture may be prepared, when the initial isolate fails to show conidial morphology. Characteristics that should be observed are septate versus nonseptate hyphae, hyaline or dematiaceous hyphae and the types, size, shape and arrangement of conidia.

Serologic Tests

Tests for antibody have an established diagnostic use in coccidioidomycosis, paracoccidioidomycosis, and in some patients with histoplasmosis. Detection of polysaccharide cryptococcal antigen in serum and CSF by latex agglutination is a method of choice for the rapid diagnosis of meningitis and disseminated infection caused by *C. neoformans*. Latex agglutination test kits for detecting *Candida* antigens in serum are also commercially available.

Discussion

1. **Define the term fungi.**

   Fungi are a group of non-motile eukaryotic organisms which exist as saprophytes, parasites or commensals.

2. **What are dimorphic fungi?**

   Fungi that have two morphologic forms such as a mold and a yeast, which develop under different growth conditions, e.g., *Histoplasma capsulatum* forms hyphae *in vitro* at room temperature, and yeast in tissues when cultured at 35–37°C on enriched media.

3. **Enumerate dimorphic fungi.**

   - *Histoplasma capsulatum*
   - *Sporothrix schenkii*
   - *Blastomyces dermatitidis*
   - *Coccidioides immitis*
   - *Paracoccidioides brasiliensis*
   - *Penicillium marneffei*

4. **What percentage of KOH is used for detecting fungal elements in keratinized tissues?**

   A 10–20% solution of KOH is used.

5. **What are the advantages of KOH preparation for detection of fungi?**
   - Preparation with KOH clears the tissue and cellular debris from all types of clinical specimens without damaging the fungal cells.
   - A definitive diagnosis of blastomycosis, coccidioidomycosis, paracoccidioidomycosis or rhinosporidiosis can be made.
   - Tentative diagnosis can be derived from the presence of fungal elements compatible to the etiologic agents of aspergillosis, dermatophytosis, sporotrichosis, mucormycosis or cryptococcosis.

6. **What is the disadvantage of KOH preparation?**
   In KOH preparation, crystals can form on standing so that interpretation of the smear becomes difficult.

7. **What is the mechanism of action of calcofluor white?**
   Calcofluor white binds to polysaccharide present in the chitin of the fungus or to cellulose, and fungal elements fluoresce apple green or blue-white, depending on the combination of filters used.

8. **Which is the best stain for studying the tissue response to fungal agents?**
   Haematoxylin and eosin stain.

9. **Which stain is best special stain for screening purpose?**
   GMS stain.

10. **What are the advantages of histopathologic procedures for diagnosis of mycoses?**
    - Histopathologic procedures are rapid and relatively inexpensive.
    - Detection of fungi in the tissues and confirmation of tissue invasion are helpful in diagnosing many opportunistic fungal infections, e.g., aspergillosis, mucormycosis, etc.
    - Fixed histopathologic specimens often may be the only available material for diagnosis.
    - Certain mycoses, e.g., rhinosporidiosis, lobomycosis and *Pneumocystis jirovecii* infection can only be diagnosed by histologic studies.

11. **Why cycloheximide is added to SDA medium?**
    Cyloheximide is added to inhibit saprophytic fungi.

12. **Enumerate fungi whose growth is inhibited by cycloheximide.**
    - *Cryptococcus neoformans*
    - *Pseudallescheria boydii*
    - *Aspergillus* spp.
    - *Fusarium* spp.
    - *Candida* spp.

13. **Why test tube agar slants are preferred for isolation of fungi as compared to agar plates?**
    Test tube agar slants are preferred because of following reasons:
    - There are less chances of contamination.
    - They are more resistant to desiccation during protracted incubation.
    - They require less space.

14. **What precautions should be taken while using test tube agar slants?**
    - The culture tube should be large enough (15 × 2 cm) to provide a wide surface area for growth.
    - The screw caps should be left loosened during incubation to permit an adequate supply of oxygen or use sterile cotton plugs.

15. **What precautions should be taken while taking nail clippings?**
    - Nails should first be cleaned with 70% alcohol.
    - Nail clippings should be taken from discoloured, dystrophic or brittle parts of nails.

16. **What are the limitations of serological tests for diagnosis of mycoses?**
    - Cross reaction may occur with other fungi because of complex and crude nature of fungal antigen extract.
    - Some patients may have antibodies in the absence of infection because they have been previously exposed to the fungus either as a saprophyte or as commensal.
    - Some patients may have little or no detectable antibody response because of underlying disease (impaired immunity).

17. **Broad-based budding yeast cells are seen in which fungal infection?**
    Blastomycosis.

18. **Name the most common fungus causing orbital cellulitis in a patient with diabetic ketoacidosis.**
    Mucor.

19. **Barrel-shaped arthroconidia are seen in which fungal infection?**
    Coccidioidomycosis.

Candida albicans

Introduction

Candida albicans is an oval or spherical budding yeast cell, 3–5 μm in diameter. It produces pseudohyphae when the buds continue to grow but fail to detach, producing chains of elongated, cells that are pinched or constricted at the septation between cells. It also can produce true hyphae. The yeast is a common commensal of the gastrointestinal tract, mucous membranes and skin. Since *Candida* is normally present on skin and mucosa, therefore, it is significant only when it is present in large numbers. In addition, presence of pseudohyphae indicates colonization. Gram-stained smears from lesions, exudates, and skin and nail scrapings show budding Gram-positive yeast cells and pseudohyphae.

Candida albicans is the commonest cause of candidiasis (moniliasis). Candidiasis is an opportunistic endogenous infection. Predisposing factors for candidiasis are AIDS, diabetes mellitus, neutropaenia and prolonged administration of antimicrobial agents.

Cultural Characteristics

Sabouraud dextrose agar (SDA)

C. albicans grows well on SDA. Cream-coloured, smooth, pasty colonies appear in 1–2 days at 25–37°C (Colour Plate VIII, Fig. 46). Lactophenol cotton blue (LCB) preparation and Gram-stained smears show budding yeast cells and pseudohyphae (Colour Plate VIII, Fig. 47).

Test for Presumptive Identification of *C. albicans*

Corn meal agar

C. albicans produces large spherical thick-walled, usually single terminal chlamydoconidia.

Germ tube test

A germ tube is a filamentous outgrowth from a yeast cell.

The filament lacks a constriction at the point of origin which differentiates it from the pseudohyphae.

Method

- Take 0.5 ml of pooled human serum into a small test tube.
- Using a sterile wire, inoculate the serum with a yeast colony from the culture plate. Place the tube in a water bath or incubator at 35–37°C for 2–3 hours.
- Using a sterile wire loop or Pasteur pipette, transfer a drop of the serum yeast culture to a glass slide and cover with a coverslip.
- Examine the preparation under low and high power objectives for germ tube.

C. albicans can also be differentiated from other species by sugar fermentation and sugar assimilation reactions.

Discussion

1. **Is *Candida albicans* a yeast or yeast-like?**

   It is yeast-like.

2. **Enumerate simple tests for the identification of *Candida albicans*.**

   Two simple tests for the identification of *C. albicans* are:

   - Germ tube test
   - Formation of chlamydoconidia on corn meal agar

3. **What important precaution should be taken while performing germ tube test?**

   To perform germ tube test, light suspension of yeast cells should be taken. Germ tube test is negative, if heavy suspension of yeast cells is used.

4. **Enumerate *Candida* spp. which are positive for germ tube test.**

   - *C. albicans*
   - *C. dubliniensis*

5. **Enumerate lesions produced by *C. albicans*.**

- *Mucocutaneous lesions:* Oral thrush, vulvovaginitis, conjunctivitis, balanitis and keratitis.
- *Skin and nail infections:* Paronychia, infection of the skin at moist sites and napkin dermatitis in infants.
- *Systemic candidiasis:* It may lead to urinary candidiasis, pulmonary candidiasis, hepatobiliary candidiasis, endocarditis, meningitis, arthritis, osteomyelitis and candidaemia.

6. **Enumerate species of *Candida*.**

- *C. albicans*
- *C. glabrata*
- *C. dubliniensis*
- *C. krusei*
- *C. tropicalis*
- *C. guilliermondii*
- *C. kefyr*
- *C. parapsilosis*

7. **What is the significance of pseudohyphae of *C. albicans*?**

Presence of pseudohyphae in tissues indicates colonization.

8. **Which species of *Candida* shows positive urease test?**

C. krusei.

Cryptococcus neoformans

Introduction

Cryptococcus neoformans is a true yeast. It causes crypto-coccosis, an opportunistic mycosis usually affecting the lungs, brain and meninges and occasionally other parts of the body. On the basis of cryptococcal polysaccharide antigen, there are five serotypes of *C. neoformans* (A to D and AD). Most infections are caused by serotypes A and D.

Direct Microscopy

India ink preparation

The direct microscopy of CSF, mixed with a drop of India ink shows round budding yeast cells, 4–10 μm in diameter. The organisms are surrounded by a wide refractile gelatinous capsule that may be twice the size of the yeast cells. In India ink preparation, it appears as a clear halo around the yeast cells (Colour Plate I, Fig. 7).

Gram staining

In cryptococcal meningitis, the yeasts are often detected in a Gram-stained preparation of CSF sediment. They are Gram-positive but stain poorly and unevenly. In a Giemsa-stained preparation, the capsule surrounding *C. neoformans* can be seen as a clear unstained area. The histopathological examination of biopsy material can be done by staining with Mayer's mucicarmine (Colour Plate VIII, Fig. 48), PAS, GMS and H&E staining.

Cultural Characteristics

Sabouraud dextrose agar

C. neoformans produces moist, white, cream-coloured mucoid colonies usually after 2–3 days of incubation (Colour Plate VIII, Fig. 49). When examined microscopically, the yeast cells are capsulated but the capsules are often smaller than when seen in specimens. Occasionally, capsules are absent. Hyphae or pseudohyphae are not normally produced. *C. neoformans* is urease positive.

Niger seed agar/bird seed agar/caffeic acid agar

C. neoformans possesses the enzyme phenol oxidase, and testing for its presence is another means of accurate identi-fications. *C. neoformans* produces black colonies on these media (Colour Plate VIII, Fig. 49).

Discussion

1. **Enumerate true yeasts.**
   - *Cryptococcus neoformans*
   - *Rhodotorula*
   - *Saccharomyces cerevisae*

2. **Define the term yeasts.**

   Yeasts are round, oval or elongated unicellular fungi which reproduce by simple budding.

3. **How can you differentiate pathogenic *C. neoformans* from nonpathogenic species?**

   Pathogenic *C. neoformans* can be differentiated from nonpathogenic species by its ability to:
   – grow at 37°C,
   – hydrolyse urea,
   – produce black colonies on niger seed agar and caffeic acid agar, and
   – produce disease in mice on intracerebral and intra-peritoneal inoculation.

4. **Name three varieties of *C. neoformans*.**
   - *C. neoformans* var. *neoformans*.
   - *C. neoformans* var. *gattii*.
   - *C. neoformans* var. *grubii*.

5. **Name the reservoir of *C. neoformans*?**

   Pigeon droppings provide a reservoir of the organisms.

6. **Does *C. neoformans* infect the birds?**

No, *C. neoformans* does not appear to infect the birds, probably because of their high body temperature (40°C), but survives passage through their gut.

7. **Name staining techniques to demonstrate *C. neoformans* capsule in biopsy materials.**

- Mayer's mucicarmine stain
- PAS
- GMS

8. **Enumerate the lesions produced by *C. neoformans*.**

- Pulmonary lesions
- Meningitis

9. **What is the basis of serotyping of *C. neoformans*?**

Cryptococcal polysaccharide antigen.

10. **How many serotypes of *C. neoformans* are there?**

Five serotypes (A to D and AD)

11. **Which tests can detect cryptococcal capsular polysaccharide antigen in serum and CSF?**

Latex agglutination and ELISA tests.

Aspergillus

Introduction

Aspergillus species are saprophytic moulds. *Aspergillus fumigatus* is the commonest human pathogen. Other species causing infection include *A. niger*, *A. flavus*, *A. terreus* and *A. nidulans*. Aspergillosis is caused by inhalation of *Aspergillus* conidia or mycelial fragments which are present on vegetation, decaying matter, soil and air.

Direct microscopy

10% KOH preparation

KOH preparation of sputum, bronchoalveolar lavage and other specimens reveal non-pigmented septate hyphae, 3–5 μm in diameter with characteristic dichotomous branching. The hyphae have a tendency to branch repeatedly. The branches arise at an angle of approximately 45°. In a majority of lesions, only hyphal forms are seen.

Histological sections

These can be stained with H&E and GMS and examined for characteristic hyphae (Colour Plate VIII, Fig. 50).

Cultural Characteristics

SDA

Colonies on SDA appear after incubation for 1–2 days at 25°C. The isolate is identified on the basis of growth characteristics and microscopic morphology. LCB mount shows branching and septate hyphae. From the latter arise conidiophores, the ends of which are expanded to form vesicles. The vesicle bears phialides which arise directly from the vesicle (uniseriate) or from sterile cells called metulae (biseriate).

Aspergillus fumigatus

The colonies of *A. fumigatus* are granular to cottony and usually have some shades of green, green-grey or green-brown pigmentation. Microscopically, the conidiophores are smooth, relatively short (usually less than 300 μm long), and 5–10 μm in diameter. The phialides are uniseriate, close together, forming only on upper two-thirds of the vesicle, parallel to the axis of conidiophore. Conidia are round, smooth, or slightly rough and 2–3.5 μm in diameter (Fig. 52.1A).

Aspergillus flavus

The colonies of *A. flavus* are granular to woolly and have some shade of yellow or yellow-brown. Microscopically, the conidiophores are long (400–800 μm), the vesicle are 25–45 μm in diameter. The phialides may arise directly from the vesicle from three-fourths or the entire circumference of the vesicle (uniseriate) or from sterile cells called metulae (biseriate). Both these conditions may exist in the same head (Fig. 52.1B). Conidia are spherical, smooth, or slightly roughened with maturity and form long chains (Fig. 52.1B).

Aspergillus niger

The surface of the colonies of *A. niger* is covered by a dense aggregate of jet black conidia. The underside of the colony is buff or yellow-grey, distinguishing *A. niger* from the dematiaceous fungi. Microscopically, the vesicles are globose and measure 30–75 μm in diameter. Phialides arise from metulae (biseriate) from the entire circumference of the vesicle. Conidiation is extremely profuse, to the extent that the vesicles are obscured by dense aggregates of 3–5 μm diameter, spherical, black conidia that become roughened with maturity (Fig. 52.1C).

Aspergillus terreus

The colonies of *A. terreus* are cinnamon buff, brown or orange-brown. Radial folds emanating from the centre of the colony are often observed. Microscopically, the vesicles are relatively small (10–16 μm in diameter) flask-shaped or hemispherical. Phialides arise from metulae (biseriate) on the upper half only. Conidia are smooth, elliptical, measure 2–2.5 μm in diameter (Fig. 52.1D).

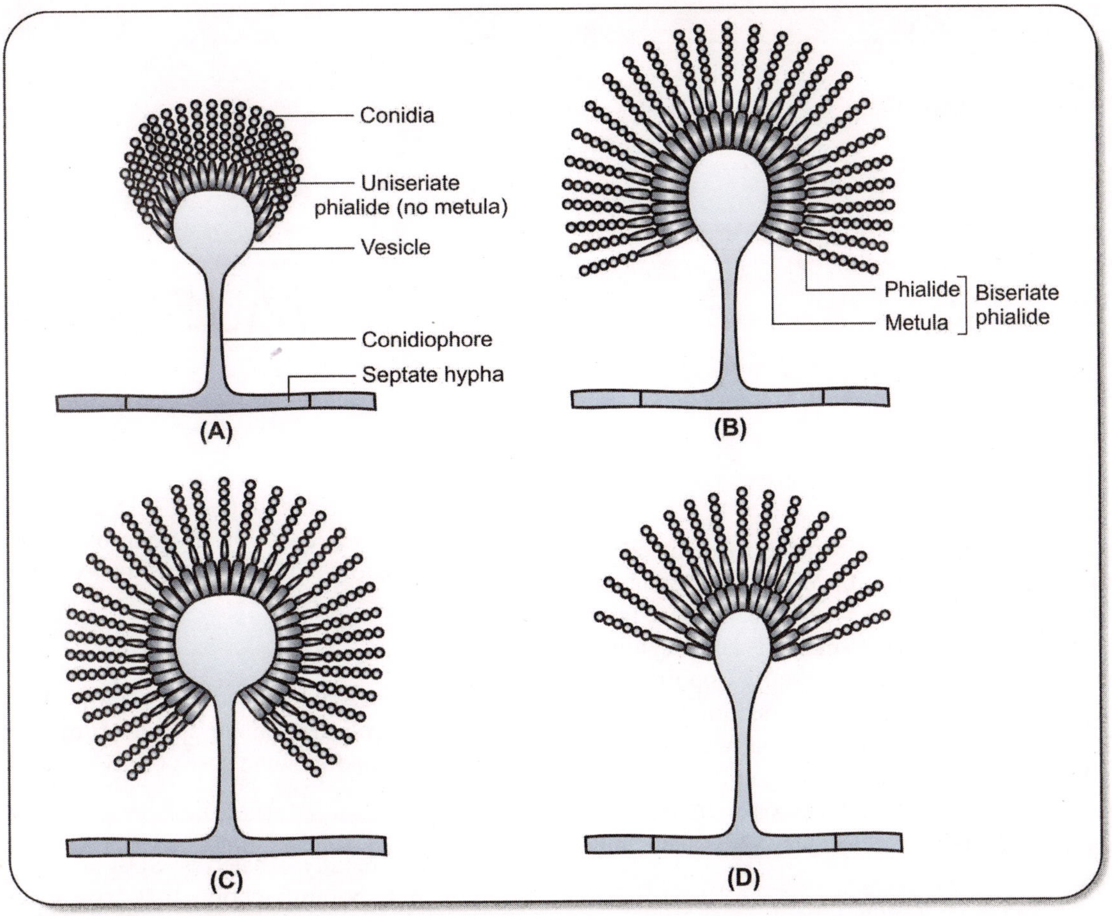

Fig. 52.1. *Aspergillus* spp.: (A) *A. fumigatus*, (B) *A. flavus*, (C) *A. niger*, and (D) *A. terreus*.

Aspergillus nidulans

A. nidulans may rarely be recovered from the cases of human infections. Phialides arise from metulae (biseriate) on their upper half surface. *A. nidulans* may form sexually derived ascospores contained within sac-like structures called cleistothecia.

Discussion

1. **Which species of *Aspergillus* is the commonest human pathogen?**

   A. fumigatus

2. **Enumerate the lesions produced by *Aspergillus*.**
   - Allergic bronchopulmonary aspergillosis
   - Intracavitary aspergilloma (fungus ball)
   - Invasive aspergillosis
   - Endocarditis
   - Paranasal granuloma

3. **Which SDA medium is used for growth of *Aspergillus*?**

   SDA without cycloheximide is used and incubated at 25°C.

4. **Name toxin produced by *Aspergillus flavus*.**

   Aflatoxin.

5. **What do you mean by term 'uniseriate' and 'biseriate'?**
   - *Uniseriate:* When phialides arise directly from the vesicle.
   - *Biseriate:* When phialides arise from sterile cells called metulae.

6. **Name species of *Aspergillus* which are biseriate.**
   - *A. niger*
   - *A. terreus*
   - *A. nidulans*

7. **Name uniseriate species of *Aspergillus*.**

   A. fumigatus.

8. **Enumerate characteristic features of *Aspergillus* hyphae.**
   - Hyphae are non-pigmented.
   - They are septate, 3–5 μm in diameter with characteristic dichotomous branching.
   - The branches arise at an angle of approximately 45°.

Mucoraceae

Introduction

Mucormycosis is an opportunistic infection caused by saprophytic fungi, notably species of *Mucor*, *Rhizopus* and *Lichtheimia* (*Absidia*) of the family Mucoraceae. These fungi are common saprophytes of soil, manure and decaying vegetables, and fruits. These are essentially opportunistic fungi. The major predisposing factors to mucormycosis are diabetes mellitus, leukaemia or lymphoma and immuno-suppression. The characteristic pathological changes in mucormycosis are suppuration and necrosis. Invasion of thrombosed blood vessels by the fungus is a conspicuous feature.

Direct Microscopy

KOH preparation

KOH preparation of scrapings from the lesions, pus, sputum and nasal discharge shows irregularly branched, nonseptate, thin-walled very broad hyphae (7–15 µm in diameter). True septa are rarely seen in the hyphae but under low magnification, crossfolds in the walls of the hyphae may resemble septa.

Histological sections

The fungi are deeply stained with routine H&E stain. On the other hand, colouration by special fungal stains such as Gridley, PAS and in some cases GMS may be very poor.

Cultural Characteristics

Fungi can be readily isolated on SDA at 37°C. *Rhizopus* has rhizoids and sporangiophores that arise in groups directly above the rhizoids. *Mucor* does not possess rhizoids and shows branched sporangiophores arising randomly along aerial mycelium. *Lichtheimia* has rhizoids and branched sporangiophores that arise from the aerial mycelium in between the rhizoids (Fig. 53.1).

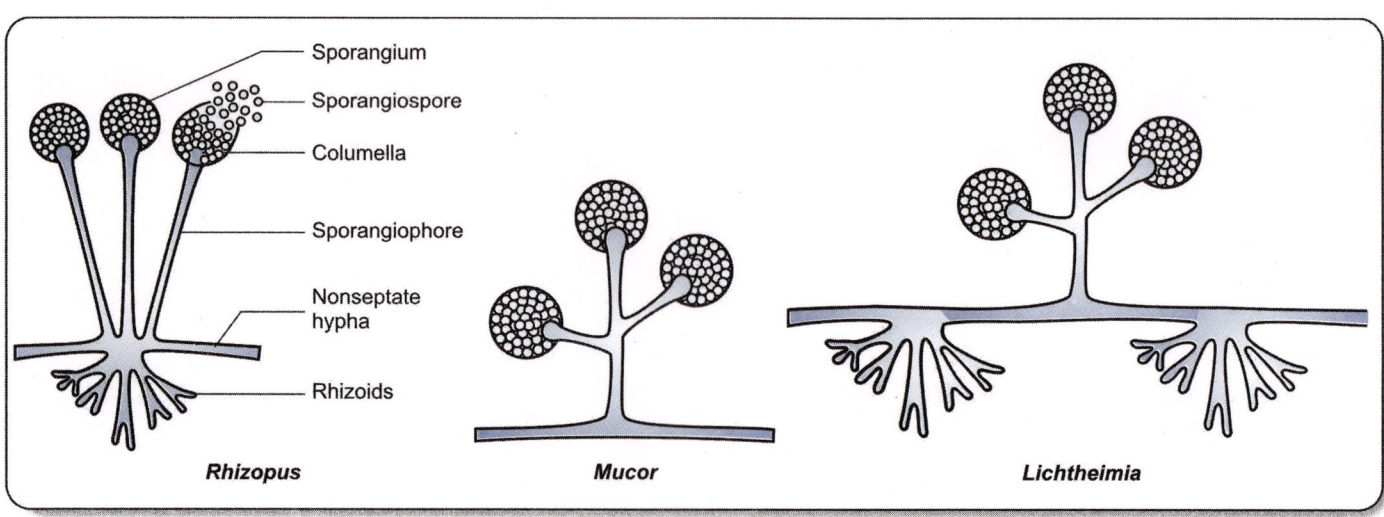

Sporangium
Sporangiospore
Columella
Sporangiophore
Nonseptate hypha
Rhizoids

Rhizopus   *Mucor*   *Lichtheimia*

Fig. 53.1. *Rhizopus, Mucor* and *Lichtheimia.*

Discussion

1. **Name fungi which can invade blood vessels.**
   - *Aspergillus*
   - *Mucor*
   - *Rhizopus*
   - *Lichtheimia*

2. **Enumerate pathogenic lesions produced by Mucor-mycetes.**
   - Rhinocerebral mucormycosis
   - Pulmonary mucormycosis
   - Gastrointestinal mucormycosis
   - Disseminated mucormycosis
   - Dermal mucormycosis
   - Subcutaneous mucormycosis

3. **How will you differentiate between aspergillosis from mucormycosis in tissue sections?**

   In tissue sections, aspergillosis can be easily differentiated from mucormycosis in its uniform dichotomous pattern of branching, the presence of many septa and its much easier detection by the special stains than the routine H&E stain.

4. **Enumerate predisposing factors of mucormycosis.**
   - Diabetes mellitus
   - Metabolic acidosis
   - Leukaemia
   - Lymphoma
   - Immunosuppression
   - Widespread use of broad-spectrum antibiotics, steroids and antimetabolites.

5. **Which type of mucormycosis is most serious and fulminating?**

   Rhinocerebral mucormycosis

6. **Which mucormycete does not possess rhizoids?**

   Mucor

7. **Which fungus has sporangiophores arising in groups directly above the rhizoids?**

   Rhizopus

8. **Describe the characteristic features of hyphae of Mucormycetes.**

   Hyphae are large ribbon-like irregularly branched, non-septate, broad and thin-walled. Hyphae may appear folded, twisted and distorted.

9. **Which is the best stain for diagnosis of mucormycosis?**

   H&E stain. Hyphae are deeply stained with haematoxylin.

Dermatophytes

Introduction

Dermatophytes infect keratinized tissues of the skin, hair and nails. Dermatophytosis, tinea or ringworm is the most common type of superficial mycosis seen in human beings. Dermatophytosis is caused by 41 species of dermatophytes which belong to three genera (*Trichophyton*—24, *Microsporum*—16, and *Epidermophyton*—1). On the basis of their natural habitat and host preferences, they are classified into three groups—geophilic, zoophilic and anthropophilic species.

Direct Microscopy

KOH preparation

KOH preparation of skin scrapings, hairs and nail clippings reveals branching septate hyphae or chains of arthroconidia. Three types of hair infection may be distinguished in wet mounts—ectothrix, endothrix and favic-type hair invasion.

- *Ectothrix:* In this, the fungus is present on the surface of the hair shaft (Fig. 54.1A). It is caused by *M. audouinii*, *M. canis* and *T. mentagrophytes*.
- *Endothrix:* In this, the arthroconidia are present within the hair completely filling the hair shaft without a conspicuous external sheath of arthroconidia (Fig. 54.1B). This is caused by *T. tonsurans*, *T. violaceum* and *T. soudanense*.
- *Favus:* In this, there is sparse hyphal growth and formation of air spaces within the hair shaft (Fig. 54.1C). This is caused by *T. schoenleinii*.

   Demonstration of fungus in nails may be possible only after clearing with KOH for a day or two.

Culture

Species identification is possible only by culture examination. Keratinous material is inoculated on SDA with chloramphenicol and cycloheximide and incubated at 27–30°C for

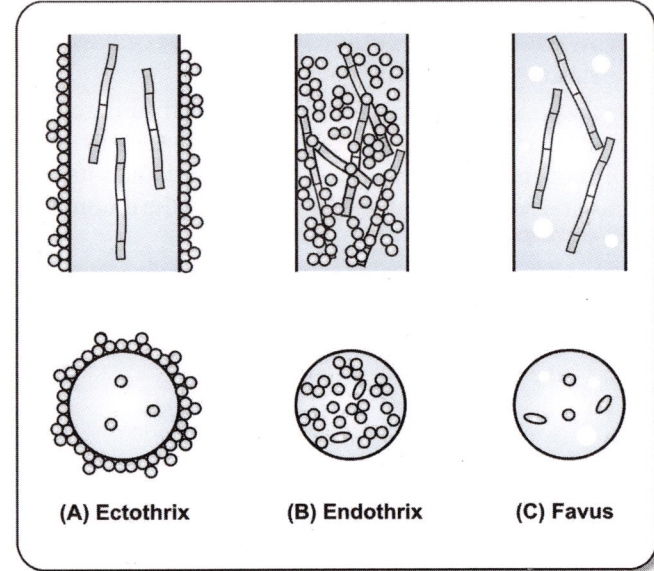

(A) Ectothrix   **(B) Endothrix**   **(C) Favus**

Fig. 54.1. Hair invasion of dermatophytes in longitudinal and transverse sections.

three weeks. Identification of dermatophytes is based on colonial morphology, colour, pigment production and production of microconidia and macroconidia (Fig. 54.2).

Trichophyton

Colonies may be powdery, velvety or waxy with pigmentation characteristic of different species. Macroconidia are usually rare but microconidia are abundant. The latter are arranged in clusters along the hyphae or borne on conidiophores. Macroconidia have smooth, thin walls, and variable in shape (cylindrical, fusiform or clavate), vary in number of septa (2–8), and in size (20–50 × 4–6 μm). They are borne singly or in clusters. Fungi of this genus can infect skin, hair and nails.

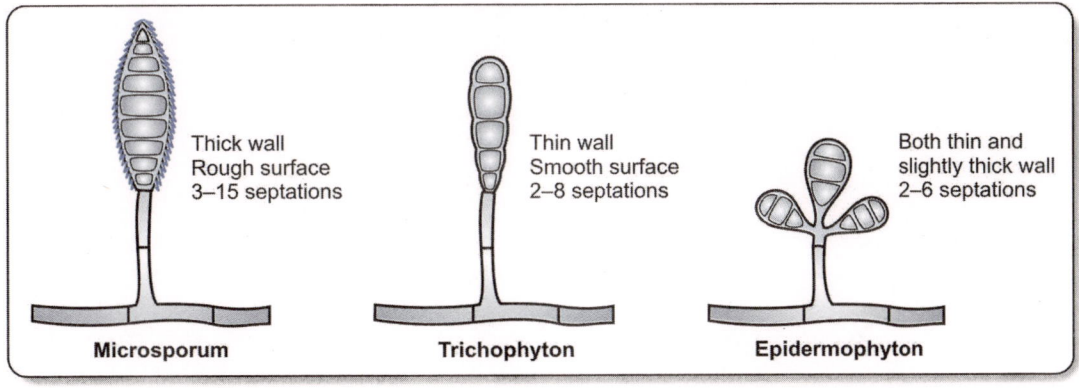

Fig. 54.2. Macroconidia in the three genera of dermatophytes.

Microsporum

Colonies of the fungi of this genus are cottony, velvety or powdery with white to brown pigmentation. Macroconidia are very numerous and microconidia are relatively scanty. Macroconidia are thick-walled and rough, vary in shape (fusiform to obovate), number of septa (3–15), and size (5–100 × 3–8 μm). They infect skin and hair but not the nails.

Epidermophyton

Colonies are powdery and greenish-yellow. Microconidia are absent and macroconidia are club-shaped. They have 2–6 septa, are 20–40 × 6–8 μm in size, thin- and slightly thick-walled and are borne singly or in clusters. It infects skin and nails but not hair.

Discussion

1. **Define dermatophytosis.**

   Dermatophytosis is superficial mycosis seen in human beings. It infects keratinized tissues of the skin, hair and nails.

2. **Define dermatomycosis.**

   The infection of skin caused by non-dermatophytic fungi and the cutaneous manifestations of systemic mycoses are known as dermatomycosis.

3. **Enumerate three genera of dermatophytes.**
   - *Trichophyton*
   - *Microsporum*
   - *Epidermophyton*

4. **Which factor is considered to differentiate three genera of dermatophytes?**

   The differentiation of the three genera is based mainly on the nature of macroconidia.

5. **In which genus of dermatophytes, macroconidia are usually rare?**

   In *Trichophyton*, macroconidia are usually rare.

6. **Club-shaped macroconidia are present in which genus of dermatophytes?**

   Club-shaped macroconidia are present in *Epidermophyton*. They are borne singly or in clusters.

7. **On which basis, dermatophytes are classified into three groups?**

   On the basis of natural habitat and host preferences, the dermatophytes are classified into three groups—geophilic, zoophilic, anthropophilic.

8. **Enumerate anthropophilic dermatophytes.**
   - *T. rubrum*
   - *M. audouinii*
   - *E. floccosum*

9. **Define dermatophytid or id reaction.**

   Hypersensitivity to fungal antigens may lead to secondary eruptions occurring in sensitized patients because of circulation of allergenic products from the primary site of infection. It is known as dermatophytid or id reaction.

10. **Define characteristic lesions of ringworm or tinea.**

    The lesions are circular which spread with an erythematous border with variable degree of scaling and inflammation.

11. **Enumerate dermatophytes causing endothrix.**
    - *T. tonsurans*
    - *T. violaceum*
    - *T. soudanense*

12. **Which species of *Trichophyton* most commonly infects man?**

    T. rubrum

13. **Enumerate pigmented dermatophytes.**
    - *T. rubrum*
    - *T. violaceum*
    - *M. canis*

14. **Which dermatophyte is positive for urease test?**

    T. mentagrophytes

Section
6

Virology

- Diagnostic approach to viral infections

Diagnostic Approach to Viral Infections

Specimen Collection

Specimens for the diagnosis of viral infections include throat swab, nasopharyngeal swab, bronchial lavage, blood, bone narrow, rectal swab, stool, urine, sterile body fluids, tissues, skin smears, CSF and serum. Specimens should be collected as early as possible following the onset of disease.

Specimen Transport

Viral transport media are used to transport swab, tissues, scrapings or fluid specimens. Transport media contain protein, such as serum, albumin or gelatin and antimicrobials to prevent contamination by bacteria and fungi. Following transport media are used:

- Hanks balanced salt solution.
- Eagles tissue culture medium.
- Leibovitz-Emory medium.

Specimen Processing

All specimens for isolation of virus should be processed immediately. In case of delay, the specimen should be stored in viral transport medium at 4°C. Processing should be done in a biological safety cabinet. Prior to processing, requisition form should be seen for following information: date and time of specimen collection, source of specimen, clinical history and suspected viruses. Laboratory diagnosis of viral infections can be carried out by the following methods:

- Direct detection of virus, viral antigen or viral genome.
- Virus isolation.
- Detection of specific antiviral antibodies.
- Cytological or histological examination of cells from the site of infection.

Direct Detection of Virus, Viral Antigen or Viral Genome

Electron microscopy (EM)

Electron microscopy is one of the most useful tools for the direct demonstration of viruses in clinical specimen. On the basis of their distinctive appearances, most of the viruses can be assigned to the correct family. Viruses that are difficult to culture (rotaviruses, astroviruses) can be recognized by electron microscopy. The clinical material can be negatively stained with potassium phosphotungstate or uranyl acetate and scanned by EM. Clinical applications of electron microscopy include detection of rotavirus and hepatitis A virus in faecal specimens, poxviruses in vesicle fluid and herpesvirus in brain biopsy tissue.

Immunoelectron microscopy

EM, as a diagnostic tool, has low sensitivity. For satisfactory results, the specimen should contain 10^7 virions per ml. The sensitivity of electron microscopy can be increased by mixing specific antibody with the specimen to aggregate the virus particles. These aggregates can be sedimented by centrifugation, negatively stained and observed under EM.

Fluorescence microscopy

Virions or viral antigens can be detected in frozen tissue sections, acetone-fixed cell smears, cells from virus infected cultures or vesicle fluid by direct or indirect fluorescent antibody technique. Fluorescence microscopy of brain biopsy can be used for the diagnosis of herpes simplex encephalitis, subacute sclerosing panencephalitis (a late sequelae of measles), and for the verification of rabies in the brain of animals suspected to be rabid. This method is also useful for the rapid diagnosis of respiratory infections caused by

Virology

6

paramyxoviruses, orthomyxoviruses, adenoviruses and herpesviruses.

Light microscopy

Viral antigens in infected cells can be detected by immuno-peroxidase staining. Tissue section or smear of infected cells is stained with antibody coupled to horseradish peroxidase. Hydrogen peroxide together with a benzidine derivative is then added. It forms a coloured insoluble precipitate which can be seen under ordinary light microscope.

Serological tests

Viral antigens may be detected by direct and indirect ELISA, radioimmunoassay and latex agglutination.

Nucleic acid probes

Enzyme-labelled or radiolabelled nucleic acid (DNA or RNA) sequences complementary to unique regions in nucleic acid sequences of most viruses are now manufactured commercially. These labelled complementary sequences are known as nucleic acid probes. Two strands of the target DNA molecule in the clinical specimens are first separated by boiling, then, following cooling, allowed to hybridize with a labelled single-stranded DNA or RNA probe present in excess. Depending on the type of label attached to the probe, hybridized-labelled probe can be detected by radiography, gamma counting or a simple colorimetric evaluation (dot-blot hybridization). By use of nucleic acid probes, cytomegalo-virus, papillomavirus and Epstein-Barr virus have been identified. *In situ* hybridization may be used to detect integrated or nonintegrated copies of viral genome in persistent infections or viral cancers. Southern blot hybridization and northern blot hybridization can be used for detection of DNA and RNA respectively.

Polymerase chain reaction (PCR)

It is a DNA amplification system that allows molecular biologists to produce microgram quantities of DNA from pico-gram amounts of starting material. It is based on repeated cycles of high temperature template denaturation, oligo-nucleotide primer annealing and polymerase mediated extension. With the revolutionary PCR technique, a target DNA sequence can be amplified at least 100,000 folds in just a few hours, a sharp contrast to the days required for conventional amplification method (culture). Thus viral DNA extracted from a very small number of virions or infected cells can be amplified to the point where it can readily be identified using labelled probes in a hybridization assay. For the detection of viral RNA, it is first converted into DNA by reverse transcriptase. PCR can be used for diagnosis of infections caused by HIV-1, HIV-2, HTLV-1, cytomegalo-virus, human papillomavirus, herpes simplex viruses, HBV, HCV, HDV, HEV, rubella virus, Epstein-Barr virus, varicella-zoster virus, human herpes virus 6 and 7, parvovirus B19,

enteroviruses, coxsackieviruses, echoviruses, rhinoviruses, measles virus and rotavirus.

Virus Isolation

Most of the viruses can be cultivated in laboratory animals, chick embryos and cell cultures.

Laboratory animals

Suckling mice less than 24-hour-old are used for the isolation of arboviruses, rabies virus, and some of the group A cox-sackieviruses. These are inoculated intracerebrally and/or intraperitoneally, then observed for up to 2 weeks for the development of pathognomonic signs before sacrificing the animal for histological examination of affected organs.

Chick embryos

Embryonated eggs offer several sites for the cultivation of viruses. Chorioallantoic membrane (CAM), allantoic cavity, amniotic cavity and yolk sac (Fig. 55.1) of 8–11-day-old eggs are inoculated and incubated for 2–9 days. The duration of incubation depends on the virus type and route of inoculation. Viruses may kill the embryo or may produce visible lesions like pocks and haemagglutinating activity in the harvested amniotic and allantoic fluid. These effects help in the identification of the virus. Many viruses can be grown in eggs, but it is now rarely used other than for the demonstration of poxviruses and the propagation of orthomyxoviruses and paramyxoviruses.

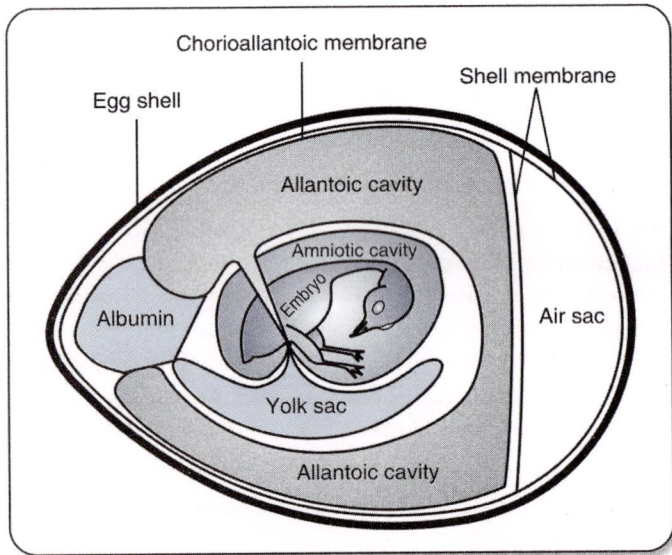

Fig. 55.1. Cross-section of an embryonated hen's egg.

Cell culture

This is the type of culture routinely employed for diagnostic virology and for studying virus–cell interactions. Cell culture is of three types:

- Primary cell culture
- Finite (diploid) cell strains
- Continuous cell lines

Detection of Virus Growth in Cell Culture

Virus growth in cell culture can be detected by the following methods.

1. Cytopathic effect (CPE)

Many viruses produce morphological changes in the cultured cells in which they grow. These changes are known as cytopathic effects (CPE) and viruses causing CPE are known as cytopathogenic viruses. Most CPE can be readily observed in unfixed and unstained monolayer of cells under low power of microscope. But fixation and staining of monolayer is essential in order to see details such as inclusion bodies and syncytia. Conventional haematoxylin and eosin is most suitable for this purpose. Fluorescent antibody staining is widely used to recognize viral antigens in such cultured cells. Following are the main types of CPE.

Rounding of cells

Viral replication may lead to nuclear pyknosis, rounding, refractility, degeneration and eventually complete or partial detachment of infected cells from the glass. This is seen in picornaviruses.

Rounding and aggregation

Some viruses may lead to cell rounding and aggregation into grape-like clusters which detach from the glass, leaving clear areas. It is seen in adenoviruses.

Syncytium formation

Some viruses (measles, respiratory syncytial virus, HIV) lead to syncytium formation in which infected cells fuse with neighbouring infected or uninfected cells to form giant cells containing several (up to 100) nuclei.

Inclusion bodies

These are intranuclear or intracytoplasmic aggregates of products of viral replication such as virus particles ready for release, over-production of a particular viral protein or proteins or some aberrant cellular structure such as clumped chromatin. They can be seen in stained preparation under a light microscope. They may be present in the cytoplasm or in the nucleus, or both of infected cells and may be acidophilic or basophilic, single or multiple, large or small and round or irregular. Vaccinia and rabies viruses produce intracytoplasmic inclusion bodies, and adenoviruses and herpesviruses produce intranuclear inclusions. Inclusion bodies of measles virus are seen in both the locations.

2. Haemadsorption

Some orthomyxoviruses (influenza) and paramyxoviruses (parainfluenza, measles and mumps) code for red cell agglutinins which are incorporated into the cell membrane during infection, so that erythrocytes adhere to the infected cells. This adherence of erythrocytes to the infected cells is known as haemadsorption. It can be used to recognize infection with non-cytocidal viruses, as well as the early stage of cytocidal viruses. Sometimes virus can be detected by haemagglutination in the medium (culture fluid).

3. Interference

The multiplication of one virus in a cell usually inhibits the multiplication of a second virus, called the challenge virus, when it is added to the culture. This is because the first virus interferes with the replicative process of the challenge virus and is known as interference challenge test. This can be used for the detection of the growth of a non-cytopathogenic virus in cell culture. A cell culture is inoculated with suspected clinical sample and incubated for several days. Then a standard dose of a known cytopathogenic challenge virus is introduced into the culture and after incubation, culture is observed for the CPE of challenge virus. If virus from original inoculum was replicating within the cells, replication of the challenge virus will be prevented and no CPE will be seen in the culture.

4. Transformation

Tumour-forming (oncogenic) viruses induce cell transformation and loss of normal contact inhibition, so that growth appears in a piled-up fashion producing microtumours. Some herpesviruses, adenoviruses, hepadnaviruses, papovaviruses and retroviruses (human T cell lymphotropic virus type 1) can transform cells.

5. Fluorescent antibody testing

Cells from virus infected cultures can be stained with fluorescein-conjugated antiserum and seen under fluorescence microscope for virus antigens. Both direct (DFA) and indirect (IFA) fluorescent antibody methods are useful in the identification of viral culture isolates. DFA testing is the most convenient method for identifying many viral isolates. It provides a complete identification in less than one hour.

6. Immunoperoxidase staining

Direct immunoperoxidase (DIP) staining method may also be used in identification of viruses isolated in cell culture.

7. Detection of enzymes

The virus isolate can be identified by detection of viral enzymes, such as reverse transcriptase in retroviruses, in the culture fluid.

8. Electron microscopy

Viruses have distinctive appearances and can be detected by electron microscopy of ultra-thin sections of infected cells.

Detection of Specific Antiviral Antibodies

Using panels of known antigens, a number of serological techniques may be used to detect specific viral antibodies. Paired sera should be collected from the patient, the 'acute-phase' serum sample collected as early as possible in the illness and the 'convalescent-phase' sample collected at least 2 weeks later. Antibodies in the serum samples can be detected by ELISA, RIA, western blot, latex agglutination, virus neutralization, haemagglutination inhibition, immunofluorescence, immunodiffusion and complement fixation tests.

Cytological or Histological Examination of Cells from the Site of Infection

Virus-induced histopathology (multinucleate giant cells and inclusion bodies) may be recognized by light microscopy.

Discussion

1. **Enumerate indications for laboratory diagnosis of viral infections.**
   - To detect emergence of drug-resistant mutants and for drug sensitivity testing.
   - To diagnose a disease for which antiviral chemotherapy is available.
   - Screening of blood donors for HIV, hepatitis B and C viruses
   - Early detection of dangerous epidemics like yellow fever, poliomyelitis, encephalitis, etc.
   - For proper management of the patient.

2. **Enumerate viruses which can be detected in urine.**
   - Cytomegalovirus
   - Mumps
   - Rubella
   - Measles
   - Polyomaviruses
   - Adenoviruses

3. **Enumerate viruses which can be detected in vesicular lesions of skin and mucous membrane.**
   - Herpes simplex
   - Varicella-zoster
   - Enteroviruses

4. **Which swab should not be used for detection of herpes simplex virus (HSV) and why?**
   Calcium alginate swab. Because it is toxic to herpes simplex virus.

5. **Within how many hours specimens for viral isolation should be processed?**
   Twelve to twenty four hours.

6. **How do you store the specimens for viral isolation in case of delay in virus culture?**

For storage up to 5 days, hold specimens at 4°C, and prolonged storage should be at –20°C or –70°C.

7. **Which serum should be added in viral transport media and why?**
   Foetal calf serum, because it is less likely to contain inhibitors, such as antibody.

8. **Which antimicrobials are added in viral transport medium?**
   - Vancomycin
   - Gentamicin
   - Amphotericin B

9. **Which animals are still used in isolation of arboviruses and coxsackieviruses?**
   Suckling mice.

10. **Which virus can be isolated in organ cultures of human embryo trachea?**
    Coronavirus.

11. **Enumerate viruses which cannot be cultivated in laboratory animals, chick embryo or cell culture.**
    - Hepatitis B virus
    - Rotavirus
    - Papillomavirus
    - Some enteric viruses

12. **Enumerate various routes of inoculation in chick embryo.**
    - Chorioallantoic membrane (CAM)
    - Amniotic cavity
    - Allantoic cavity
    - Yolk sac

13. **Name chick embryo vaccines.**
    - Yellow fever (17D strain)
    - Rabies (Flury vaccine)

14. **Enumerate viruses which can be propagated in amniotic cavity.**
    - *Influenzavirus A, B* and *C*

15. **Classify various cell cultures.**
    - Primary cell cultures
    - Finite (diploid) cell cultures
    - Continuous cell cultures

16. **Enumerate various continuous cell cultures.**
    - HeLa
    - HEp-2
    - KB
    - McCoy
    - Detroit 6
    - Vero
    - BHK-21
    - Chang C/I/L/K

17. **How many subcultures of finite (diploid) cell cultures are possible before the cells die off?**

Twenty to fifty.

18. **What is the source of HEp-2 continuous cell cultures?**

Human epithelioma of larynx

19. **Which indicator is added in growth media for virus isolation?**

Phenol red

20. **Enumerate viruses which show syncytium formation in cell culture.**

- Measles
- Respiratory syncytial virus
- HIV

21. **Define inclusion bodies.**

Inclusion bodies are intranuclear or intracytoplasmic aggregates of products of viral replication such as viral particles, viral proteins or some aberrant cellular structure such as clumped chromatin.

22. **Enumerate viruses which produce intracytoplasmic inclusion bodies.**

- Vaccinia virus
- Rabies virus

23. **Enumerate viruses which can be detected by haemadsorption in cell culture.**

- Influenza
- Parainfluenza
- Measles
- Mumps

24. **Name viruses which are usually detected by electron microscopy.**

- Rotavirus
- Hepatitis A virus
- Poxviruses
- Herpesvirus

25. **What do you mean by term "feeding" in virology?**

Feeding means removal of old medium followed by the addition of fresh culture medium.

26. **Which two media are used for cell culture?**

- Growth medium
- Maintenance medium

27. **How maintenance medium is different from growth medium?**

Maintenance medium is similar to growth medium but contains less serum and is used to keep cells in a steady state of metabolism.

28. **What is the temperature of incubation of cell cultures for isolation of viruses?**

35–37°C

29. **What is the temperature of incubation of cell cultures for isolation of rhinoviruses?**

33°C

30. **Enumerate intracytoplasmic inclusion bodies seen in viral infections.**

Intracytoplasmic inclusion bodies seen in viral infections are given in Table 55.1.

Table 55.1. Intracytoplasmic inclusion bodies seen in viral infections

Inclusion bodies	Virus
Negri bodies	Rabies virus
Guarnieri bodies	Vaccinia
Bollinger bodies	Fowlpox
Molluscum bodies	Molluscum contagiosum

31. **In which viral infection, inclusion bodies are present in cytoplasm as well as nucleus?**

Measles

32. **How do you differentiate variola pocks from vaccinia pocks on the CAM of chick embryo?**

Variola pocks are small, shiny, white, convex, non-necrotic, non-haemorrhagic lesions, while vaccinia pocks are large, irregular, flat, greyish, necrotic lesions, some of which are haemorrhagic.

33. **Name the smallest viruses.**

Parvoviruses (about 20 nm in diameter).

34. **Name the largest viruses.**

Poxviruses (about 300 nm in diameter).

35. **Name viruses which carry two identical copies of its genome?**

Retroviruses.

36. **Name viruses which do not withstand freeze-drying.**

Polioviruses.

37. **Name viruses which are relatively resistant to chlorination.**

Polioviruses and hepatitis A virus.

38. **Which human viral disease can be prevented by active immunization after acquisition of infection?**

Rabies.

39. **Name hepatitis viruses which may cause hepato-cellular carcinoma.**

Hepatitis B virus and hepatitis C virus.

40. **Name hepatitis virus which has DNA genome.**

Hepatitis B virus.

41. **Name hepatitis viruses transmitted by faecal-oral route.**

Hepatitis A virus and hepatitis E virus.

42. **Which human hepatitis viruses can be cultivated in cell culture?**
   - Hepatitis A virus
   - SEN virus (SEN-V)

43. **Name viruses which may be transmitted by transfusion and transplantation.**
   - Hepatitis B virus
   - Hepatitis C virus
   - Hepatitis D virus
   - Human immunodeficiency virus
   - Human T cell lymphotropic virus-1
   - Cytomegalovirus.

44. **Name hepatitis viruses which may be transmitted by parenteral and sexual routes.**
   - Hepatitis B virus
   - Hepatitis C virus
   - Hepatitis D virus
   - Hepatitis G virus

45. **In which viral disease, inclusion bodies resemble owl's eye?**
   Cytomegalovirus infection.

46. **Name live virus vaccines.**
   - Smallpox
   - Yellow fever
   - Oral polio vaccine (Sabin vaccine)
   - Measles
   - Mumps
   - Rubella
   - Varicella.

47. **Which virus can remain latent in ganglia for many years?**
   Herpesviruses.

48. **Glandular fever is caused by which virus?**
   Epstein-Barr virus.

49. **Shingles is caused by which virus?**
   Varicella-zoster virus.

50. **Name the malignancies associated with Epstein-Barr virus.**
   - Burkitt's lymphoma
   - Nasopharyngeal carcinoma
   - B cell lymphoma

51. **Epidemic keratoconjunctivitis is caused by which virus?**
   Adenoviruses.

52. **Herpangina is caused by which virus?**
   Coxsackieviruses group A.

53. **Enumerate viruses causing aseptic meningitis.**
   - Enteroviruses (echoviruses, polioviruses, coxsackieviruses)
   - Mumps
   - Herpes simplex
   - Varicella-zoster
   - Measles
   - Adenoviruses
   - Arboviruses

54. **Which *Enterovirus* was associated with a pandemic of acute hemorrhagic conjunctivitis in 1969?**
   Enterovirus 70.

55. **Enumerate rabies vaccines.**
   - Neural vaccines
     - Semple vaccine
     - Beta-propiolactone vaccine
     - Suckling mouse brain vaccine
   - Non-neural vaccines
     - Duck egg vaccine
     - Cell culture vaccines
       * Human diploid cell (HDC) vaccine
       * Purified chick embryo cell (PCEC) vaccine
       * Purified Vero cell (PVC) vaccine

56. **Which viral infection is associated with hydrophobia?**
   Rabies.

57. **What are the dose, route of inoculation, site and schedule of post-exposure prophylaxis of rabies cell culture vaccine?**
   Five or six doses given intramuscularly in the deltoid region in 1.0 ml volume on days 0, 3, 7, 14, 30 and 90 after exposure are recommended. The last dose is optional.

58. **What are Koplik's spots?**
   They are small, 1–3 mm in diameter, bluish white spots surrounded by erythema. They can be seen on the buccal mucosa and are pathognomonic of measles.

59. **Name late complication of measles.**
   Subacute sclerosing panencephalitis.

60. **While attempting to isolate filoviruses, what should be the biosafety level?**
   Biosafety level 4.

61. **Name the most common prion disease in humans.**
   Creutzfeldt-Jakob disease.

62. **Which is the most prevalent subtype of group M of HIV-1 in India?**
   Subtype C.

63. **What is the duration of window period in HIV infection?**
   4–12 weeks.

64. **What is the risk of acquisition of HIV infection from needle-stick injury from HIV-positive person?**
   0.3%.

65. **Blood bank screening for HIV was initiated in which year?**

1985.

66. **Which is the commonest mode of transmission of HIV?**

Sexual.

67. **What is the efficiency of transmission of HIV by blood transfusion?**

>90%.

68. **What is the efficiency of transmission of HIV by the sexual route?**

0.1–1% per episode.

69. **Which is the commonest opportunistic infection in AIDS patients in India?**

Tuberculosis.

70. **Which virus is associated with erythematous eruption of the cheeks (slapped cheek)?**

Erythrovirus (*Parvovirus* B19).

71. **What is the sequence of manifestations seen in measles?**

Fever → Koplik's spots → Rash.

72. **Which hepatitis virus is associated with highest mortality in pregnancy?**

Hepatitis E virus.

73. **Acute hepatitis B is best diagnosed by which serological marker?**

IgM anti-HBc antibody.

74. **Which hepatitis virus is the most common cause of transfusion-associated hepatitis?**

Hepatitis B virus.

75. **Which hepatitis virus is the most common cause of hepatocellular carcinoma?**

Hepatitis B virus.

76. **Which hepatitis virus has the maximum potential for chronicity?**

Hepatitis C virus.

77. **What is the schedule of hepatitis B vaccination?**

Recombinant yeast hepatitis B vaccine adsorbed with aluminium hydroxide as adjuvant, stored in cold not frozen, and are injected intramuscularly into the deltoid region in a course of three doses given at 0, 1, 6 months.

78. **Define non-responder in hepatitis B vaccination.**

The non-responder is one who does not show sero-conversion even after 6 doses of vaccination, i.e., two series of vaccination.

79. **Which marker rises following hepatitis B vaccination?**

Anti-HBs antibody.

80. **Which day is celebrated as world AIDS day?**

December 1st

81. **Which state in India has the highest HIV prevalence?**

Manipur.

82. **Which NACO strategy is used for screening of HIV in blood bank?**

Strategy I.

83. **Name one tick-borne arboviral infection.**

Kyasanur forest disease.

84. **Hand-foot-and-mouth disease is caused by which virus?**

It is usually caused by types 5 and 16 of group A cox-sackieviruses.

85. **How do you differentiate smallpox and chickenpox rashes?**

Smallpox rashes have centrifugal distribution, while chickenpox rashes have centripetal distribution.

Section 7

Recent Advances

- Molecular biology

Molecular Biology

NUCLEIC ACID PROBES

Principle

The basic principle behind nucleic acid probe technology is hybridization of characterized nucleic acid probe to a specific nucleic acid sequence in a test specimen followed by detection of the paired hybrid.

The hybridization reaction consists of four components:

- The probe
- The target (which is contained in the sample)
- The reporter molecule
- The hybridization method

Probe

A nucleic acid probe is a sequence of single-stranded nucleic acid that can hybridize specifically with its complementary strand via nucleic acid–base pairing. A probe may be constructed to detect either DNA or RNA. All micro-organisms, simple or complex, contain some unique sequences of DNA or RNA within their genome that distinguish them from all other organisms. The method of developing a nucleic acid probe (either DNA or RNA) is to cut or isolate those sequences from the nucleic acid of the cell using a set of enzymes known as restriction endonucleases, reproduce them in large quantities and attach a reporter molecule to them so that they can be incorporated into a hybridization process. The probe may be synthetically produced from oligo-nucleotide of specific sequences.

Target

The nucleic acid in the sample is referred to as the target. The sample can consist of a suspension of an unknown organism (for culture confirmation) or a clinical specimen such as sputum or stool.

Reporter molecule

The label on the probe, whether it is a radioisotope or an enzyme, is referred to as the reporter molecule. It helps to detect the hybridization reaction that may have occurred between probe and target. These include:

- Radioactive labels
  - ^{32}P
  - ^{125}I
  - ^{35}S
- Digoxigenin
- Chemiluminescence label
- Biotin-avidin
- Enzymes
  - Alkaline phosphatase
  - Horseradish peroxidase

Hybridization

This is the process whereby two single strands of nucleic acid come together to form a stable double-stranded molecule. However, they will bind and stay together, only if the sequences of bases along each stretch of nucleic acid are complementary. Hybridization is accomplished in tubes or by spotting the unknown organisms on a filter paper such as nitrocellulose paper, lysing them to release DNA, and denaturing in mild alkali to single strands. The probe can then be added and after thorough washing to remove any unbound probe, the tube or probe is examined for evidence of hybridization. Depending upon the label (reporter molecule) hybridization can be detected by autoradiography, spectrophotometers or luminometers. Formalin-fixed, paraffin-embedded tissues can also be probed particularly for viral DNA sequences.

Applications of Nucleic Acid Probes

- Rapid identification of organisms with long incubation time.

Recent Advances

7

- Direct detection of organisms in clinical specimens (Table 56.1).
- Confirmation of cultural isolates.
- Detection of non-viable organisms.
- Identification of toxins, virulence factors and resistance markers.

Table 56.1. Microorganisms where nucleic acid probes have been applied to diagnostic microbiology

Culture confirmation and identification	Direct detection in clinical specimens
Bacteria	**Bacteria**
• *Mycobacterium tuberculosis*	• *Mycobacterium tuberculosis*
• *M. avium*	• *Neisseria gonorrhoeae*
• *M. avium* complex	• *Chlamydia trachomatis*
• *Neisseria gonorrhoeae*	• *Legionella pneumophila*
• *Chlamydia trachomatis*	• *Mycoplasma pneumoniae*
• *Haemophilus influenzae*	• *Bordetella pertussis*
• *Listeria monocytogenes*	• *Gardnerella vaginalis*
• *Campylobacter* spp.	• *Streptococcus pyogenes*
• *Enterococcus* spp.	
• *Streptococcus agalactiae*	**Fungi**
	• *Candida* spp.
Fungi	**Protozoa**
• *Blastomyces dermatitidis*	• *Trichomonas vaginalis*
• *Coccidioides immitis*	
• *Histoplasma capsulatum*	**Viruses**
• *Cryptococcus neoformans*	• Enteroviruses
Viruses	• Human papillomavirus
• Human papillomavirus	

BLOTTING

Blotting techniques are named according to the target molecule, which can be DNA, RNA and proteins.

Western Blotting

In this technique, partially purified microbial preparation is first heated with a detergent such as sodium dodecyl sulphate (SDS). The SDS helps to release individual proteins from complex proteins. The proteins are separated according to their molecular weight on polyacrylamide gel by electrophoresis. The lower molecular weight proteins move readily through the gel matrix to the bottom of the gel. The separated proteins form invisible 'bands' in the gel. Now these separated protein bands on the surface of the gel are transferred to nitrocellulose membrane by blotting or electrophoresis. Nitrocellulose membrane is cut into strips after washing. A number of commercial kits for western blotting contain nitrocellulose membrane strips on which the protein antigens of interest have been electrophoretically separated.

Test procedure

- The nitrocellulose membrane is immersed in diluted patient serum and incubated. Specific antibodies in sample, if present, will bind to protein bands on the surface of nitrocellulose membrane during incubation.
- After incubation, the nitrocellulose membrane is thoroughly washed to remove unbound antibodies.
- After washing, the nitrocellulose membrane is incubated with enzyme tagged-antihuman gammaglobulin. Enzyme substrate is subsequently added which indicates positive test. The substrate changes colour in the presence of enzyme and permanently stains the nitrocellulose membrane. The position of the band on the membrane indicates the antigen (protein) with which the antibody has reacted.

Applications

- Supplemental test for HIV infection.
- Diagnosis of Lyme disease.
- Diagnosis of congenital syphilis.

Southern Blotting

DNA fragments obtained by restriction endonuclease enzyme are separated on the gel by electrophoresis. The separated DNA fragments are transferred to nitrocellulose membrane by blotting. The DNA bound to the membrane is denatured to single-stranded form and allowed to react with radioactive single stranded DNA probes. Hybridization, if occurs, is further detected by autoradiography.

Northern Blotting

In this technique, RNA mixture is separated by gel electrophoreses, blotted and identified by using radiolabelled probe.

Polymerase Chain Reaction (PCR)

Kary Mulis invented this method in 1989. He was awarded Nobel Prize in 1993. Polymerase chain reaction is a primer-mediated, temperature-dependent technique for the enzymatic amplification of a specific sequence (target sequence) to such an extent that it can be detected. The technique can be used to detect very small amounts of specific nucleic acid material in clinical specimens where bacterial, viral or fungal agents are thought to play a causative role. The fundamental basis of this technology is that each pathogenic organism possesses a unique 'signature sequence' in its DNA or RNA composition by which it can be identified. It is based on repeated cycles of high temperature template denaturation, oligonucleotide primer annealing, and polymerase mediated extension (Fig. 56.1).

To multiply a strip of genetic material, four ingredients are placed together in a small vial:

1. Target DNA.
2. Short strands of DNA called primers which tag the section to be copied.
3. Polymerase—an enzyme that promotes gene replication in all living cells.
4. Nucleotides—the building blocks for making DNA.

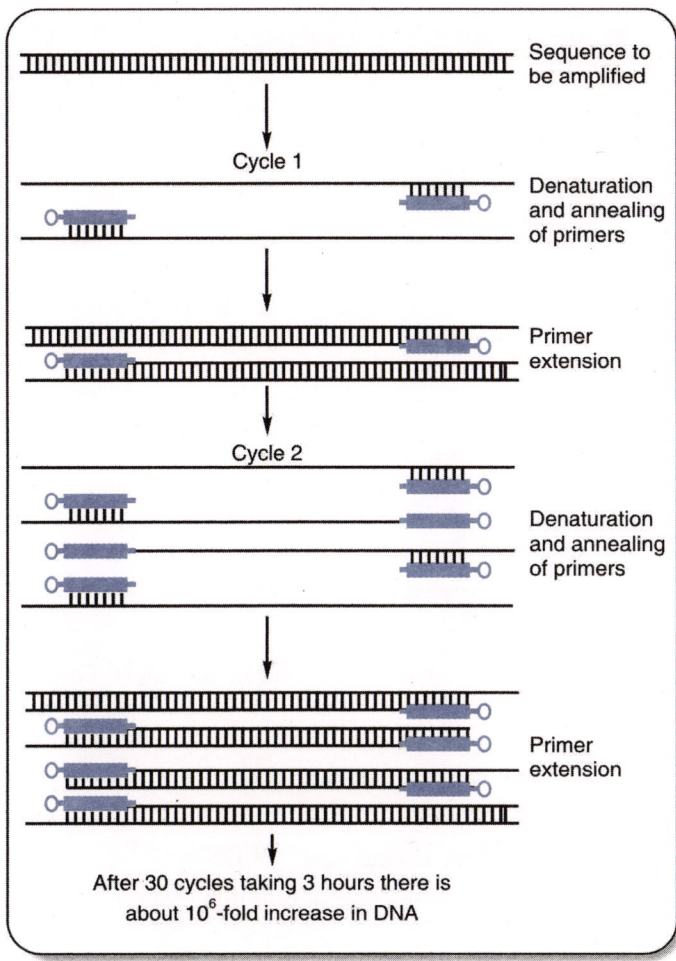

Fig. 56.1. Polymerase chain reaction.

Table 56.2. Programming of cycles in polymerase chain reaction

Step	Temperature	Time	Cycle
Initial denaturation	94°C	5 minutes	First cycle
Denaturation	94°C	30 seconds	
Annealing of primers	55°C	1 minute	30 cycles
Primer extension	72°C	1 minute	
Final primer extension	72°C	7 minutes	Last cycle

Amplified sequences of target DNA can be detected by a variety of methods. If enough amplified DNA is present, it can be visualized by:

1. Gel electrophoresis and ethidium bromide staining.
2. Southern blot and dot-blot analysis with either radioactive or nonradioactive probes.
3. Oligomer restriction.
4. Oligomer hybridization.
5. Reverse dot-blot.

Reverse Polymerase Chain Reactions

Instead of *Taq* polymerase described above, *Tth* polymerase obtained from *Thermus thermophilus* may be used. The *Tth* enzyme possesses both DNA polymerase and reverse transcriptase activities at high temperature. This allows both cDNA synthesis from mRNA followed by PCR amplification.

Applications of PCR

The development of PCR or gene amplification method is a major methodological breakthrough in molecular biology. Within a short span, this method has found its way into nearly every type of laboratory from forensic to ecology and from diagnosis to pure research.

In diagnosis of infections

This technique is used in diagnosis of infections caused by viruses, bacteria, fungi and protozoa.

In diagnosis of inherited disorders

The PCR technology is being widely used to amplify gene segments that contain known mutations for diagnosis of inherited diseases such as sickle cell anaemia, β-thalassaemia, cystic fibrosis, etc. PCR is especially useful for prenatal diagnosis of inherited diseases, where cells obtained from the foetus by amniocentesis are very few.

In cancer detection

Identification of mutations in oncosuppressor genes such as retinoblastoma gene can help to identify individuals at high risk of cancer.

In medicolegal cases

PCR allows DNA in a single cell, hair follicle or sperm to be amplified enormously and analyzed. The pattern obtained is then compared with that of various suspects.

PCR is carried out in three steps:

1. Heat at 94°C is applied to the target DNA, breaking the bonds that hold the strands together. This is known as **denaturation**.
2. The temperature is then reduced to 55°C, promoting the primers to attach themselves to either end of the target strip. This is known as **annealing** of primers.
3. Then polymerase enzyme triggers the formation of new DNA strand from the nucleotides. Extension of the primers is done by a thermostable *Taq* polymerase (purified from *Thermus aquaticus*, a thermophilic bacterium that lives in hot springs at temperatures of 70–75°C). This is known as **primer extension**. When the temperature is again raised the new strands separate and the process begins again.

These three steps are repeated again and again by manipulating the temperature, a process that is automated by the PCR machine (Table 56.2). A cycle takes about 3–5 minutes and after 30 cycles, taking about 3 hours, a single copy of DNA can be increased up to 1,000,000 copies, a sharp contrast to the days required by conventional amplification method (culture).

Discussion

1. **Enumerate basic steps of nucleic acid probe technology.**
   - Preparation and labelling of single-stranded nucleic acid probe.
   - Preparation of single-stranded target nucleic acid.
   - Hybridization of target and probe nucleic acid.
   - Detection of hybridization.

2. **Enumerate various reporter molecules used for labelling probes.**
   - Radioactive (^{32}P, ^{125}I, ^{35}S)
   - Biotin-avidin
   - Digoxigenin
   - Chemiluminescent labels
   - Fluorescein labels

3. **Enumerate viruses which can be detected directly in the specimens using probes.**
   - Enteroviruses
   - Human papillomaviruses
   - Herpes simplex viruses

4. **Enumerate gels which can be used to separate RNA/DNA.**
   - Agarose
   - Acrylamide

5. **What is the function of sodium dodecyl sulphate (SDS) in Western blotting?**

   SDS is a detergent. It releases individual proteins from complex proteins (denatures protein).

6. **Who discovered Southern blotting?**

   EM Southern.

7. **Enumerate methods to transfer DNA, RNA or protein to nitrocellulose membrane.**
   - Electrophoresis
   - Blotting

8. **Which chemical is used to stain the DNA fragments separated by gel electrophoresis?**

   Ethidium bromide

9. **What is the role of restriction endonuclease enzymes in molecular biology?**

   Restriction endonucleases cut the double-stranded DNA at specific sequences and produce DNA fragments of varying length.

10. **Who invented polymerase chain reaction (PCR)?**

    Kary Mulis in 1989.

11. **Enumerate three basic steps of a PCR cycle.**
    - Denaturation
    - Annealing
    - Primer extension

12. **How much time is taken in one cycle of PCR?**

    Three to five minutes.

13. **Define polymerase chain reaction.**

    Polymerase chain reaction is a primer-mediated, temperature-dependent technique for the enzymatic amplification of a specific sequence to such an extent that it can be detected.

14. **At what temperature, annealing of primers occurs?**

    55°C.

15. **In how many cycles of PCR, good amplification of DNA is obtained?**

    30 cycles.

16. **How many copies of DNA are obtained after 30 cycles of PCR?**

    10^6 copies from a single copy of DNA.

17. **Enumerate various methods of detection of amplified DNA.**
    - Gel electrophoresis and ethidium bromide staining.
    - Southern blot and dot-blot analysis with either radioactive or nonradioactive probes.
    - Oligomer restriction.
    - Oligomer hybridization.
    - Reverse dot-blot.

18. **Enumerate various amplification techniques.**
    - PCR   Polymerase chain reaction
    - LCR   Ligase chain reaction
    - SDA   Strand displacement amplification
    - bDNA   Branched chain hybrid capture
    - CPT   Cycling probe technology
    - TMA   Transcription mediated amplification
    - NASBA   Nucleic acid sequence based amplification
    - 3SR   Self-sustaining sequence replication

Section
8

Spots

- Spots

Spots

1. McIntosh and Fildes' Anaerobic Jar

This is most reliable and widely used anaerobic jar. It is cylindrical vessel made of glass or metal with a metal lid, which is held firmly in place by a clamp. The lid has two tubes with taps, one acting as gas inlet and the other as the outlet (Fig. 57.1). On its undersurface, it carries a gauze sachet carrying alumina pellets coated with palladium. It acts as a room temperature catalyst for the conversion of hydrogen and oxygen into water. It acts as a catalyst, as long as the sachet is kept dry.

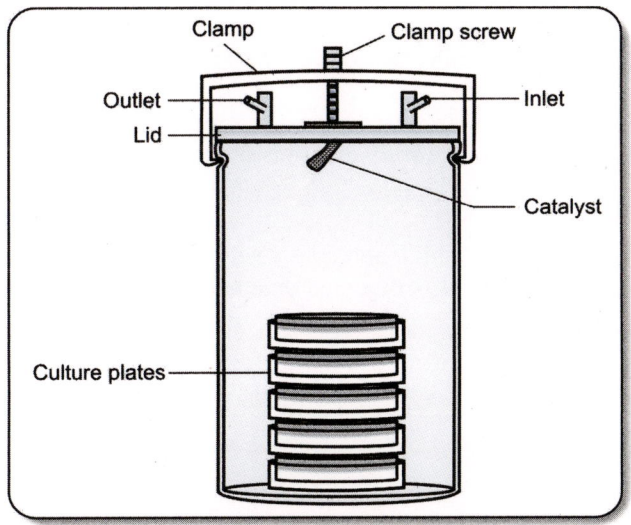

Fig. 57.1. McIntosh and Fildes' anaerobic jar.

Inoculated culture plates are placed inside the jar and the lid is clamped tight. The outlet tube is connected to a vacuum pump and the air inside is evacuated. The outlet tap is then closed and the inlet tube connected to a hydrogen supply. Hydrogen is drawn in rapidly. As soon as this inrush of gas has ceased, the inlet tap is also closed. After about 5 minutes, inlet tap is again opened. There occurs again an immediate inrush of hydrogen since the catalyst creates a reduced pressure within the jar due to the conversion of hydrogen and leftover oxygen into water. The jar is left connected to hydrogen supply for about 5 minutes, then the inlet tap is closed and the jar is placed in the incubator, catalysis will continue until all the oxygen in the jar has been used up.

Indicator

Chemical indicator

Methylene blue indicator is used for verifying the anaerobic condition in the jar. When it is placed in an anaerobic environment it is reduced from its coloured oxidized form to a colourless reduced leuco-compound.

Biological indicator

In place of chemical indicator, a culture plate inoculated with strict anaerobe such as *Clostridium tetani* and strict aerobe such as *Pseudomonas aeruginosa* may be used as biological indicator. Growth of strict anaerobe and no growth of strict aerobe indicates that anaerobiasis has been maintained.

2. GasPak Envelope

The GasPak is now the method of choice for preparing anaerobic jar (Fig. 57.2). The GasPak is commercially available as a disposable envelope containing chemicals which generate hydrogen and carbon dioxide on the addition of water. After the inoculated plates are kept in the jar, the GasPak envelope with water added, is placed inside and lid screwed tight. Hydrogen and carbon dioxide are liberated and the presence of a cold catalyst in the envelope permits the combination of hydrogen and oxygen to produce an anaerobic environment.

Advantages

- Operation of the jar is quick and simple.
- There is no need of vacuum pump and cylinders of compressed gas.

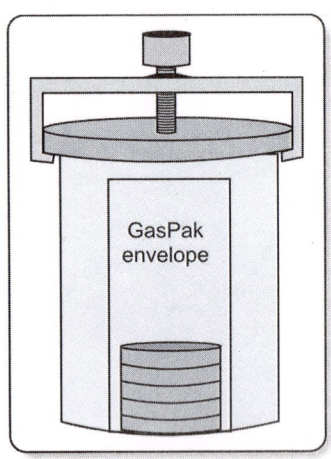

Fig. 57.2. GasPak anaerobic jar.

3. VDRL Slide

It is a glass slide with 12 paraffin rings of approximately 15 mm diameter (Fig. 57.3). It is used to do VDRL test for diagnosis of syphilis. Slide tests require a small quantity of antigen or antibody as compared to tube tests. Positive or negative reactions can be detected under microscope.

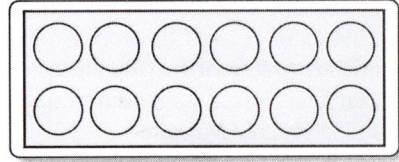

Fig. 57.3. VDRL slide.

4. Seitz Filter (Asbestos Filter)

This is made up of a disc of asbestos (magnesium trisilicate). It is supported on a perforated metal disc within a metal funnel. The latter with filter disc fitted is sterilized by autoclaving. It is then fitted onto a sterile flask through a silicone rubber bung (Fig. 57.4). The fluid to be sterilized is put into the funnel

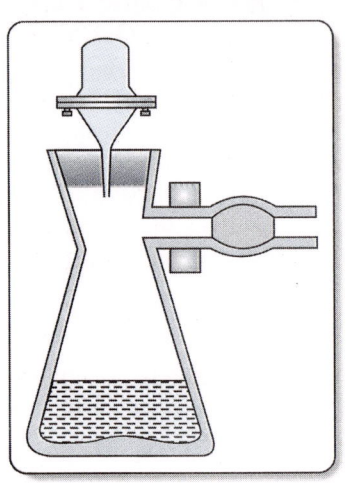

Fig. 57.4. Seitz filter.

and flask connected to the exhaust pump through its side tap. Sterilized fluid is collected from the flask and filter disc is discarded after use. These discs are available with different grades of porosity. *Serratia marcescens* and *Pseudomonas diminuta* have been used to test the efficacy of filter.

Uses

- It is used to sterilize liquids such as sera and solutions of heat-labile substances such as sugars and urea, for preparation of media.
- It is also useful for separation of bacteriophages and bacterial toxins from bacteria and for the isolation of organisms which are scanty in fluids.

5. Swab Stick

It is a thin wire or stick with cotton wrapped at one end. It is kept in a cotton-plugged test tube (Fig. 57.5) and is sterilized in hot air oven at 160°C for one hour or 180°C for 20 minutes.

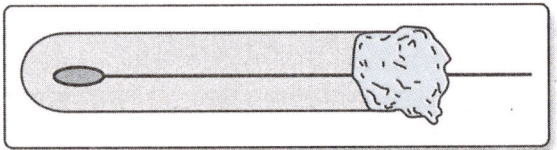

Fig. 57.5. Swab stick.

Uses

- It is used for collection of clinical specimens like pus or other discharge.
- It is also used for preparing lawn culture on Mueller-Hinton agar to find out the antibiotic sensitivity pattern of bacteria.

6. Nichrome Loop

The loop is flat, circular and completely closed with 2–4 mm internal diameter. It is mounted on a handle (Fig. 57.6). The

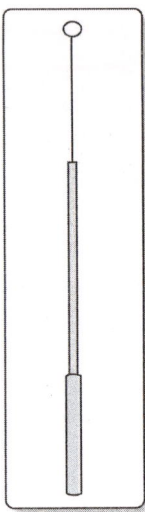

Fig. 57.6. Nichrome loop.

loop is sterilized by holding it almost vertical in a Bunsen burner flame until red hot. Owing to the high cost of platinum, loops for routine work are made of nichrome, No. 24 SWG.

Uses

- It is used for inoculating various clinical specimens on solid or liquid media.
- It is used in streak culture and stroke culture.
- It is used to put up biochemical reactions.

7. Cavity Slide

This is a glass slide with a cavity. It is used to determine the motility of bacteria by hanging drop preparation.

8. Microtitre Plate

It is a plastic plate with 96 wells (8 × 12) (Fig. 57.7). It is made up of polystyrene. It is used because small quantity of antigen or antibody are required to conduct the test.

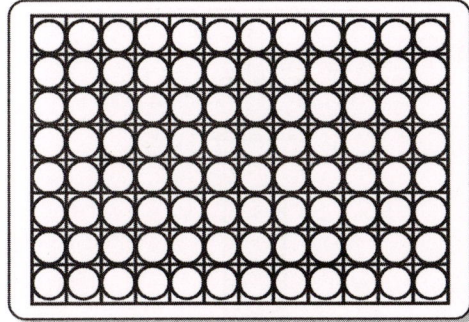

Fig. 57.7. Microtitre plate.

Uses

- It may be used to conduct ELISA test.
- It may be used to conduct Weil-Felix agglutination reaction and haemagglutination test.

9. Antibiotic Sensitivity Plate

Kirby-Bauer disc diffusion method

The petri dish usually contains Mueller-Hinton agar. Inoculation is done on the dried surface of agar plate by streaking the swab three times over the entire agar surface. Antibiotic discs are placed on this plate. Usually, not more than 7 discs are placed on one plate of 100 mm diameter. The plate is incubated at 35–37°C for 16–18 hours. Next day by using a transparent plastic ruler, the zones of complete growth inhibition around each of the discs are carefully measured (Fig. 14.1). The interpretation of zone size into susceptible, moderately susceptible or resistant is based on interpretation chart (Table 14.1).

10. Blood Culture Bottle

It is a glass bottle with a capacity of 150–200 ml. It contains

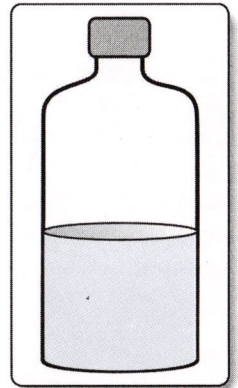

Fig. 57.8. Blood culture bottle.

metallic screw cap covered with sterilized paper (Fig. 57.8). It contains 50–100 ml volume of liquid culture medium (glucose broth, bile broth or brain heart infusion broth). 5–10 ml of blood is collected aseptically from antecubital vein and inoculated in blood culture bottle through a hole in screw cap. This is followed by incubation of bottle at 37°C. Depending upon the organisms suspected, subcultures are made on appropriate culture plates at variable intervals. This method is used for blood culture of patients suffering from pyrexia of unknown origin and septicaemic patients.

11. Castaneda Blood Culture Medium

This blood culture bottle contains both liquid serum dextrose broth and solid serum dextrose agar media (Fig. 57.9). The blood is inoculated into the broth and bottle incubated in the upright position. For subculture, the bottle is tilted, so that the broth flows over the surface of agar slant. It is again incubated in upright position. In positive cases, colonies appear on the slant. This is most definitive method for the diagnosis of brucellosis.

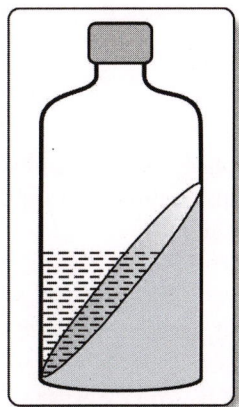

Fig. 57.9. Castaneda blood culture bottle.

Advantages

This technique reduces the chances of contamination and risk of infection to laboratory personnel.

12. Clot Culture

Clot culture is helpful for diagnosis of typhoid fever. With strict aseptic precautions, 5 ml blood is withdrawn from the patient into a sterile test tube and allowed to clot. The separated serum is removed for serological test. The clot is broken up with a sterile glass rod and added to a bottle of bile broth containing streptokinase. Streptokinase causes rapid clot lysis with release of bacteria trapped in the clot.

Advantages

- Clot culture with streptokinase yields a higher rate of isolation than whole blood culture as the bactericidal action of the serum is obviated.
- Sample of serum is available for serological tests.

13. Craigie's Tube

This consists of large tube containing semisolid agar (0.2–0.3%) with monophasic antiserum. Within the agar, a small tube, which is open at both the ends, is placed with its upper end projecting well above the surface (Fig. 57.10). The isolated bacterium is inoculated into the inner tube and after 8–16 hours incubation, subculture is taken from the surface of medium in the outer tube.

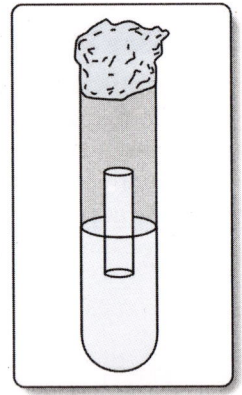

Fig. 57.10. Craigie's tube.

Uses

- It demonstrates motility of the organisms
- The definitive identification of a diphasic *Salmonella* is made by using this tube.

14. BCG Vaccine

It is a live-attenuated vaccine introduced by Calmette and Guerin. This is a strain of *Mycobacterium bovis* attenuated by repeated subcultures, every 3 weeks, for 230 subcultures on slices of potato soaked in autoclaved bile containing glycerol (5%) over a period of 13 years. BCG vaccine is available in liquid form and freeze-dried (lyophilized) form. The lyophilized vaccine is reconstituted with sterile physiological saline to make a final concentration of 0.1 mg in 0.1 ml of the vaccine. Once reconstituted, vaccine should be utilized within

3–6 hours. Following injection of 0.1 ml of vaccine intradermally, the organisms grow to a limited extent in the tissues. This vaccine should be administered soon after birth failing which it may be given at any time during the first year of life. The protective efficacy of BCG vaccine varies from 80% to a total absence of protection. The present consensus is that BCG **does** protect from tuberculosis.

Uses

- BCG vaccine induces active immunity to tuberculosis.
- It stimulates T lymphocytes which offer some protection against leprosy and leukaemia also.
- It is believed to prevent meningeal, skeletal and miliary form of tuberculosis to a large extent.

15. Tuberculin Syringe

It is 1 ml glass syringe. Sterilized plastic syringes are also available (Fig. 57.11).

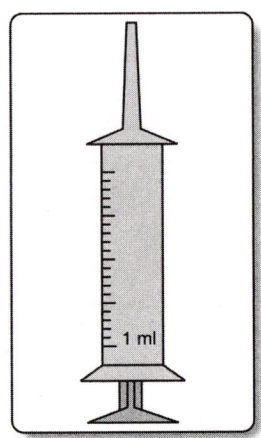

Fig. 57.11. Tuberculin syringe.

Uses

- It is used to conduct Mantoux test.
- It can be used to inject insulin.
- It can be used to inject antigen to conduct various skin hypersensitivity tests.
- It can be used to inject small amount of test material into animal.

16. Glass Syringes

Glass syringes are available in different capacities and these are sterilized in hot air oven (160°C for 1 hour).

Uses

- These are used to withdraw blood or fluids from patients for conducting diagnostic tests.
- These are also used to withdraw blood from animals to prepare blood agar plate.
- These are used to give intramuscular or intravenous injections to patients.

17. Plastic Syringes

Sterilized plastic syringes are also available. These are sterilized by gamma irradiations. This method of sterilization is known as **cold sterilization**. They can be used for all those procedures where we use glass syringes.

18. Disinfectants

Disinfectants are antimicrobial agents used to kill potentially infectious agents present on inanimate objects. Antiseptics (mild disinfectant) are non-toxic antimicrobial agents that may be applied topically to the body surface either to kill or inhibit the growth of pathogenic organisms. The disinfectants and antiseptics may be dispensed in bottle showing its identity. It may be phenol, cresol, Dettol, glutaraldehyde, formalin, etc.

Uses

- Glutaraldehyde is used for sterilization of heat-sensitive instruments like cystoscope, bronchoscope, thermometers, etc.
- Formalin is used for fumigation of operation theatres, wards, laboratories, etc.
- Dettol may be used for cleaning wound.

19. Shell Vial Culture Tube

Shell vial is a round tube with a flat bottom and contains a coverslip on which the cells are grown (Fig. 57.12). Specimens are inoculated onto the shell vial cell monolayer. The shell vial culture technique can be used to detect most viruses that grow in conventional cell culture. Coverslips are stained using virus-specific immunofluorescent conjugates. Typical fluorescing inclusions confirm the presence of virus.

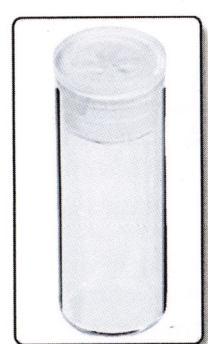

Fig. 57.12. Shell vial culture tube.

Advantages

- Most viruses are detected within 24 hours.
- It can be used for isolation of *Chlamydia trachomatis*.

20. Tissue Culture Bottle

It may be made up of glass or plastic (Fig. 57.13). It contains tissue culture medium. The medium is buffered with bicarbonate to give a pH of 7.2–7.4 and phenol red is added

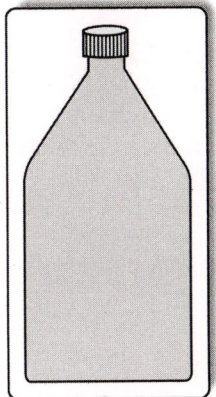

Fig. 57.13. Tissue culture bottle.

as a pH indicator. Antimicrobial agents are added to prevent bacterial and fungal contamination.

Uses

- They are used for propagation of cell cultures.
- Cytopathic effect of viruses can be observed in the cultured cells.

21. Bijou Bottle

It is a small screw-capped round glass bottle available in 15 ml capacity (Fig. 57.14).

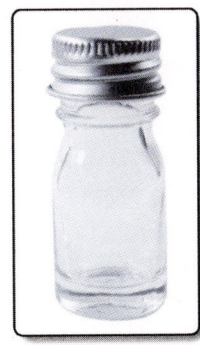

Fig. 57.14. Bijou bottle.

Uses

- It is used to maintain stock culture of bacteria.
- It may be used for transportation of bacterial culture.

22. Dark-field Condenser

Dark-field condenser is used for dark-field microscopy. By means of condenser the specimen is illuminated by oblique light only. The rays do not enter the tube of the microscope, and in consequence, do not reach the eye of the observer unless they are scattered by objects (e.g., bacteria) of different refractive index from the medium, in which they are suspended. As a result, the organisms appear brightly illuminated against a dark background. It renders visible delicate organisms such as *Treponema pallidum*.

23. Petri Dishes

Petri dishes of glass and plastic are routinely used in laboratory. After washing, glass petri dishes are sterilized in hot air oven at 160°C for one hour. The melted medium is poured in sterilized petri dishes and left undisturbed until the medium has set. Plastic petri dishes are available in two varieties, i.e., disposable and reusable. Disposables are discarded after single use. Reusables are washed, sterilized by autoclaving and reused.

Uses

- They are used to prepare various solid culture media.
- They may be used for gross examination of stool sample.
- They are used to put up slide culture test for fungi.

24. Test Tubes Stoppered with Cotton-Wool Plug

Test tubes of glass are routinely used in laboratory. They are available in different capacities. After washing and drying, they are stoppered with cotton-wool plugs and sterilized in hot air oven at 160°C for 1 hour. After each use, they are discarded in jar containing disinfectant after removing the cotton plugs.

Uses

- They are used for pouring liquid media.
- They are used for preparation of solid media in the form of slopes, e.g., Christensen medium and Simmon's citrate medium.
- They are used to put up biochemical reactions.

25. Lovibond Comparator

This is used to measure the pH of different media. Two tubes are marked as 'C' for control and 'T' for test. Approximately 5 ml of medium is taken in both the tubes. Now 0.2 ml of phenol red solution is added in tube 'T'. After mixing, the colour of tube 'T' is compared with control tube 'C' in lovibond comparator (Fig. 57.15). For alkaline pH 1 N NaOH and for acidic pH 0.1 N HCl is added in a dropwise manner so as to finally get the desired pH.

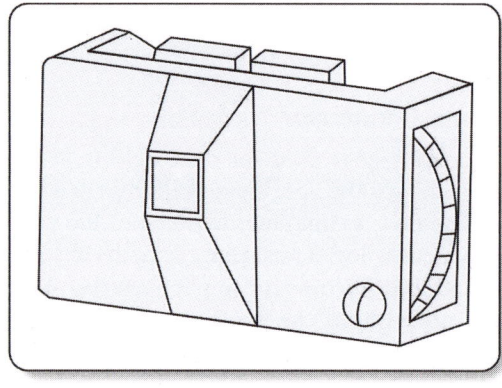

Fig. 57.15. Lovibond comparator.

26. Indicators

Indicators may be dispensed in test tube showing their identity. These are phenol red indicator, Andrade's indicator, bromothymol blue indicator, etc.

Phenol red indicator

This is routinely used in bacteriology for the comparison of pH of standard media. It has a pH range of 6.8–8.4. It is yellow at pH 6.8 and purple pink at pH 8.4.

Andrade's indicator

This is added in sugar media to detect acid production during the fermentation of sugars. It has a pH range of 5.0–8.0. It is yellow at alkaline pH and red at acidic pH.

Bromothymol blue indicator

This is used in Simmon's citrate medium to indicate the utilization of citrate. It has a pH range of 6.0–7.6. It is yellow in acidic pH and blue at alkaline pH.

27. National institute of Health Swab (NIH Swab)

NIH swab consists of a glass rod at one end of which a piece of transparent cellophane (with sticky surface out) is wrapped and held in place with a rubber band. The other end of the glass rod is fixed in a rubber stopper and kept in a test tube (Fig. 27.5). The cellophane part is used for swabbing by rolling over the perianal skin. Then the cellophane is detached, spread over glass slide and examined microscopically. This procedure should be repeated on three successive days. Eggs of *Enterobius vermicularis* which are deposited in large numbers on the perianal skin at night can be demonstrated.

28. *Ascaris lumbricoides* (Roundworm)

Adult worm

The body of *A. lumbricoides* is cylindrical tapering gradually at the anterior end and somewhat less so at the posterior end. White longitudinal streaks can usually be seen along the entire length of the pinkish cream body of the parasite (Fig. 57.16).

Male worm

It measures 15–30 cm in length and 3–4 mm in diameter. The posterior end is curved ventrally to form a hook. The ejaculatory duct along with the anus open into the cloaca from which arises a pair of copulatory spicules of equal size.

Female worm

It is longer and stouter than the male worm and measures 25–40 cm in length and 5 mm in diameter. The tail is straight and conical. The anus is subterminal and opens on the ventral surface in the form of a transverse slit. The vulva opens at the junction of the anterior and the middle thirds of the body on the midventral aspect of the worm. This part of the worm is narrower and is known as **vulvar waist**. A mature female lays nearly 200,000 eggs daily which are passed in the faeces.

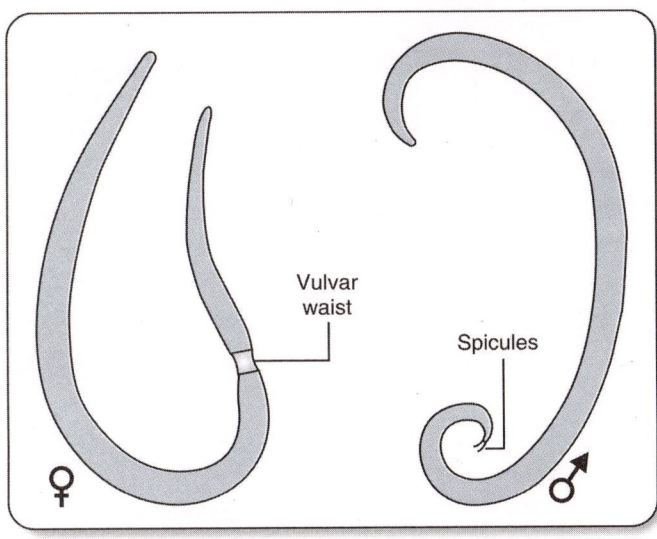

Fig. 57.16. Adult worms of *Ascaris lumbricoides*.

29. *Taenia saginata* (Beef Tapeworm; Unarmed Tapeworm of Man)

The adult worm consists of scolex (head), neck and strobila which is made up of a large number of proglottids (1,000–2,000). It is 4–6 metres or more in length. Scolex is large, quadrate without rostellum and hooklets and possesses four suckers which may be pigmented.

30. *Taenia solium* (Pork Tapeworm; Armed Tapeworm of Man)

It is 2–4 metres or more in length. Scolex is small, globular, with rostellum armed with a double row of 25–30 alternating large and small hooklets and possesses four suckers which are not pigmented. Number of proglottids is 800–1,000, which are expelled in chains of 5 or 6.

31. Hydatid Cyst

It represents larval form of *Echinococcus granulosus* (Colour Plate VIII, Fig. 51). The cyst wall consists of ectocyst and endocyst. Ectocyst is outer layer. It is tough, acellular, laminated, hyaline membrane up to 1 mm in thickness. It is elastic, therefore, when excised or ruptured, it curls on itself, thus, exposing the inner layer containing brood capsules, scolices and daughter cysts. Endocyst is inner or germinal layer. It consists of a number of nuclei embedded in a protoplasmic mass. It measures 22–25 µm in thickness. It gives rise to ectocyst on outside and brood capsules and scolices on inside (Colour Plate VIII, Fig. 52). It also secretes hydatid fluid. Hydatid fluid is clear, colourless or pale yellow with specific gravity 1.005–1.010. It is antigenic, therefore, it is used for Casoni test.

32. Casoni Antigen

Antigen for the Casoni test is sterile hydatid fluid drawn from the unilocular hydatid cysts from sheep, pig, cattle or man. The fluid is filtered, tested for sterility and stored in sealed ampoules under refrigeration. It is used in Casoni test which is an immediate hypersensitivity skin test for diagnosis of hydatid cyst. For the test, 0.2 ml of the antigen is injected intradermally in one arm. For control, an equal amount of sterile normal saline is injected intradermally on the other arm. The control fades almost immediately, while the tested site in positive case develops a large wheal measuring 5 cm or more in diameter with multiple pseudopodia within 30 minutes. This test has a low sensitivity (55–70%) and gives false positive reactions in patients suffering from other cestode infections.

33. *Fasciola hepatica* (Sheep Liver Fluke; Common Liver Fluke)

It is a large leaf-shaped fluke measuring 30 × 13 mm and brown to pale grey in colour. It is bilaterally symmetrical with three body layers, but has no true body cavity. At the anterior end, there is distinct conical projection. The posterior end is broadly pointed. The oral sucker is situated in the conical projection at the anterior end. The ventral sucker is 1.6 mm in diameter and is situated nearby in a line with two shoulders.

Appendices

- Appendix I   pH indicators
- Appendix II   Greek alphabet
- Appendix III   International System of Units (SI)—SI prefixes
- Appendix IV   Notifiable infectious diseases

                      Old nomenclature of a few organisms

- Appendix V   Characteristic colonial appearance

                      Characteristic appearance of bacteria in stained smear

- Appendix VI   Differentiation of bacteria of Enterobacteriaceae by biochemical tests
- Appendix VII   Overview of microbiology, mycology and parasitology

APPENDIX I

pH Indicators

	pH range	Colour change
Phenol red	6.8–8.4	Yellow to red
Neutral red	6.8–8.0	Red to yellow
Methyl red	4.4–6.2	Red to yellow
Cresol red	7.2–8.8	Yellow to red
Congo red	3.0–5.0	Blue-violet to red
Bromothymol blue	6.0–7.6	Yellow to blue
Bromocresol purple	5.2–6.8	Yellow to purple
Thymol blue	8.0–9.6	Yellow to blue
Thymol blue (acid range)	1.2–2.8	Red to yellow
Litmus	4.5–8.3	Red to blue
m-Cresol purple	7.6–9.2	Yellow to purple
Andrade's indicator	5.0–8.0	Pink to yellow

APPENDIX II

Greek Alphabet

	Small	Capital
Alpha	α	A
Beta	β	B
Gamma	γ	Γ
Delta	δ	Δ
Epsilon	ε	E
Zeta	ζ	Z
Eta	η	H
Theta	θ	Θ
Kappa	κ	K
Lambda	λ	Λ
Mu	μ	M
Xi	ξ	Ξ
Pi	π	Π
Rho	ρ	P
Sigma	σ	Σ
Phi	ϕ	Φ
Chi	χ	X
Psi	ψ	Ψ
Omega	ω	Ω

APPENDIX III

International System of Units (SI)—SI Prefixes

Factor	Prefix	Symbol
10^{-18}	atto	a
10^{-15}	femto	f
10^{-12}	pico	p
10^{-9}	nano	n
10^{-6}	micro	μ
10^{-3}	milli	m
10^{-2}	centi	c
10^{-1}	deci	d
10	deca	da
10^{6}	mega	M
10^{9}	giga	G
10^{12}	tera	T
10^{15}	peta	P
10^{18}	exa	E

APPENDIX IV

Notifiable Infectious Diseases

- Cholera
- Plague
- Anthrax
- Diphtheria
- Tetanus
- Leptospirosis
- Relapsing fever
- Typhus fever
- Meningococcal septicaemia
- Leprosy
- Tuberculosis
- Typhoid fever
- Malaria
- Smallpox
- Measles
- Mumps
- Rubella
- Rabies
- Acute poliomyelitis
- Viral haemorrhagic fever
- Acute encephalitis

Old Nomenclature of a Few Organisms

Old nomenclature	New nomenclature
Klebs-Loeffler bacillus	*Corynebacterium diphtheriae*
Preisz-Nocard bacillus	*Corynebacterium pseudotuberculosis*
Friedlander's bacillus	*Klebsiella pneumoniae*
Eberth-Gaffky bacillus or Eberthella typhi	*Salmonella* serotype Typhi
Whitmore's bacillus	*Burkholderia pseudomallei*
Pfeiffer's bacillus	*Haemophilus influenzae*
Koch-Weeks bacillus	*Haemophilus aegypticus*
Bordet-Gengou bacillus	*Bordetella pertussis*
Donovan's bacillus	*Klebsiella granulomatis*
Hansen bacillus	*Mycobacterium leprae*

APPENDIX V

Characteristic Colonial Appearance

Appearance	Organisms
Oil-paint	*Staphylococcus aureus*
Draughtsman or carrom coin	*Streptococcus pneumoniae*
Daisy head	*Corynebacterium diphtheriae* biotype gravis
Frog's egg	*C. diphtheriae* biotype intermedius
Poached egg	*C. diphtheriae* biotype mitis
Fried egg	*Mycoplasma*
Medusa head	*Bacillus anthracis*
Bisected pearls or mercury drops	*Bordetella*
Aluminium paint (confluent growth)	*Bordetella*
Rough, buff and tough	*Mycobacterium tuberculosis*
Pitting or corroding	*Eikenella corrodens*
Molar tooth	*Actinomyces israelii*

Characteristic Appearance of Bacteria in Stained Smear

Appearance	Organisms
Rail road track or school of fish	*Haemophilus aegyptius*
Thumb print	*Bordetella*
Fish in stream	*Vibrio cholerae*
Safety pin	*Yersinia pestis*
Drumstick	*Clostridium tetani*
Bamboo stick	*Bacillus anthracis*
Bunch of grapes	*Staphylococcus aureus*
Lanceolate or flame-shaped	*Streptococcus pneumoniae*
Kidney shaped	*Neisseria gonorrhoeae* and *N. meningitidis*
Chinese letter arrangement	*Corynebacterium diphtheriae*
Cigar bundle	*Mycobacterium leprae*
Sun ray	*Actinomyces*

APPENDIX VI

Differentiation of Bacteria of Enterobacteriaceae by Biochemical Tests

Biochemical tests	Escherichia coli	Edwardsiella	Citrobacter freundii	Klebsiella pneumoniae	Entero-bacter	Salmonella	Shigella	Hafnia	Serratia	Proteus	Provi-dencia	Morganella	Yersinia entero-colitica
Indole	+	+	−	−	−	−	v	−	−	v	+	+	v
MR	+	+	+	−	−	+	+	−	−	+	+	+	+
VP	−	−	−	+	+	−	−	+	+	−	−	−	v
Citrate	−	−	+	+	+	v	−	+	+	v	v	−	−
Urease	−	−	v	+	v	−	−	−	−	+	v	+	+
H₂S	−	+	+	−	−	+	−	−	−	+	−	−	−
Motility	+	+	+	−	+	+	−	+	+	+	+	+	+ at 22°C
Growth in KCN	−	−	+	+	+	−	−	+	+	+	+	+	−
PPA	−	−	−	−	−	−	−	−	−	+	+	+	−
Gelatin (22°C)	−	−	−	−	v	−	−	−	+	+	−	−	−
Malonate	−	−	v	+	v	−	−	v	−	−	−	−	−
Lysine decarboxylase	v	+	−	v	v	+	−	+	+	−	−	−	−
Arginine decarboxylase	v	−	v	−	v	+	v	v	−	−	−	−	−
Ornithine decarboxylase	v	+	v	−	+	+	−	+	+	v	−	+	+
ONPG	+	−	+	+	+	−	−	+	+	−	−	−	+
Acid from													
Glucose	+	+	+	+	+	+	v	+	v	+	v	+	−
Lactose	+	−	v	+	+	−	−	−	v	−	−	−	−
Sucrose	v	−	v	+	+	−	−	−	+	v	v	−	+
Mannitol	+	−	+	+	+	+	v	+	+	−	−	−	+

(v – variable)

APPENDIX VII

Overview of Microbiology, Mycology and Parasitology

Strict aerobes

- *Mycobacterium tuberculosis*
- *Pseudomonas aeruginosa*
- *Burkholderia*
- *Bordetella pertussis*

Strict anerobes

- *Clostridium tetani*
- *C. difficile*
- *Bacteroides fragilis*
- *Peptostreptococcus*
- *Anaeroplasma*

Microaerophilic bacteria

- *Campylobacter*
- *Helicobacter*
- *Actinomyces*
- *Borrelia*
- *Leptospira*

Clostridia which can grow in microaerophilic condition

- *Clostridium perfringens*

Non-motile clostridia

- *Clostridium perfringens*
- *C. tetani* type VI

Microorganism which survives pasteurization by Holder method

- *Coxiella burnetii*

Microorganisms that normally do not invade the bloodstream

- *Clostridium tetani*
- *C. perfringens*
- *Corynebacterium diphtheriae*
- *Shigella* spp.

Microorganisms which readily undergo antigenic variation

- *Borrelia recurrentis*
- *B. duttonii*
- *Neisseria gonorrhoeae*
- *N. meningitidis*
- *Trypanosoma brucei gambiense*
- *Influenza virus*
- *Human immunodeficiency viruses*

Lactose-fermenting bacilli

- *Escherichia*

- *Klebsiella*
- *Enterobacter*
- *Citrobacter*
- *Vibrio vulnificus*

Late lactose-fermenters

- *Shigella sonnei*
- *Vibrio cholerae*

Oxidase-positive bacteria

- *Neisseria meningitidis*
- *N. gonorrhoeae*
- *Vibrio*
- *Pseudomonas*
- *Aeromonas*
- *Pleisomonas*
- *Campylobacter*
- *Helicobacter*
- *Alkaligenes*
- *Burkholderia* (except *B. mallei* and *B. maltophila*)
- *Haemophilus influenzae*
- Brucellae
- *Bordetella pertussis* (weakly positive)

Non-motile Gram-positive rods

- *Corynebacterium diphtheriae*
- *Nocardia*
- *Clostridium perfringens*
- *Bacillus anthracis*

Pigment producers

- *Pseudomonas aeruginosa*—blue green pigment
- *Serratia*—red pigment
- *Staphylococcus aureus*—yellow pigment
- Photochromogenic and scotochromogenic mycobacteria—bright yellow or orange

Urease-positive organisms

- *Proteus*
- *Klebsiella*
- *Ureaplasma*
- *Helicobacter*

Obligate intracellular organisms

- Bacteria
  - All rickettsiae
  - All Chlamydiaceae
  - *Mycobacterium leprae*
- Viruses
  - All are obligate intracellular parasites

- Protozoa
  - *Plasmodium*
  - *Babesia*
  - *Leishmania*
  - *Trypanosoma cruzi*—amastigote form
  - *Toxoplasma gondii*

Organisms that are found extracellular in the body but cannot be cultured on inert media

- *Treponema pallidum*
- *Pneumocystis jirovecii*

Organisms that cause congenital malformations (Mnemonic: TORCH)

- **T**   *Toxoplasma gondii*
- **Other**   *Treponema pallidum*
- **R**   *Rubella*
- **C**   Cytomegolovirus
- **H**   Herpes virus

Bacteria entering the body by inhalation

- *Mycobacterium* spp.
- *Nocardia* spp.
- *Mycoplasma pneumoniae*
- *Legionella* spp.
- *Bordetella* spp.
- *Chlamydia psittaci*
- *Streptococcus* spp.

Organisms entering the body through needle-stick injury

- Hepatitis B virus
- Hepatitis C virus
- Human immunodeficiency virus
- *Staphylococcus aureus*
- *Pseudomonas* spp.

Sexually-transmitted bacteria

- *Neisseria gonorrhoeae*
- *Treponema pallidum*
- *Chlamydia trachomatis*

Microorganisms showing bipolar staining

- *Yersinia pestis*
- *Yersinia pseudotuberculosis*
- *Pasteurella* spp.
- *Francisella tularensis*
- *Burkholderia pseudomallei*
- *Haemophilus ducreyi*

Five most common causes of meningitis

- *Haemophilus influenzae*
- *Neisseria meningitidis*
- *Streptococcus pneumoniae*
- Group B streptococci
- *Listeria monocytogenes*

Fungus infection in which isolation and other procedures should be carried out in safety cabinet and petri dish should not be used for the isolation of the fungus

- *Coccidioides immitis*

Catalase negative member of family Enterobacteriaceae

- *Shigella dysenteriae* type-I

Bacterium which infects erythrocytes

- *Bartonella bacilliformis*

Microorganisms causing pseudomembranous colitis

- *Clostridium difficile*
- *Clostridium perfringens*
- *Staphylococcus aureus*

Parasites causing anaemia

- *Plasmodium* spp.
- *Babesia microti*
- *Leishmania donovani*
- *Schistosoma haematobium*
- *Ancylostoma duodenale*
- *Necator americanus*
- *Diphyllobothrium latum*
- *Trichuris trichiura*

Parasites causing infection of eye

- *Acanthamoeba* spp.
- *Toxoplasma gondii*
- *Onchocerca volvulus*
- *Encephalitozoon* spp.
- *Toxocara* spp.
- *Loa loa*
- *Echinococcus granulosus*
- *Trypanosoma cruzi*
- *Nosema* spp.
- *Angiostrongylus cantonensis*
- *Dirofilaria conjunctivae*
- *Taenia solium*

Parasites causing CNS infection

- Protozoa
  - *Entamoeba histolytica*
  - *Acanthamoeba* spp.
  - *Plasmodium falciparum*
  - *Trypanosoma brucei gambiense*
  - *T. b. rhodesiense*
  - *T. cruzi*
  - *Naegleria fowleri*
  - *Balamuthia mandrillaris*
  - *Toxoplasma gondii*
  - *Microsporidia*
- Cestodes
  - *Taenia solium*
  - *T. multiceps*

- *Echinococcus granulosus*
- *E. multilocularis*
- *E. vogeli*
- *Spirometra* spp.
- Trematodes
  - *Schistosoma japonicum*
  - *Paragonimus westermani*
- Nematodes
  - *Trichinella spiralis*
  - *Strongyloides stercoralis*
  - *Gnathostoma spinigerum*
  - *Toxocara canis*
  - *Angiostrongylus cantonensis*
  - *Toxocara cati*

Parasites associated with malignancy

- *Schistosoma haematobium*
- *Opisthorchis viverrini*
- *Clonorchis sinensis*

Parasites causing skin ulcers

- *Leishmania tropica*
- *L. braziliensis*
- *L. major*
- *L. mexicana* complex
- *L. peruviana*
- *Dracunculus medinensis*

Parasites causing blood and mucus in stool

- *Entamoeba histolytica*
- *Schistosoma japonicum*
- *S. mansoni*
- *Trichuris trichiura*
- *Balantidium coli*

Parasites showing antigenic variation

- *Trypanosoma brucei gambiense*
- *T. b. rhodesiense*
- *Plasmodium* spp.
- *Giardia lamblia*

Parasites causing autoinfection

- *Strongyloides stercoralis*
- *Enterobius vermicularis*
- *Taenia solium*
- *Hymenolepis nana*
- *Cryptosporidium parvum*
- *Capillaria philippinensis*

Parasites causing opportunistic infection in AIDS cases

- *Toxoplasma gondii*
- *Isospora belli*
- *Entamoeba histolytica*
- Free-living protozoa
- *Leishmania* spp.

- *Cryptosporidium parvum*
- *Microsporidia*
- *Giardia lamblia*
- *Cyclospora cayetanensis*
- *Strongyloides stercoralis*

Parasites causing pneumonia, pneumonitis, or Loeffler's syndrome

- Migrating larvae of:
  - *Ascaris lumbricoides*
  - *Ancylostoma duodenale*
  - *Necator americanus*
  - *Strongyloides stercoralis*
- Eggs of *Paragonimus westermani*
- *Echinococcus granulosus*
- *Entamoeba histolytica*
- *Cryptosporidium parvum*

Parasites causing larva migrans

- Cutaneous larva migrans
  - *Ancylostoma braziliense*
  - *A. caninum*
  - *Bunostomum phlebotomum*
  - *Uncinaria stenocephala*
  - *Gnathostoma spinigerum*
  - *G. doloresi*
  - *G. hispidum*
  - *G. nipponicum*
- Visceral larva migrans
  - *Toxocara canis*
  - *T. cati*
  - *Angiostrongylus cantonensis*
  - *Gnathostoma spinigerum*
  - *Anisakis simplex*

Parasites causing tropical eosinophilia

- *Wuchereria bancrofti*
- *Brugia malayi*

Obligate intracellular parasites

- *Plasmodium* spp.
- *Babesia* spp.
- *Leishmania* spp.
- *Trypanosoma cruzi* (amastigote form)
- *Toxoplasma gondii*
- *Microsporidia*

Parasites residing in lymphatic system

- *Wuchereria bancrofti*
- *Brugia malayi*
- *B. timori*

Parasites found in urine

- *Trichomonas vaginalis*
- *Wuchereria bancrofti*

- *Schistosoma haematobium*
- *Dioctophyma renale*

Parasites found in CSF

- *Trypanosoma brucei gambiense*
- *T. b. rhodesiense*
- *Acanthamoeba* spp.
- *Angiostrongylus* spp.
- *Naegleria fowleri*
- *Balamuthia* spp.

Parasites found in sputum

- *Paragonimus westermani*
- *Entamoeba histolytica*
- Fragments of laminated membrane and free scolices of *Echinococcus granulosus*
- Rarely, migrating larvae of
  - *Ascaris lumbricoides*
  - *Ancylostoma duodenale*
  - *Necator americanus*
  - *Strongyloides stercoralis*
- *Capillaria aerophila*

Parasites found in peripheral blood film

- Protozoa
  - *Plasmodium* spp.
  - *Babesia* spp.
  - *Leishmania* spp.
  - *Trypanosoma brucei gambiense*
  - *T. b. rhodesiense*
  - *T. cruzi*
- Nematodes
  Microfilariae of:
  - *Wuchereria bancrofti*
  - *Brugia malayi*
  - *B. timori*
  - *Loa loa*
  - *Mansonella ozzardi*

Parasites transmitted by sexual contact

- *Trichomonas vaginalis*
- *Giardia lamblia*
- *Entamoeba histolytica*

Parasites transmitted congenitally

- *Toxoplasma gondii*
- *Microsporidia*
- *Plasmodium* spp.
- *Trypanosoma cruzi*

Parasites transmitted by blood transfusion

- *Plasmodium* spp.
- *Trypanosoma cruzi*
- *Babesia* spp.

Parasites entering through skin

Direct
- *Ancylostoma duodenale*
- *A. caninum*
- *A. braziliense*
- *Necator americanus*
- *Schistosoma japonicum*
- *Strongyloides stercoralis*
- *Schistosoma haematobium*
- *S. mansoni*

Through blood-sucking insects
- Protozoa
  - *Leishmania* spp.
  - *Plasmodium* spp.
  - *Trypanosoma* spp.
  - *Babesia* spp.
- Nematodes
  - *Wuchereria bancrofti*
  - *Brugia malayi*
  - *B. timori*
  - *Mansonella streptocerca*
  - *M. ozzardi*
  - *M. perstans*
  - *Dirofilaria* spp.
  - *Loa loa*
  - *Onchocerca volvulus*

Acid-fast oocysts and eggs

- Oocysts
  - *Cryptosporidium parvum*
  - *Cyclospora cayetanensis*
  - *Isospora belli*
- Eggs
  - *Schistosoma intercalatum*

Skin tests showing immediate hypersensitivity in

- Hydatid disease
- Schistosomiasis
- Strongyloidiasis
- Filariasis

Skin tests showing delayed hypersensitivity in

- Leishmaniasis

Oviparous nematodes

- Laying unsegmented eggs
  - *Ascaris lumbricoides*
  - *Trichuris trichiura*
- Laying eggs with segmented ova
  - *Ancylostoma duodenale*
  - *Trichostrongylus* spp.
  - *Necator americanus*
  - *Ternidens deminutus*
- Laying eggs containing larva
  - *Enterobius vermicularis*

Ovoviviparous nematodes
- *Strongyloides stercoralis*

Viviparous nematodes
- *Dracunculus medinensis*
- *Brugia malayi*
- *B. timori*
- *Trichinella spiralis*
- *Wuchereria bancrofti*

Sheathed microfilariae found in blood
- *Wuchereria bancrofti*
- *Brugia malayi*
- *B. timori*
- *Loa loa*

Unsheathed microfilariae

Found in blood
- *Mansonella ozzardi*
- *M. perstans*
- *Dirofilaria* spp.

Found in skin
- *M. streptocerca*
- *Onchocerca volvulus*

Largest protozoal parasite inhabiting large intestine of man
- *Balantidium coli*

Smallest tapeworm infecting humans
- *Hymenolepis nana*

Largest nematode parasitizing human intestine
- *Ascaris lumbricoides*

Smallest nematode known to cause infection in man
- *Strongyloides stercoralis*

Largest trematode known to cause infection in man
- *Fasciolopsis buski*

Amoebae forming cysts in tissues
- *Acanthamoeba* spp.
- *Balamuthia mandrillaris*

Parasite causing fat-coloured and frothy stool
- *Giardia lamblia*

Parasite in urethral and vaginal discharge, and prostatic secretions
- *Trichomonas vaginalis*